Recent Advances in
OPHTHALMOLOGY–14

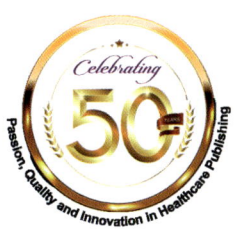

Recent Advances in
OPHTHALMOLOGY–14

Editors

HV Nema MS
Former Professor and Head
Department of Ophthalmology
Institute of Medical Sciences, Banaras Hindu University
Varanasi, Uttar Pradesh, India

Nitin Nema MS DNB
Professor
Department of Ophthalmology
Sri Aurobindo Institute of Medical Sciences
Indore, Madhya Pradesh, India

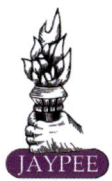

JAYPEE BROTHERS MEDICAL PUBLISHERS
The Health Sciences Publisher
New Delhi | London | Panama

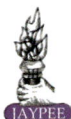 **Jaypee Brothers Medical Publishers (P) Ltd**

Headquarters
Jaypee Brothers Medical Publishers (P) Ltd
4838/24, Ansari Road, Daryaganj
New Delhi 110 002, India
Phone: +91-11-43574357
Fax: +91-11-43574314
Email: jaypee@jaypeebrothers.com

Overseas Offices
J.P. Medical Ltd
83 Victoria Street, London
SW1H 0HW (UK)
Phone: +44 20 3170 8910
Fax: +44 (0)20 3008 6180
Email: info@jpmedpub.com

Jaypee-Highlights Medical Publishers Inc
City of Knowledge, Bld. 235, 2nd Floor
Clayton, Panama City, Panama
Phone: +1 507-301-0496
Fax: +1 507-301-0499
Email: cservice@jphmedical.com

Jaypee Brothers Medical Publishers (P) Ltd
Bhotahity, Kathmandu, Nepal
Phone: +977-9741283608
Email: kathmandu@jaypeebrothers.com

Website: www.jaypeebrothers.com
Website: www.jaypeedigital.com

© 2019, Jaypee Brothers Medical Publishers

The views and opinions expressed in this book are solely those of the original contributor(s)/author(s) and do not necessarily represent those of editor(s) of the book.

All rights reserved. No part of this publication may be reproduced, stored or transmitted in any form or by any means, electronic, mechanical, photocopying, recording or otherwise, without the prior permission in writing of the publishers.

All brand names and product names used in this book are trade names, service marks, trademarks or registered trademarks of their respective owners. The publisher is not associated with any product or vendor mentioned in this book.

Medical knowledge and practice change constantly. This book is designed to provide accurate, authoritative information about the subject matter in question. However, readers are advised to check the most current information available on procedures included and check information from the manufacturer of each product to be administered, to verify the recommended dose, formula, method and duration of administration, adverse effects and contraindications. It is the responsibility of the practitioner to take all appropriate safety precautions. Neither the publisher nor the author(s)/editor(s) assume any liability for any injury and/or damage to persons or property arising from or related to use of material in this book.

This book is sold on the understanding that the publisher is not engaged in providing professional medical services. If such advice or services are required, the services of a competent medical professional should be sought.

Every effort has been made where necessary to contact holders of copyright to obtain permission to reproduce copyright material. If any have been inadvertently overlooked, the publisher will be pleased to make the necessary arrangements at the first opportunity. The **CD/DVD-ROM** (if any) provided in the sealed envelope with this book is complimentary and free of cost. **Not meant for sale.**

Inquiries for bulk sales may be solicited at: jaypee@jaypeebrothers.com

Recent Advances in Ophthalmology–14
First Edition: **2019**
ISBN: **978-93-5270-901-4**
Printed at Sanat Printers

Dedicated to
Loving memory of Pratibha

Editorial Board

Devindra Sood MD
Director
Glaucoma Imaging Centre
New Delhi, India

Frank Goes MD
Director
Oagchirurgie-Oagheelkunde
Antwerp, Belgium

Jorge L Alïö MD PhD
Director
Vissum Institute of Ophthalmology
Universidad Miguel Hernández
Alicante, Spain

Jyotirmay Biswas
MS FMRF FNAMS FIC (Path) FAICO
Director
Department of Uveitis and Ocular Pathology
Sankara Nethralaya
Chennai, Tamil Nadu, India

Lingam Gopal MS FRCS
Associate Professor and Consultant
Department of Ophthalmology
National University Health System
Singapore
Department of Vitreoretinal Services
Sankara Nethralaya
Chennai, Tamil Nadu, India

Suresh R Chandra MD
Professor
Department of Ophthalmology and Visual Sciences
University of Wisconsin School of Medicine and Public Health
Madison, Wisconsin, USA

Contributors

Alejandra E Rodriguez PhD
Biologist
Research and Development Department
VISSUM Innovation and Cornea and
Ocular Surface Department
VISSUM Corporation, Alicante, Spain

Annamalai Odayappan DO DNB
Medical Consultant
Glaucoma Services
Aravind Eye Hospital
Puducherry, India

Arpitha Pereira DOMS DNB FICO
Senior Resident
Narayana Nethralaya Eye Institute
Bengaluru, Karnataka, India

Arup Chakrabarti MS
Chief
Cataract and Glaucoma Services
Chakrabarti Eye Care Center
Thiruvananthapuram, Kerala, India

Avinash Pathengay MD FRCS
Director
Academy for Eye Care Education
Consultant
Vitreo-Retina and Uveitis Service
LV Prasad Eye Institute
Visakhapatnam, Andhra Pradesh, India

Casey J Randleman
Premed MSc Student
Emory University
Atlanta, GA, USA

Chaitra Jayadev DOMS FVR FICO PhD
Vitreoretinal Consultant
Narayana Nethralaya Eye Institute
Bengaluru, Karnataka, India

D Ramamurthy MD FNAMS
Director
The Eye Foundation
Coimbatore, Tamil Nadu, India

Gitansha Shreyas Sachdev MS FICO
Consultant
Cataract and Refractive Services
The Eye Foundation
Coimbatore, Tamil Nadu, India

Hemlata Gupta DNB FNAMS
Senior Consultant
Cataract and Refractive Services
Centre for Sight
New Delhi, India

Hima Pendharkar DMRD DNB
(Radiodiagnosis) DM (Diagnosis and
Interventional Neuroradiology)
Associate Professor
Department of Neuroimaging and
Interventional Radiology
National Institute of Mental Health and
Neurosciences
Bengaluru, Karnataka, India

Jayesh Vazirani MS
Director
Excel Eye Care: Center for Excellence in
Cornea and Ocular Surface Disorders
Ahmedabad, Gujarat, India

Jorge L Alió MD PhD
Director
Vissum Institute of Ophthalmology
Universidad Miguel Hernández
Alicante, Spain

Lingam Gopal MS FRCS
Associate Professor and Consultant
Department of Ophthalmology
National University Health System
Singapore
Department of Vitreoretinal Services
Sankara Nethralaya
Chennai, Tamil Nadu, India

M Ravishankar DO DHM
Senior Consultant
Rajan Eye Care Hospital Pvt Ltd
Chennai, Tamil Nadu, India

MG Pavan Kumar DO
Fellow
Glaucoma Services
Aravind Eye Hospital
Puducherry, India

Mahipal S Sachdev MD
Chairman and Medical Director
Centre for Sight
New Delhi, India

Maithri Arun Kumar DNB
Senior Resident
MN Eye Hospital
Chennai, Tamil Nadu, India

Malarchelvi Palani MS DO DNB FICO FTERF
Consultant
MN Eye Hospitals
Chennai, Tamil Nadu, India

Manila Khatri MS
Senior Resident Ophthalmology
Government Medical College
Virat Eye Care Centre
Shahdol, Madhya Pradesh, India

Maria A Amesty MD PhD
Medical Director
Ocular Plastic, Reconstructive, Lacrimal
and Orbital Surgery Department
VISSUM Corporation, Alicante, Spain

Meena Chakrabarti MS
Senior Consultant
Chakrabarti Eye Care Center
Thiruvananthapuram, Kerala, India

Mohan Rajan MBBS DO Dip NB FMRF
MNAMS MCh FACS FRCS PhD
Chairman and Medical Director
Rajan Eye Care Hospital Pvt Ltd
Chennai, Tamil Nadu, India

Murali Ariga MS DNB FAICO (Glaucoma)
Director, Swamy Eye Clinic
Head, Glaucoma Services
MN Eye Hospitals
Head, Department of Ophthalmology
Sundaram Medical Foundation
Chennai, Tamil Nadu, India

Nikunj Tank DO DNB
Cataract Fellow
Sitapur Eye Hospital
Sitapur, Uttar Pradesh, India

Olena Al-Shymali MD
Clinical Resarch Fellow
Research and Development Department
VISSUM Innovation and Department of
Cornea, Cataract and Refractive Surgery
VISSUM Corporation, Alicante, Spain

Partha Biswas MS
Chairman, ARC, AIOS
Director, BB Eye Foundation
Kolkata, West Bengal, India

Prakrati Gupta MS
Consultant, VST Centre for Glaucoma
LV Prasad Eye Institute
Hyderabad, Telangana, India

Prashob Mohan MS
Consultant Cornea
Giridhar Eye Institute
Kochi, Kerala, India

Pratheeba Nivean MS DO
Consultant, Glaucoma and Oculoplasty
MN Eye Hospital
Chennai, Tamil Nadu, India

Contributors XI

Purvi R Bhagat MS DO
Associate Professor, Glaucoma Clinic
M & J Western Regional Institute of Ophthalmology
Civil Hospital and BJ Medical College
Ahmedabad, Gujarat, India

Rajesh Babu B MS FMRF MSc CEH
Director
Drishti Eye Hospital
Bengaluru, Karnataka, India

Rajiv Choudhary MS
Director, Rajas Eye Hospital
Indore, Madhya Pradesh, India

Rashmi Deshmukh MS DNB FAICO
Associate Consultant
Cornea, Cataract and Refractive Services
Centre for Sight
New Delhi, India

Rengaraj Venkatesh DNB
Head of Department and Consultant
Department of Glaucoma Services
Aravind Eye Hospital and Postgraduate Institute of Ophthalmology
Puducherry, India

Sandeep Saxena MS FRCS Ed FRCS FRCOphth FAICO FAMS
Professor and Chief of Retina Service
Department of Ophthalmology
King George's Medical University
Lucknow, Uttar Pradesh, India

Santosh GK Gadde DNB FVR
Vitreoretinal Consultant
Narayana Nethralaya Eye Institute
Bengaluru, Karnataka, India

Saurabh Mistry DNB
Fellow, Medical Research Foundation
Sankara Nethralaya
Chennai, Tamil Nadu, India

Sharat Hegde MS
Consultant
Vitreo-Retina and Uveitis Service
LV Prasad Eye Institute
Visakhapatnam, Andhra Pradesh, India

Shivani Dixit MS
Glaucoma Specialist
Sitapur Eye Hospital
Sitapur, Uttar Pradesh, India

Shreyansh Doshi DNB
Consultant
Vitreo-Retina and Uveitis Service
LV Prasad Eye Institute
Visakhapatnam, Andhra Pradesh, India

Sirisha Senthil MS FRCS
Consultant
VST Centre for Glaucoma
LV Prasad Eye Institute
Hyderabad, Telangana, India,

Sneha Batra MS (Gold Medalist) FICO
Fellow (Phacorefractive Surgery and Medical Retina)
BB Foundation
Kolkata, West Bengal, India

Soosan Jacob MS FRCS DNB
Director and Chief
Dr Agarwal's Refractive and Cornea Foundation (DARCF)
Senior Consultant, Cataract and Glaucoma Services
Dr Agarwal's Group of Eye Hospitals
Chennai, Tamil Nadu, India

Sriram DO DNB
Junior Consultant
Rajan Eye Care Hospital Pvt Ltd
Chennai, Tamil Nadu, India

Sudharshan S MS
Consultant, Department of Uveitis and Ocular Pathology, Sankara Nethralaya
Chennai, Tamil Nadu, India

Suhas Haldipurkar DOMS FAICO
Medical Director, Laxmi Eye Institute
Navi Mumbai, Maharashtra, India

Zain Khatib MS DNB
Clinical Assistant, Laxmi Eye Institute
Navi Mumbai, Maharashtra, India

Preface

Like previous volumes, the RAO-14 contains chapters on selected topics on cornea, glaucoma, cataract, and retina. Corneal ectasia after LASIK is not a rare complication. It causes visual disablement and great dissatisfaction to the patient. Authors have described risk factors for the development of post-Lasik ectasia and suggested methods to prevent it. Once the complication occurs, it should be treated early. The management strategies include contact lens, intracorneal rings, collagen cross-linking and keratoplasty.

Of late, renewed interest has been generated in Lamellar Keratoplasty (LK) and many forms of LK have been introduced. Deep Anterior Lamellar Keratoplasty (DALK), Superficial Anterior Lamellar Keratoplasty (SALK) or Tucked-In Lamellar Keratoplasty (TILK) is indicated in stromal pathology with healthy endothelium. These procedures have least risk of rejection. On the other hand, Descemet Stripping Automated Endothelial Keratoplasty (DSAEK), Descemet's Membrane Endothelial Keratoplasty (DMEK), and Pre-Descemet's Endothelial Keratoplasty (PDEK) are performed in diseased endothelium with healthy stroma. Authors have described three innovative techniques to better visualize and support the graft. These include— (1) Endoilluminator-assisted PDEK, (2) Air pump-assisted PDEK and (3) Host Descemetic scaffolding to support the graft.

Keratopigmentation or tattooing was a popular technique to mask corneal opacities in the past. However, the practice of tattooing has been greatly reduced after the introduction of keratoplasty. Alio and coworkers have devised special instruments and use micronized mineral pigments and claim "Keratopigmentation is a modern surgery that provides an excellent solution for patients where other treatment options are not suitable."

Blood supply to optic nerve plays a vital role in the pathogenesis of glaucoma. The difference between arterial blood pressure and intraocular pressure (IOP) is defined as ocular perfusion pressure (OPP). There are published reports that patients with glaucoma have low OPP as compared to normal individuals. The quantification of blood flow in the eye can provide evidence about the pathological changes in optic nerve head. The cause of reduction of OPP is not known but seems to be vascular dysregulation or insufficient autoregulation. Authors have described both invasive and noninvasive methods of assessment of the ocular blood flow as well as local and systemic factors which influence it. They feel that data are not sufficient to validate use of ocular blood flow assessment for the treatment and prognosis of glaucoma.

Selective Laser trabeculoplasty is considered a relatively safe procedure in the management of glaucoma. Authors have briefly described the mechanism of action, indications and contraindications, advantages and disadvantages, complications and outcome of the technique.

Management of intractable glaucoma poses a great challenge to ophthalmologists. Glaucoma drainage device (GDD) forms a new bypass pathway for the aqueous humor. It is a useful device for the management of intractable glaucoma as it drains the aqueous from the anterior chamber into the subconjunctival space. GDDs are of three types—setons, valved implant and nonvalved implant. Authors have described step-by-step surgical procedure of implantation of the implant and its early and late complications.

There are a number of factors which influence the outcome of IOL implantation. One of the most important factors is the correct calculation of power of IOL. Ultrasound has been used for measurement of ocular parameters for the calculation of IOL power for quite a long time. However, these calculations do not reach within 0.50 diopters of the target refraction in 25% of cases, and some of the eyes present significant refractive surprise. Recently, biometers using optical partial coherence interferometry or optical low coherence reflectometry have been introduced. These biometers are user-friendly and accurate. Mohan and Chakrabarti presented a detailed account of advances in the calculation of IOL power determination.

Cataract operation is the most common surgery performed worldwide. Several measures have been adopted to make it safe and improve its outcome even in complicated cases. Chapters like Custom Cataract Surgery, Astigmatism Management in Cataract Surgery, Posterior Capsular Rupture Recognition and Management, Femtosecond Laser-assisted Cataract Surgery in Posterior Polar Cataracts, Pseudoexfoliation Cataract: Management and Phacoemulsification in Subluxated Lenses are included in this volume for the benefit of young ophthalmic surgeons so that they may become more careful and meticulous in performing the surgery in difficult patients. It is not rare to witness loss of capsular support in cataract surgery. The surgeon cannot implant IOL in the bag. The scleral fixed IOL is the right answer in such a situation.

It has become a fashion to cite clinical trials extensively without clearly understanding their application in real-life situations. Lingam Gopal deserves compliments for discussing how to adopt the results of trials in the management of retinal vascular diseases.

Optical Coherence Tomography Angiography (OCTA) is a noninvasive, high resolution imaging technique that provides angiographic maps of retina and choroid to study the blood circulation. It can diagnose ischemia of choriocapillaris and choroidal neovascular membrane (CNVM). Since OCTA presents a 3D view of tissues, it can detect minor abnormalities of the retina and choroid. In a comprehensive chapter, Chaitra and colleagues have described principle and procedure of OCTA and discussed the findings in normal retina and common retinal diseases such as diabetic retinopathy, retinal vascular occlusions, CNVM and age-related macular degeneration. OCTA can also be used to evaluate inflammatory diseases of retina and choroid, and intraocular tumors.

The chapter on the role of spectral domain-optical coherence tomography (SD-OCT) in the evaluation of diabetic retinopathy highlights the importance of examination of vitreomacular interface and inner and outer layers of retina. A relationship between disruption of ellipsoid zone and visual acuity has been found.

In this volume, the readers can also derive benefit from interesting chapters on Necrotizing Retinopathies, Nyctalopia, Ocular Burns and Cerebral Angiography.

We know that in the past few decades tremendous progress has been made in all fields of ophthalmology. This volume presents information on some of the advances. Hopefully, the postgraduate students, residents and general ophthalmologists will utilize the knowledge effectively for the better care of their patients.

HV Nema
Nitin Nema

Acknowledgments

We are indebted to all contributors for submitting their chapters well in time in spite of their preoccupations and other commitments. Authors' cooperation in correction of proofs and replacement of photographs is laudable.

Credit goes to Shri Jitendar P Vij (Group Chairman), Mr Ankit Vij (Managing Director) and Ms Chetna Malhotra Vohra (Associate Director–Content Strategy) for their interest in Recent Advances in Ophthalmology series. We appreciate the hard work of Ms Nikita Chauhan (Senior Development Editor) for elimination of plagiarism and staff of M/s Jaypee Brothers Medical Publishers (P) Ltd, New Delhi for nice production of the book.

Contents

1. **Management of Post-LASIK Ectasia**   1
   Partha Biswas, Sneha Batra
   - Epidemiology   1
   - Presenting Features   2
   - Investigations Helpful in the Diagnosis of PLE   2
   - Risk Factors for PLE   5
   - Pathogenesis   9
   - Histopathology   11
   - Management   12
   - Prevention   16

2. **Recent Advances in Lamellar Keratoplasty**   23
   Casey J Randleman, Soosan Jacob
   - Recent Advances in Endothelial Keratoplasty   23
   - Recent Advances in Anterior Lamellar Keratoplasty   32

3. **Keratopigmentation: An Innovative Surgical Option for Therapeutic and Cosmetic Purposes**   39
   Olena Al-Shymali, Alejandra E Rodriguez, Maria A Amesty, Jorge L Alió
   - Instruments, Pigments, and Technologies Involved in Keratopigmentation   40
   - Keratopigmentation Surgical Techniques   42
   - Indications   45
   - Ophthalmological Assessment   46
   - Contraindications to Keratopigmentation   47
   - Outcomes   48
   - Complications   49

4. **Ocular Blood Flow in Glaucoma**   53
   Murali Ariga, Pratheeba Nivean, Malarchelvi Palani, Maithri Arun Kumar
   - Assessment of Ocular Blood Flow   53
   - Scanning Laser Ophthalmoscopic Angiography   54
   - Color Doppler Imaging   55
   - Laser Doppler Velocimetry   57
   - Laser Doppler Flowmetry   58
   - Retinal Vessel Analyzer   58

- Retinal Oximetry 58
- Doppler Optical Coherence Tomography 59
- Optical Coherence Tomography Angiography 59
- Factors that Affect Ocular Blood Flow 62

5. Selective Laser Trabeculoplasty 67
Purvi R Bhagat, Shivani Dixit, Nikunj Tank

- History and Concept 67
- Mechanism of Action 67

6. Shunts in the Management of Intractable Glaucoma 74
Rengaraj Venkatesh, Annamalai Odayappan, MG Pavan Kumar

- Types of Glaucoma Drainage Devices 74
- Current Drainage Devices 77
- Preoperative Evaluation 80
- Choosing Glaucoma Drainage Devices 81
- Surgical Procedure 81
- Placement of the Tube 85
- Site of Implantation 85
- Use of Antifibrotics 85
- Complications 85

7. Recent Advances in Intraocular Lens Power Calculation 90
Prashob Mohan, Arup Chakrabarti

- Biometry 90
- IOL Power Calculation Formulae 100

8. Custom Cataract Surgery 112
Rajiv Choudhary

- Refractive Targeting 112
- Biometry 112
- Customization of Surgical Modality 113
- Role of Microincisional Cataract Surgery in Customization 115
- Intraocular Lens Selection 115
- How to Minimize Postoperative Astigmatism and Correct Preexisting Astigmatism? 117

9. Astigmatism Management in Cataract Surgery 123
Gitansha Shreyas Sachdev, D Ramamurthy

- Preoperative Assessment 123
- Posterior Corneal Astigmatism 124
- Preoperative Corneal Marking 124
- Surgical Methods for Treating Corneal Astigmatism 126

10. Pseudoexfoliation Cataract: Management 135
Prakrati Gupta, Sirisha Senthil

- Preoperative Evaluation 135
- Pseudoexfoliation and Cataract Surgery 138
- Postoperative Complications 143

11. Femtosecond Laser-Assisted Cataract Surgery in Posterior Polar Cataracts — 147
Mahipal S Sachdev, Gitansha Shreyas Sachdev, Rashmi Deshmukh, Hemlata Gupta
- Posterior Polar Cataract *147*
- Femtosecond Laser-Assisted Cataract Surgery *149*

12. Posterior Capsular Rupture Recognition and Management — 156
Mohan Rajan, M Ravishankar, Sriram
- Improperly Managed Posterior Capsular Rupture *156*
- Early Signs of Posterior Capsular Rupture *156*
- Prevention of Posterior Capsular Rupture *158*

13. Phacoemulsification in Subluxated Lenses — 171
Suhas Haldipurkar, Zain Khatib
- Capsular Support Devices for Subluxated Lenses *171*
- Preoperative Workup *176*
- Surgical Procedure *177*

14. Scleral-Fixated Intraocular Lenses: A Review — 184
Meena Chakrabarti, Arup Chakrabarti
- Sutured Scleral Fixation *184*
- Sutureless Intrascleral Haptic Fixated Posterior Chamber Intraocular Lens *197*
- Postoperative Complications of Sutureless Scleral Fixation *204*
- Sutured versus Sutureless Scleral Fixation *205*

15. Message from Clinical Trials and How to Adopt them for Real Life Situations in Management of Retinal Vascular Disorders — 211
Lingam Gopal
- Efficacy versus Effectiveness *211*
- Bilateral Diabetic Macular Edema *218*
- Proliferative Diabetic Retinopathy *219*
- Retinal Vein Occlusions *220*
- Retinopathy of Prematurity *223*
- Neovascular Age Related Macular Degeneration *223*
- Dry Age Related Macular Degeneration *223*

16. Optical Coherence Tomography—Angiography in Retinal Diseases — 236
Chaitra Jayadev, Arpitha Pereira, Santosh GK Gadde
- Principle *236*
- Phase-Based Optical Coherence Tomography Angiography *237*
- Amplitude-Based Optical Coherence Tomography Angiography *238*
- Complex Signal-Based Optical Coherence Tomography Angiography *238*
- Image Processing *239*
- Optical Coherence Tomography Angiography of Normal Eyes *240*

- Artifacts *241*
- Optical Coherence Tomography Angiography of Retinal Disorders *243*

17. Optical Coherence Tomography in Diabetic Retinopathy 260
Manila Khatri, Sandeep Saxena
- Spectral Domain-Optical Coherence Tomography Analysis in Diabetic Retinopathy *260*
- Bioimaging Biomarkers in Diabetic Macular Edema *268*

18. Necrotizing Retinopathies 274
Rajesh Babu B, Saurabh Mistry, Sudharshan S
- Herpetic Retinitis *274*
- Historical Background *274*
- Etiology *276*
- Clinical Features *276*
- Acute Retinal Necrosis *276*
- Progressive Outer Retinal Necrosis *277*
- Surgical Management of Acute Retinal Necrosis *280*
- Cytomegalovirus Retinitis *280*
- Other Retinitis/Retinopathies *282*
- Other Rare Causes *283*

19. Nyctalopia 287
Avinash Pathengay, Sharat Hegde, Shreyansh Doshi
- Etiology *287*
- Clinical Features of Specific Disorders causing Nyctalopia *288*
- Pathophysiology *295*
- Approach to the Patient of Nyctalopia *296*
- Treatment *296*

20. Management of Ocular Burns: A Practical Approach 302
Jayesh Vazirani
- Emergency and Acute Phase Management *302*
- Ocular Surface Reconstruction and Vision Restoration after Severe Ocular Burns *305*

21. Cerebral Angiography in Neuro-Ophthalmology 309
Hima Pendharkar
- Indications for Cerebral Angiography *310*
- Contraindications *310*
- Preprocedural Workup *310*
- Procedure *311*
- Complications *312*
- Advances in Cerebral Angiography: 3D-Digital Subtraction Angiography *315*
- Case Studies *317*

Index 323

CHAPTER 1

Management of Post-LASIK Ectasia

Partha Biswas, Sneha Batra

■ INTRODUCTION

Laser-assisted in situ keratomileusis (LASIK) has become the gold standard for the treatment of refractive errors worldwide.[1] Over time, the rate of complications has been seen to be extremely low.[2] However, when these complications do occur, visual consequences can be substantial and patient dissatisfaction high, particularly because it is performed mainly as an elective cosmetic procedure, especially in young patients.

Post-LASIK ectasia (PLE) is defined as a region of abnormal steepening and increased curvature within a centrally flattened optical zone.[3] There is associated biomechanical weakening of the cornea.[4]

Seiler documented the first case report of PLE in the year 1998,[5] and it was thought at that time that an epidemic of iatrogenic keratectasia is looming over the world with increasing numbers of refractive procedures being performed worldwide without proper screening criteria in place. However, 20 years down the line, that fear has not been substantiated, and rate of PLE reported has remained low worldwide.[6,7]

Prevention and management of post-LASIK ectasia has remained a hot topic for debate, and following a famous trial in 2005 when a young man with PLE was awarded millions of dollars as compensation, a consensus group was formed by American Academy of Ophthalmology (AAO) and American Society of Cataract and Refractive Surgery (ASCRS), which enumerated the risk factors for eliminating high-risk candidates, and also certified that PLE may even occur in candidates without any known risk factor, and that it should not be considered negligence on part of the surgeon.[8]

■ EPIDEMIOLOGY

The incidence of PLE has been reported as 0.01–0.66% in various studies.[6,7] The mean duration from the initial laser procedure to detection is 15.3 months. A quarter of patients develop PLE within the first 3 months and at least half of them within 1 year of the laser procedure.[9] The earliest case was reported within one week,[10] while the latest was after 144 months.[11]

Post-LASIK ectasia was seen more frequently among males and in the younger age group, in patients with thin corneas and high refractive errors pre-operatively.[9]

▪ PRESENTING FEATURES

Any case of post-LASIK myopic regression, particularly if accompanied by a change in corneal topography, should be regarded with suspicion. Such patients should be closely followed up for at least 6 months before a decision for an enhancement procedure is taken.

Common Clinical Findings
- Progressively increasing refractive error (mainly myopia and irregular myopic astigmatism).
- Progressively decreasing best corrected visual acuity (BCVA).
- Stromal thinning (Fig. 1).
- Anterior and posterior corneal steepening.
- Vogt's striae (rarely).

Rare presentations in PLE include acute hydrops with perforated cornea,[12] and a case of globe rupture secondary to trauma.[13]

▪ INVESTIGATIONS HELPFUL IN THE DIAGNOSIS OF PLE
- Corneal topography (Figs. 2A to D).
- Anterior segment optical coherence tomography (AS-OCT) showing ectatic changes (Fig. 3).
- Ocular response analyzer (ORA) shows decreased ocular hysteresis.[14]

Randleman criteria for PLE is as follows:[15]
- Inferior topographic steepening of more than or equal to 5 diopters (D).
- Loss of more than or equal to 2 Snellen's lines of visual acuity.
- Alteration in refractive error of 2 D (spherical or cylindrical).

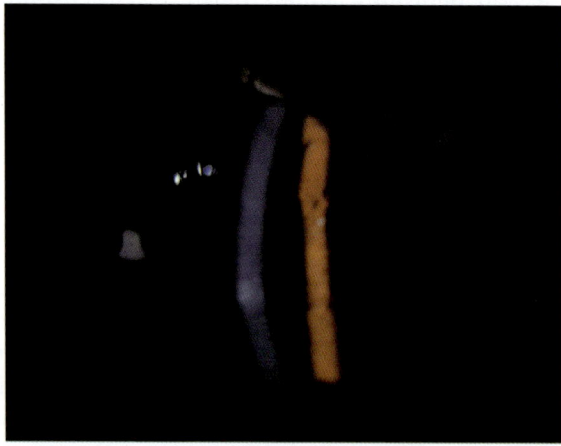

Fig. 1: Slit lamp photograph of a patient with post-laser-assisted in situ keratomileusis ectasia showing stromal thinning, ectasia, and scarring.

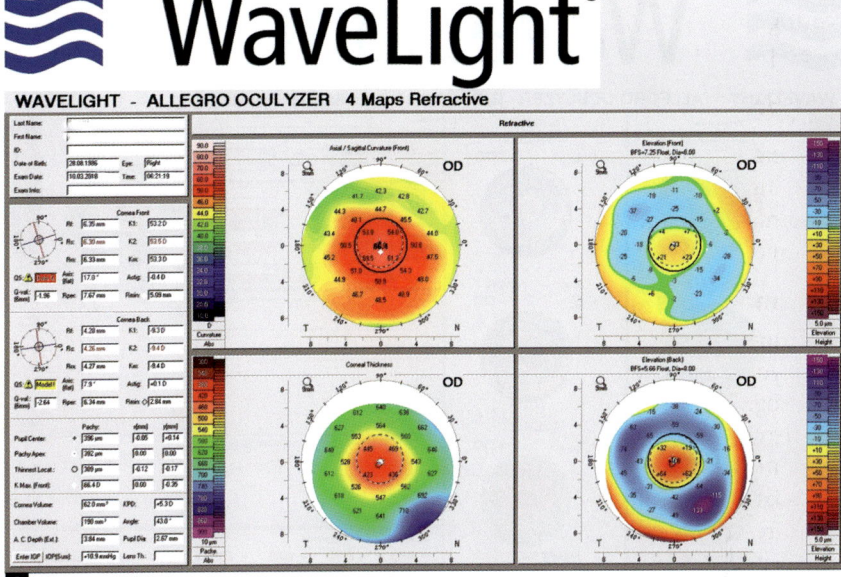

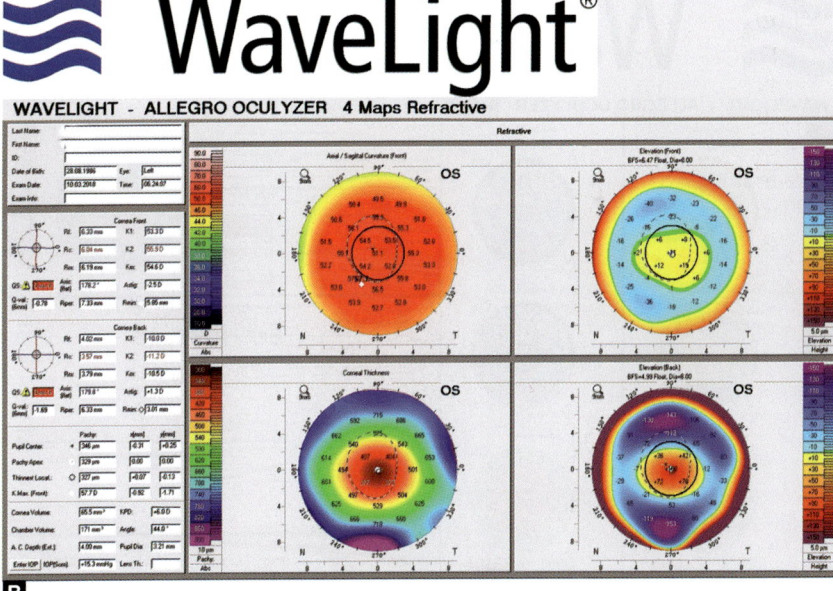

Figs. 2A and B

Padmanabhan et al. in their study suggested the following criteria as indicators of development of post-LASIK ectasia:[16]
- Increasing myopic refractive error with decrease in BCVA.
- An increase in magnitude of the highest anterior and posterior topographic elevation.

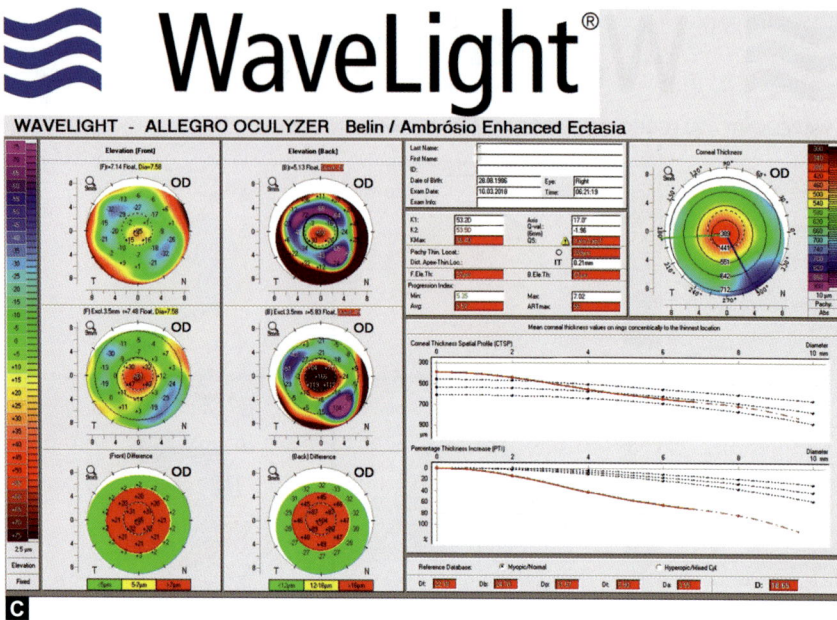

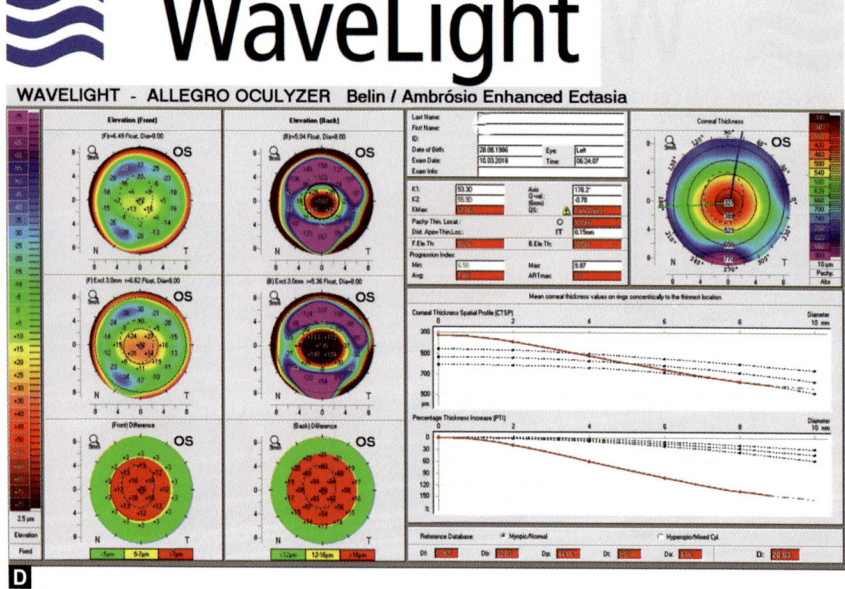

Figs. 2C and D

Figs. 2A to D: Corneal topography of a patient with post-laser-assisted in situ keratomileusis ectasia. (A and B) Refractive quad map of right and left eyes showing ectatic changes; (C and D) Belin/Ambrósio enhanced ectasia display of the same patient showing ectatic changes.

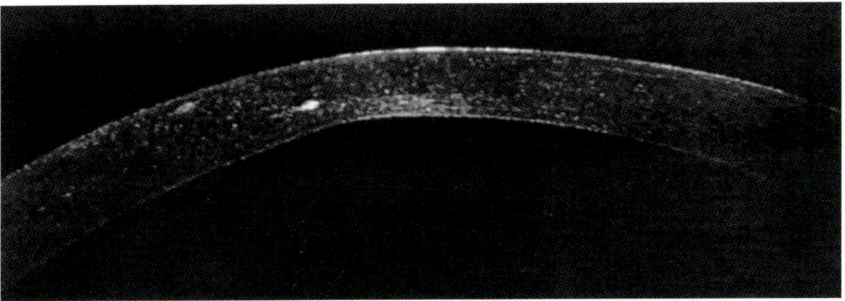

Fig. 3: Anterior segment optical coherence tomography of a patient with post-laser-assisted in situ keratomileusis ectasia showing thinning and ectatic changes.

- A shift of the location of the steepest point on the anterior cornea and that of the highest elevation of the posterior cornea towards the center of cornea.
- A reversal of the corneal asphericity towards greater prolateness.
- An increase in negative spherical aberration and coma.

They also devised a grading system for the management of PLE (Table 1).

RISK FACTORS FOR PLE

In their historic study,[9] Randleman et al. described the major etiological factors for PLE, and also devised the ectasia risk score system (ERSS) to identify the high-risk candidates before the laser procedure (Table 2).

Preoperative Topographic Pattern

In the overall subgroup analysis in the Randleman study, abnormal topography pattern was found to be the most significant factor. More than 40% of ectasia cases had grossly abnormal changes such as keratoconus and pellucid marginal degeneration (PMD).[9] These are now considered to be absolute contraindications to LASIK with medicolegal implications (Fig. 4). The following corneal topography patterns were considered:
- Normal or symmetrical
- *Suspicious*:
  - Asymmetric bow-tie:
    - Asymmetric steepening less than 1 D
    - No skewing of radial axis (SRA)
  - Inferior steep axis or SRA:
    - Significant SRA ± inferior steepening
    - More than or equal to 1 D of inferior steepening locally, but overall inferior-superior asymmetry (I-S) value less than 1.4.
- *Abnormal*: Keratoconus, PMD, or forme fruste keratoconus with an I-S value of more than or equal to 1.4.

Residual Stromal Bed

Patients with PLE have been shown to have significantly lower residual stromal bed (RSB) thickness than controls.

Table 1: Padmanabhan et al. grading system for post-LASIK ectasia.[16]

Grade	Normal	Mild	Moderate	Severe
Score	1	2	3	4
CDVA	≤0.18	0.19–0.48	0.49–0.78	>0.78
SE	+1 to –1	–1.1 to –5	–5.1 to –10	>–10
HPE	≤25	26–50	51–75	>75
$Z°_4$	≥0	<0 to ≥–0.5	<–0.5 to ≥–1	<–1
Q	≥0	<0 to ≥–1	<–1 to ≥–2	<–2

(CDVA: corrected distance visual acuity; HPE: highest posterior elevation; Q: corneal asphericity; SE: spherical equivalence; $Z°_4$: Zernike coefficient for spherical aberration)

Table 2: Randleman's ectasia risk factor score system (ERSS).[9]

Score / Parameter	IV	III	II	I	0
Corneal topography	Forme fruste keratoconus	Inferior steepening/skewed radial axis		Asymmetric bowtie	Normal/symmetric bowtie
Residual stromal bed (μ)	<240	240–259	260–279	280–299	>300
Age (years)		18–21	22–25	26–29	>30
Preoperative pachymetry (μ)	<450	451–480	481–510		>510
Preoperative refractive error (D)	>–14	>–12 to –14	>–10 to –12	>–8 to –10	–8 or less

It has been studied that posterior stroma is biomechanically weaker as compared to the anterior stroma, due to the differential distribution of keratocytes. Hence, corneal tensile strength is seen to decrease after LASIK.

In the Randleman ectasia score, all RSB thickness values less than 300 μ were considered increasingly significant in 20 μ intervals. Moreover, it has been documented that up to 33% of eyes with attempted RSB thickness of 250 μ could end up having actual RSB thickness less than 200 μ. The variability of flap thickness has been seen to occur with both mechanical microkeratomes and femtosecond lasers. Hence, it is now said that intraoperative measurement of RSB thickness is critical. It was seen in a survey among members of the International Society of Refractive Surgery or AAO in 2004, that only 31% refractive surgeons routinely measure flap or RSB thickness during surgery.[17]

It is seen that ectasia due to low RSB thickness usually occurs in the central corneal region while inferotemporal ectasia is usually seen in missed cases of forme fruste keratoconus or PMD.[18]

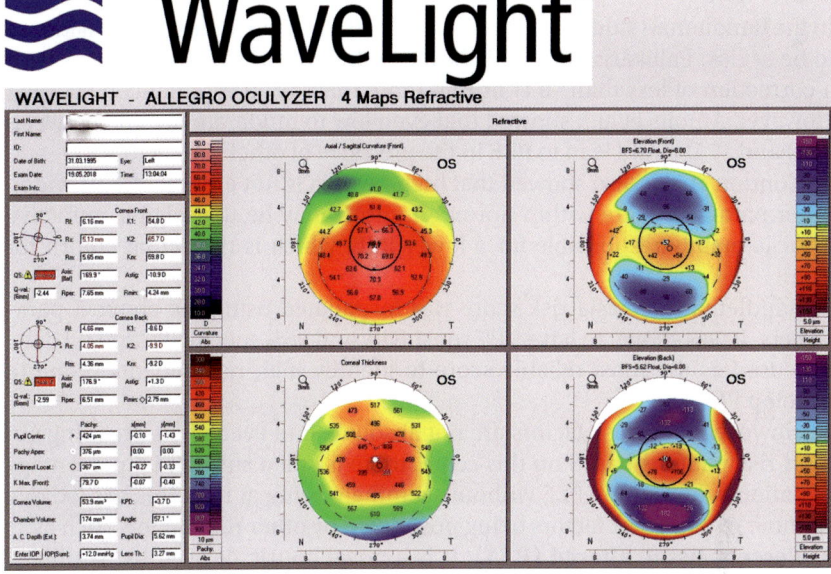

Fig. 4: Corneal topography showing ectatic changes suggestive of keratoconus—absolute contraindication for refractive surgery.

Why 250µ of RSB was Considered the Magical Cut-Off Number?

Andreasson et al.[19] found the elastic modulus of the keratoconic cornea to be 1.6–2.5 (average 2.1) times less than that of a normal cornea. Using these data, Seiler et al.[5] postulated that reduction in the load-bearing portion of a normal cornea from 525 µ to 250 µ (a factor of 2.1) might simulate the elasticity of a cornea with keratoconus and predispose to development of ectasia. This value coincides with Barraquer's early recommendation that a RSB thickness of at least 250 µ be maintained to prevent corneal ectasia after keratomileusis.[20]

Age

When ectasia cases with and without topographic abnormalities were compared, age was the only other significantly different factor. Patients without abnormal topographies were significantly younger than patients with defined topographic abnormalities. In the Randleman study, patients younger than 30 years were seen to be at risk; however, no recommendation was made on the basis of age.

Preoperative Pachymetry

The refractive error, preoperative pachymetry and RSB are interdependent factors. In the ectasia score, corneas with less than 510 µ were considered to be at risk.

High Myopia

In the Randleman study, patients with more than 8 D myopia were considered to be at risk. Pallikaris et al. had shown in their review that no subjects with a correction of less than −8 D or RSB more than 325 μ experienced ectasia.[7] However, Amoils et al.[21] showed that even low to moderate myopia between −4 D and −7 D could lead to PLE in the presence of other risk factors.

Condon et al.[22] also showed that high myopia is not a risk factor provided other parameters are within normal limits. It may be that higher refractive error is mainly responsible for a lower RSB, which is the actual culprit for PLE.

Randleman's ectasia risk score was formulated using the above 5 parameters. It was shown to have 91% sensitivity and 96% specificity, and till date, it is used as the most reliable score to identify high-risk patients prone to develop PLE.

However, these risk factors are not absolute, and even after screening out high-risk patients based on this score, there is still a substantial percentage of patients developing PLE without seemingly being at risk. This has led to a number of other risk factors being postulated by other researchers such as:

- **Percent tissue altered (PTA):** It is a novel metric devised by Santhiago et al.[23,24] which predicts high-risk patients irrespective of their topographic patterns. It is calculated as:

    PTA = (FT + AD)/CCT, where FT: flap thickness; AD: ablation depth; CCT: central corneal thickness.

    They showed that in a patient with normal corneal topography, PTA more than or equal to 40 was the most prevalent risk factor (97%), followed by age less than 30 years (63%), RSB less than or equal to 300 μ (57%) and Randleman ectasia score more than or equal to 3 (43%).

    Compared to RSB or CCT values, PTA provides a more individualized measure of biomechanical alteration because it considers the relationship between total thickness, tissue altered through ablation and flap creation, and ultimate RSB thickness. PTA was shown to have higher prevalence, higher odds ratio, and higher predictive capabilities for ectasia risk than moderate to high ectasia risk score system values.

- **Ablation ratio:** Brenner et al.[25] devised a new metric, ablation ratio, which is calculated as:

    Ablation ratio = Ablation depth/Pachymetry

    It was shown to have the strongest correlation with post-LASIK ectasia spherical equivalence.

- **Ablation depth:** The depth of ablation and increased intraocular pressure (IOP) were shown to be significant risk factors for post-LASIK ectasia in white rabbits.[26] Tatar et al.[27] also showed that deep ablation more than 75 μ is the most important risk factor for the development of PLE.

- **Choice of procedure:** About 4% cases of PLE have occurred after photorefractive keratectomy (PRK), whereas 96% cases occur after LASIK.[9] Dawson et al.[28] reported that PRK, sub-Bowman's keratomileusis (SBK) and advanced surface ablation (ASA) cause lesser reduction in the biomechanical strength of the cornea.

- **Multiple enhancements:** Multiple ablations are also thought to be an associated factor.[29] However, it is difficult to say whether it is a true risk factor or the progressive myopia in these cases was actually due to missed cases of early PLE.
- **Thicker flaps:** Thicker flap weakens the biomechanically crucial obliquely-oriented anterior stromal layer predisposing to PLE.[30]
- **Chronic rubbing of eyes:** It could be a contributory factor.[31]
- **Pregnancy:** It may induce certain hormonal changes such as production of the hormone relaxin which can induce or exaggerate pre-existing PLE.[32]
- **Other risk factors:** These include candidates with family history of keratoconus and male sex.

Belin/Ambrósio Enhanced Ectasia Display (BAD)[33]

Brazilian ophthalmologist Renato Ambrósio and Arizona's Michael Belin developed a new software incorporated in the Pentacam® machine, which uses imaging of both the anterior and posterior corneal surfaces, and uses elevation-based tomographic data, combined with pachymetric analysis to generate a more accurate screening criteria for refractive surgery. While the first set of images displays the elevation of the anterior and posterior surfaces of the cornea compared to the best fit sphere (BFS) over a central 8 mm zone, the second set of images (the enhanced elevation map) eliminates the ectatic portion of the cornea from the computation, which helps to accentuate the effect of ectasia even in minimal amount.

The lower two maps (subtraction maps) show a color coding (red/yellow/green) to differentiate between normal and ectatic corneas. The corneal thickness spatial profile (CTSP) and percentage thickness increase (PTI) graphs depict the progressive thinning of the cornea from the periphery to the thinnest point, and the percentage of increase from the thinnest point out to the periphery respectively. Ultimately, a D value (Belin-Ambrósio deviation value) is calculated, which is indicated in yellow (suspicious) when it is more than or equal to 1.6 standard deviation (SD) from the mean (Fig. 5A), and in red (abnormal) when it is more than or equal to 2.6 SD from the mean (Fig. 5B).

However, despite screening protocols with all the known risk factors in place, some patients still develop ectasia with no identifiable cause. It is now thought that an individual's intrinsic tensile strength of the cornea probably is the most crucial factor for the development of ectasia.[34-37]

PATHOGENESIS

Post-LASIK ectasia can be said to occur when the tensile strength of an individual's cornea is lowered below a certain threshold which is essential to maintain the shape of the cornea. This can occur in the following three ways:[38]

1. The cornea undergoing laser refractive procedure does not show any topographic changes, but is intrinsically weaker and prone to develop ectatic changes in the future.

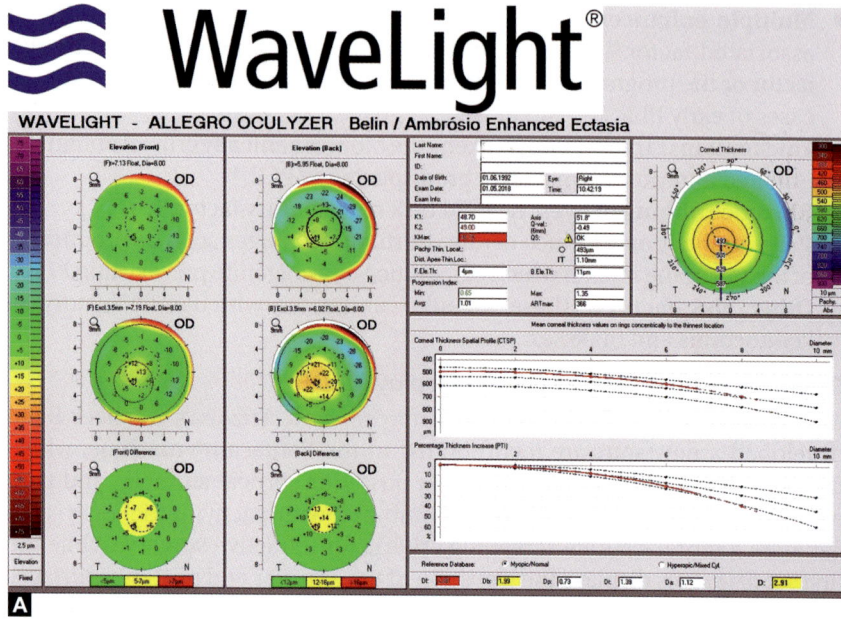

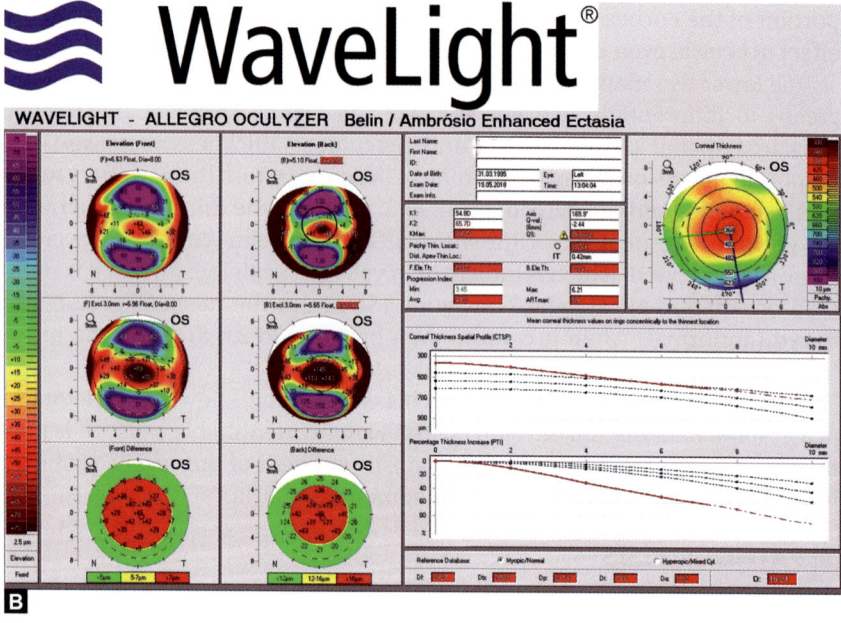

Figs. 5A and B: Belin/Ambrósio-enhanced ectasia display map. (A) Belin "suspicious" with D value in yellow range; (B) Ectatic changes with D value in red range.

2. The cornea undergoing laser shows subtle topographic changes, but seems to be stable clinically, and is weakened further by the laser procedure.
3. The cornea undergoing laser was biomechanically normal preoperatively, but an excessive amount of tissue loss weakens it beyond its threshold.

The chief alteration predisposing to PLE is seen in the anterior corneal biomechanics which precipitates thinning and compression of collagen fibrils, resulting in loss of global structural integrity.[6]

HISTOPATHOLOGY

Randleman et al.[39] described in detail the histopathological and ultrastructural changes in corneas affected by PLE. Specimens of cornea with PLE which underwent penetrating keratoplasty (PKP) were observed for histopathological changes under light microscopy, and the following features were observed:
- Corneal epithelial hypoplasia.
- Breaks in the Bowman's membrane, typically smaller than that seen in keratoconus.
- Adequate thickness of the flap.
- Adequate thickness of the hypocellular primitive stromal scar.
- Reduced thickness of the RSB.
- Large interlamellar clefts in the ectatic region of the RSB.

The specimens were also evaluated in 2.5% glutaraldehyde under transmission electron microscope (TEM), where the following changes were noted:
- Reduced thickness of the stromal lamellae.
- Reduced number of lamellae in the stroma.
- Loss of keratocyte density.[40]
- Reduced thickness of the collagen fibrils.[41]
- Presence of aggregated microfibrils in the Bowman's membrane and stroma.
- Degeneration of the proteoglycans within the collagen fibrils, which lead to degeneration of the fibrils themselves, causing disorganization of the lamellae.[41]
- Wavy and distorted stromal collagen bundles, especially in the posterior corneal region.[42]

Immunohistochemistry and Other Novel Investigations
- Increase in proteinases such as matrix metalloproteinase (MMP) 10 and 3 suggesting ongoing epithelial basement membrane lysis and remodeling.[43]
- Alpha 1-proteinase inhibitor (α1-PI) and Sp1 expression are unchanged.[44]
- In vivo confocal microscopy shows increased corneal dendritic cell density.
- Tear cytokine analysis shows altered cytokines as in dry eye suggesting a possible inflammatory role in PLE.[45]
- Significant elevation of MMP 9 and decrease in tissue inhibitor of MMP (TIMP) 1 in tear samples.[46]

Biomechanical Elasticity Theory[14]
The biomechanical theory postulates that interlamellar and interfibrillar slippage occurs postoperatively in those areas of the residual stroma which

are subjected to maximum stress. This chronic phenomenon is termed as "interfiber fracture".

Guirao, in his study, used the spherical thin-shell model to demonstrate that tissue removal from an intact cornea causes anterior shifting of the posterior corneal surface with an increase in its dioptric power.[47]

As mentioned earlier, the posterior cornea is biomechanically weaker as compared to the anterior stroma. The creation of an anterior flap disturbs this distribution as this vital part of the stroma no longer contributes to the biomechanical integrity of the cornea.[23]

MANAGEMENT

Contact Lenses

Contact lenses can be used in the earlier stages of PLE. Rigid gas permeable (RGP) lenses are the most commonly used lenses. They are very similar to those used in keratoconus patients, and lenses are custom made for every patient.[48]

Rose K lenses have been specially developed for ectatic corneas, and are now one of the most commonly used lenses worldwide (Fig. 6A). Scleral lenses have also been used in PLE patients, especially for those with irregular corneas (Fig. 6B).[49] They can be either semi-scleral (16–18 mm diameter), or full scleral lenses (18–22 mm diameter). Hybrid lenses with central RGP like features, and peripheral soft lens-like configuration, have also been developed, which have replaced piggyback lenses now (Fig. 6C). PROSE (prosthetic replacement of ocular surface ecosystem) lenses have also been tried successfully (Fig. 6D).[50]

Collagen Cross-Linking (CXL)

Collagen cross-linking is considered to be the gold standard treatment for progressive corneal ectasia, but it is associated with slow and painful recovery periods.[4]

The indications for CXL in case of PLE are as follows:
- Increase in K_{max} more than 1 D in 1 year.
- Decrease in BCVA.
- Requirement for altered contact lens fitting more than biannually.

The contraindications to CXL are as follows:
- Thinnest pachymetry less than 400 μ.
- Corneal infection.
- Autoimmune diseases.
- Pregnancy or lactation period.

The CXL protocol followed usually is the Dresden protocol[51] which includes:
- Removing the corneal epithelium over 8 mm under topical anesthesia.
- Soaking the corneal stroma in isotonic 0.1% riboflavin solution every 3 minutes for 30 minutes.
- Application of ultraviolet A light at 3 mW/cm² irradiance and 5.4 J/cm² dose for half an hour (Fig. 7).

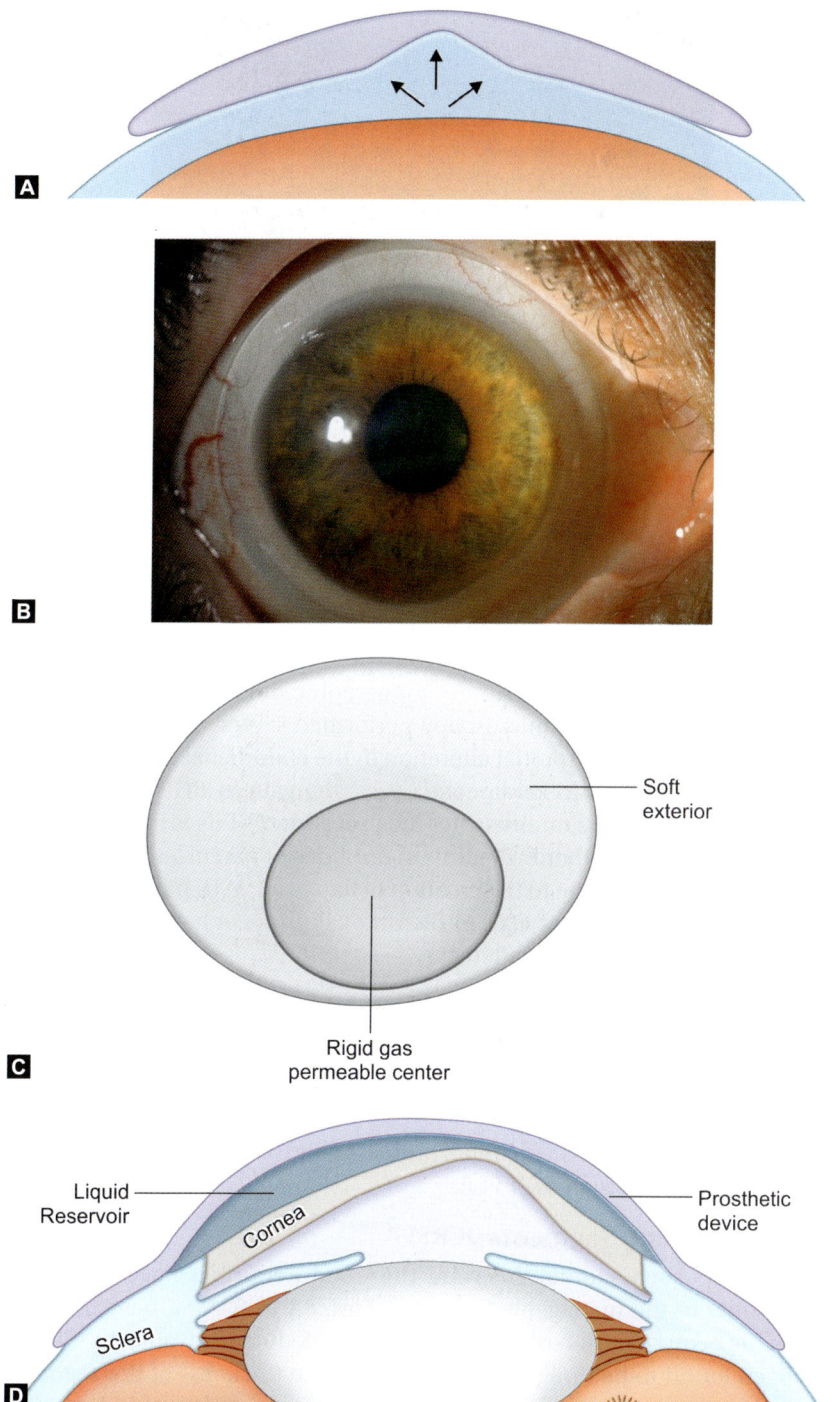

Figs. 6A to D: Contact lenses used in the management of post-laser-assisted in situ keratomileusis ectasia. (A) Rose K lens; (B) Scleral lens; (C) Hybrid lens; (D) PROSE lens.

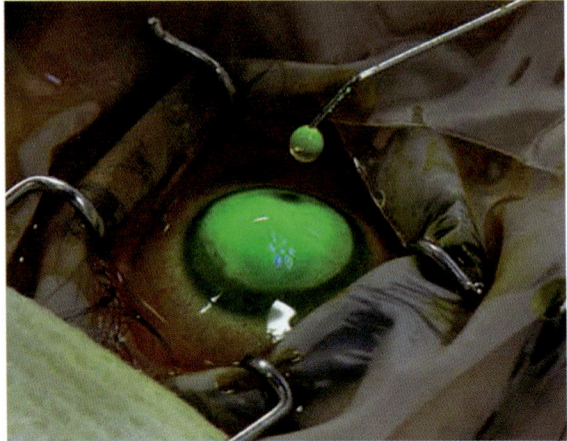

Fig. 7: Collagen cross-linking for management of post-laser-assisted in situ keratomileusis ectasia.

- Application of bandage contact lens for 3 days for rapid re-epithelialization.
- Antibiotic and steroid eye drops are given postoperatively.

Collagen cross-linking has shown long-term stability without significant side effects, and over time, it improves BCVA, decreases cylindrical power and K_{max} values, and halts progression of topographic indices and higher order aberrations.[6,52,53] Confocal microscopy performed 1 year after CXL showed good results with no substantial alteration in the endothelial cell count.[54]

However, compared to keratoconus eyes, the gain in BCVA is slow and usually not seen until 12 months after the procedure.[55] This is because cross-linking results in strengthening mainly of the anterior part of stroma, which is already compromised due to the creation of flap in a LASIK patient.[56]

Various modifications of CXL to the original protocol have been tried to increase the efficacy in PLE patients:

- Epithelium on CXL.[4]
- Under flap CXL (ufCXL): early onset mild cases of PLE treated by lifting the LASIK flap and irradiating with 18 mW/cm² UV light.[57]
- Athens protocol: Consecutive sequential topography-guided partial transepithelial PRK and CXL.[58,59]
- Combined PTK-PRK-CXL (Cretan protocol plus) has also been successfully used to stop the progress of PLE.[60]

Intracorneal Ring Segments (ICRS)

Various ICRS such as Intacs, Ferrara rings and Kera rings have been used successfully in the management of PLE (Figs. 8A to C).[61-63] These implants flatten the central portion of the cornea thereby reducing myopia. Its efficacy has been found to be directly proportional to the thickness of the segment, and inversely proportional to its diameter. The progression of PLE is often halted and a corneal transplant may no longer be required. The advantages are that it is reversible and tissue saving in nature.

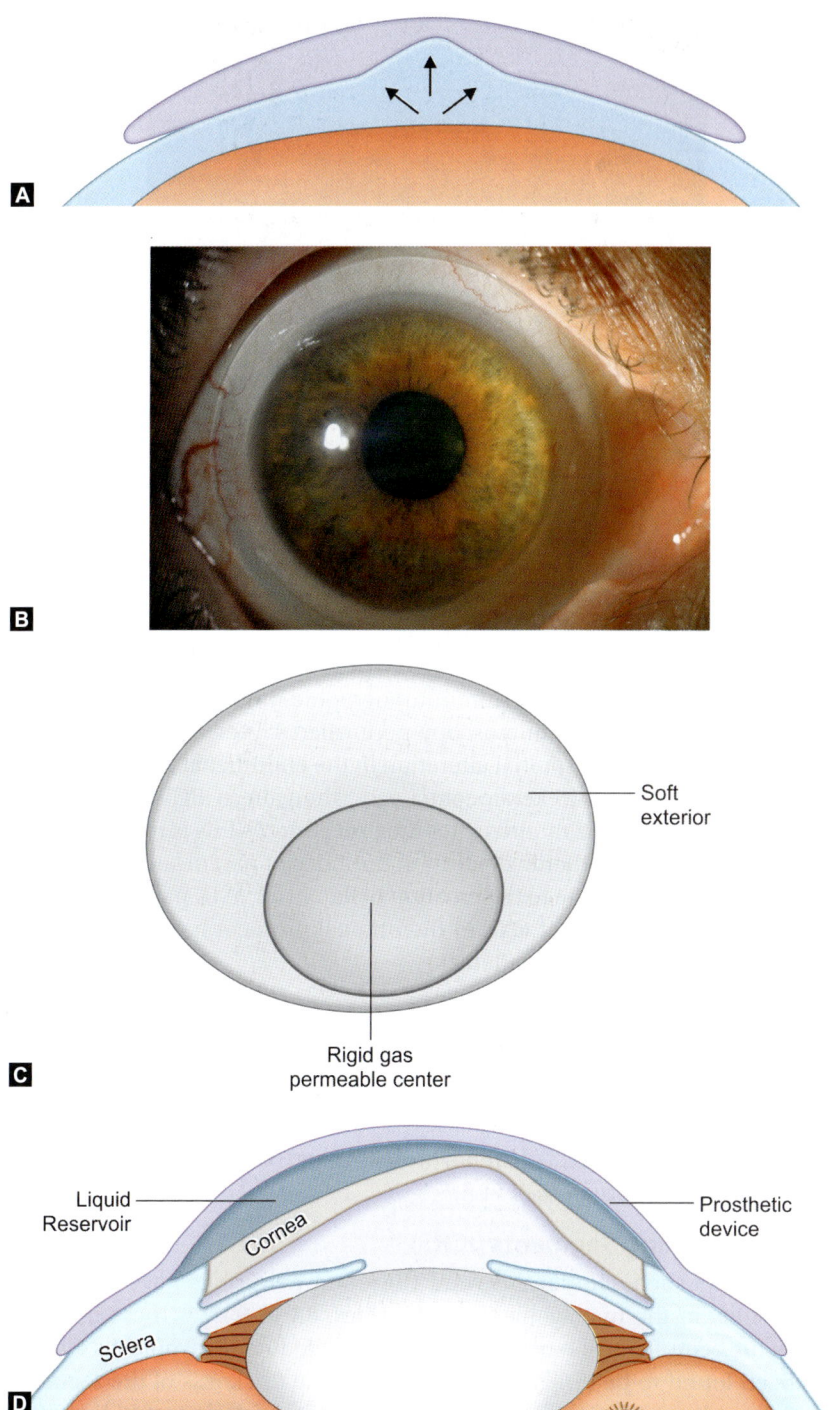

Figs. 6A to D: Contact lenses used in the management of post-laser-assisted in situ keratomileusis ectasia. (A) Rose K lens; (B) Scleral lens; (C) Hybrid lens; (D) PROSE lens.

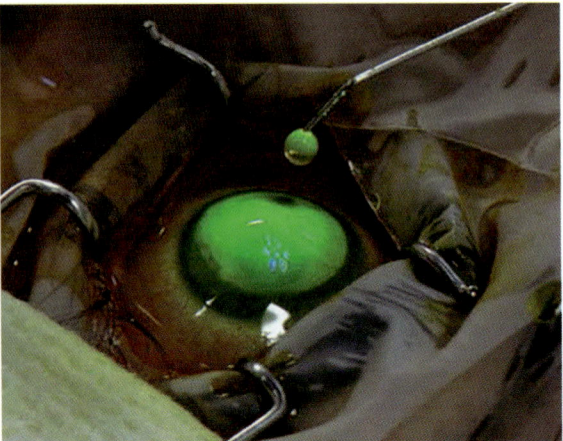

Fig. 7: Collagen cross-linking for management of post-laser-assisted in situ keratomileusis ectasia.

- Application of bandage contact lens for 3 days for rapid re-epithelialization.
- Antibiotic and steroid eye drops are given postoperatively.

Collagen cross-linking has shown long-term stability without significant side effects, and over time, it improves BCVA, decreases cylindrical power and K_{max} values, and halts progression of topographic indices and higher order aberrations.[6,52,53] Confocal microscopy performed 1 year after CXL showed good results with no substantial alteration in the endothelial cell count.[54]

However, compared to keratoconus eyes, the gain in BCVA is slow and usually not seen until 12 months after the procedure.[55] This is because cross-linking results in strengthening mainly of the anterior part of stroma, which is already compromised due to the creation of flap in a LASIK patient.[56]

Various modifications of CXL to the original protocol have been tried to increase the efficacy in PLE patients:
- Epithelium on CXL.[4]
- Under flap CXL (ufCXL): early onset mild cases of PLE treated by lifting the LASIK flap and irradiating with 18 mW/cm² UV light.[57]
- Athens protocol: Consecutive sequential topography-guided partial transepithelial PRK and CXL.[58,59]
- Combined PTK-PRK-CXL (Cretan protocol plus) has also been successfully used to stop the progress of PLE.[60]

Intracorneal Ring Segments (ICRS)

Various ICRS such as Intacs, Ferrara rings and Kera rings have been used successfully in the management of PLE (Figs. 8A to C).[61-63] These implants flatten the central portion of the cornea thereby reducing myopia. Its efficacy has been found to be directly proportional to the thickness of the segment, and inversely proportional to its diameter. The progression of PLE is often halted and a corneal transplant may no longer be required. The advantages are that it is reversible and tissue saving in nature.

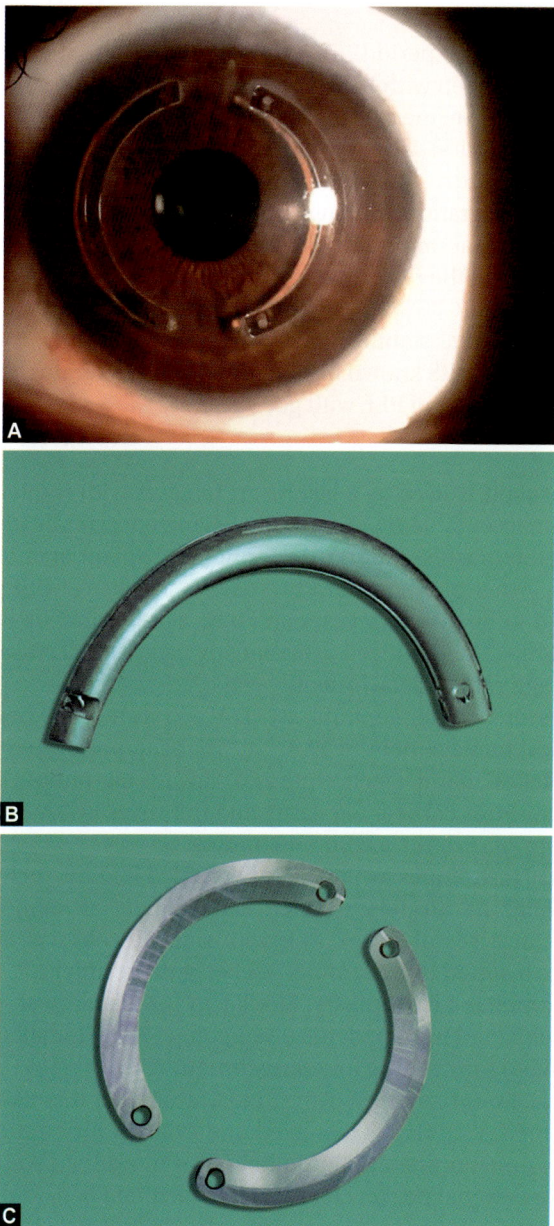

Figs. 8A to C: Intracorneal ring segments used in the management of post-laser-assisted in situ keratomileusis ectasia. (A) Intacs; (B) Ferrara rings; (C) Kera rings.

The indications of ICRS are:
- Patients with loss of more than or equal to 2 Snellen's lines of BCVA.
- Grade 4 PLE.

Contraindications to ICRS implantation are:
- Any previous ocular surgery.
- Vernal keratoconjunctivitis.

- Viral keratitis.
- Pregnancy/lactation period.

The complications seen with ICRS are:[62]
- **Intraoperative:** Segment decentration, insufficient depth of channel, superficial dissection with perforation of Bowman's membrane
- **Postoperative:** Extrusion of implant, neovascularization, infective keratitis, segment migration, melting of cornea

For PLE, implantation of a single segment in the ectatic portion is more effective in reducing the refractive error than implanting two segments.[64]

Combination of ICRS and CXL has been tried successfully for vision improvement as well as stabilization of ectasia.[65]

A new variety of ICRS known has Intacs SK (severe keratoconus) has been used in advanced cases of PLE with good results.[66]

Keratoplasty

Corneal transplant is used as a last resort in cases with intolerance to RGP lenses, and unacceptable BCVA, usually having contraindication to CXL or ICRS. PKP is the most commonly performed transplant of choice in ectasia patients. The visual prognosis in PLE cases is excellent, with graft survival rates reported to be 97% at 5 years and 92% at 10 years.[8] Its complications include graft rejection, induced astigmatism, cataract, increased IOP, endophthalmitis, and retinal detachment.

Deep anterior lamellar keratoplasty (DALK) has recently been advocated for the surgical management of PLE.[67] It has been performed in PLE cases using both Melles' manual technique and Anwar's big-bubble technique.[68,69] It effectively restores corneal regularity and improves BCVA. However, high-residual ametropia is often a common finding.

Newer surgical techniques, which have been tried for PLE, include:
- **Intralamellar keratoplasty (ILK):** Schanzlin et al. demonstrated this technique in cases of severe PLE with sagging cones; a donor stromal lenticule is inserted into a stromal pocket of the recipient.[70]
- **Tuck-in lamellar keratoplasty:** Similar to ILK; Jiang et al. used a donor lenticule obtained from patients undergoing SMILE (small incision lenticule extraction) procedure for this technique.[62]
- **Flap replacement surgery:** Titiyal et al. described this novel procedure in which the LASIK flap is dissected and excised. A donor lenticule with Descemet's membrane and endothelium removed is taken, and tucked into an intrastromal pocket created in the recipient bed, and sutured.[71]

PREVENTION

As described above, multiple etiological factors have been described for the development of PLE; however, PLE still often develops in patients who do not have any of these criteria. A review of the published literature incriminates three main culprits, which must be avoided:
- **Missed ectatic pathologies:** These can be prevented by meticulous screening using corneal topography, especially the Belin/Ambrósio dis-

play on Pentacam® which can predict corneas prone to develop ectasia in the future (Figs. 9A and 9B).
- **Multiple enhancements:** Ectatic disorders must be ruled out before retreatment is considered.
- **Thinned RSB:** RSB must be routinely measured intraoperatively since thickness of flap has been known to vary considerably even in the hands of a single surgeon.

Screening protocols must be in place in every institute where LASIK is done, and it may be individualized based on the surgeon's experience. The Randleman's ectasia score is most commonly used; however, it has been criticized as not being able to detect high-risk patients among those having normal topography.[72] Various other scoring systems have been developed;[73] however, it is essential to develop a customized screening protocol based on the laser machine being used.

Some authors have reported combined procedures which may help to prevent the development of PLE:
- **Combined LASIK and CXL (LASIK Xtra):** CXL serves as a prophylaxis against refractive regression and to prevent the development of PLE in high-risk patients. No associated decrease in visual acuity is seen. Refractive and keratometric outcomes have been shown to be comparable to or better than LASIK alone. No case of PLE has been reported in these patients.[74-78]

The following laser refractive procedures have been shown to have lesser risk of development of PLE as compared to LASIK:
- Femto-LASIK is more consistent and has more predictable flap size and depth of ablation, and it also causes limited reduction of corneal biomechanical integrity.[35]
- SMILE is thought to preserve the anterior stromal collagen which has a bigger role in the maintenance of corneal integrity.[79]
- Photorefractive keratectomy, ASA, and SBK cause lesser reduction in corneal tensile strength compared to LASIK.[28]

CONCLUSION

Post-LASIK ectasia has not emerged as the epidemic as was predicted by the critics in the early years of refractive surgery. However, even a single case can be problematic considering its medicolegal implications and the number of disability affected life years (DALYs) involved. Hence, every refractive surgeon must be aware of this important complication, and the screening protocols which have been developed for its prevention. It is also equally important to be able to detect its presence early, and provide appropriate management, since early treatment has been shown to have promising visual rehabilitative results. However, despite all screening protocols, ectasia has been seen to develop even in subjects with seemingly no risk factor. Hence, the Joint Consensus Committee of 2005 had recommended that PLE be considered a known risk factor of laser refractive procedures, which may develop despite the strictest screening protocols. The patient should be made aware of this

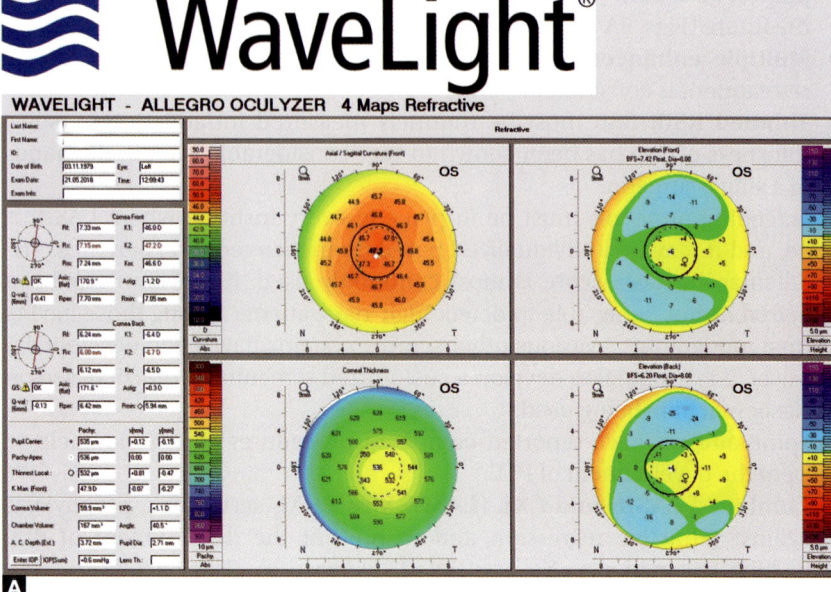

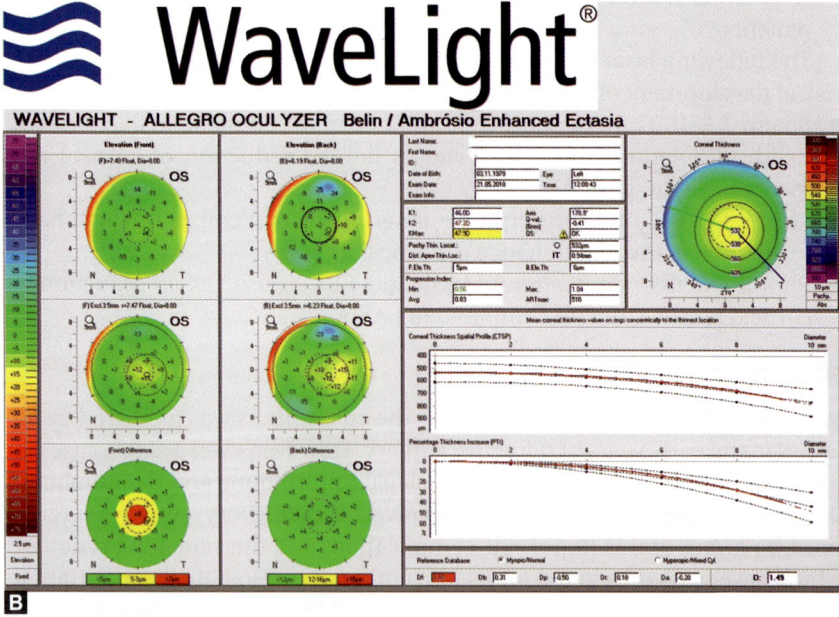

Figs. 9A and B: Corneal topography of a high-risk patient screened out for laser-assisted in situ keratomileusis. (A) Four maps refractive showing no obvious abnormality apart from high steep K (47.9 D); (B) Belin/Ambrósio display showing suspicious changes in anterior float, predictive of possible future ectasia development.

entity before the procedure, and a meticulous follow-up of high-risk patients is essential.

REFERENCES

1. Kamiya K, Igarashi A, Hayashi K, et al. A multicenter retrospective survey of refractive surgery in 78,248 eyes. J Refract Surg. 2017;33(9):598-602.
2. Karabela Y, Muftuoglu O, Gulkilik IG, et al. Intraoperative and early postoperative flap-related complications of laser in situ keratomileusis using two types of Moria microkeratomes. Int Ophthalmol. 2014;34(5):1107-14.
3. Vinciguerra P, Camesasca F, Albè E, et al. Corneal collagen cross-linking for ectasia after excimer laser refractive surgery: 1-year results. J Refract Surg. 2010;26(7):486-97.
4. Moscovici BK, Campos M. Intrastromal crosslinking in post-LASIK ectasia. Arq Bras Oftalmol. 2014;77(3):191-2.
5. Seiler T, Koufala K, Richter G. Iatrogenic keratectasia after laser in situ keratomileusis. J Refract Surg. 1998;14(3):312-7.
6. Tong JY, Viswanathan D, Hodge C, et al. Corneal collagen crosslinking for post-LASIK ectasia: an Australian study. Asia Pac J Ophthalmol. 2017;6(3):228-32.
7. Pallikaris IG, Kymionis GD, Astyrakakis NI. Corneal ectasia induced by laser in situ keratomileusis. J Cataract Refract Surg. 2001;27(11):1796-802.
8. Binder PS, Lindstrom RL, Stulting RD, et al. Keratoconus and corneal ectasia after LASIK. J Cataract Refract Surg. 2005;31(11):2035-8.
9. Randleman JB, Woodward M, Lynn MJ, et al. Risk assessment for ectasia after corneal refractive surgery. Ophthalmology. 2008;115(1):37-50.
10. Rao SN, Epstein RJ. Early onset keratectasia following laser in situ keratomileusis: case report and literature review. J Refract Surg. 2002;18(2):177-84.
11. Said A, Hamade IH, Tabbara KF. Late onset corneal ectasia after LASIK surgery. Saudi J Ophthalmol. 2011;25(3):225-30.
12. Gupta C, Tanaka TS, Elner VM, et al. Acute hydrops with corneal perforation in post-LASIK ectasia. Cornea. 2015;34(1):99-100.
13. Cheung AY, Heidemann DG. Globe rupture of a post-LASIK keratectasia eye from blunt trauma. Cornea. 2016;35(12):1662-4.
14. Condon PI. 2005 ESCRS Ridley Medal Lecture: will keratectasia be a major complication for LASIK in the long term? J Cataract Refract Surg. 2006;32(12):2124-32.
15. Randleman JB, Russell B, Ward MA, et al. Risk factors and prognosis for corneal ectasia after LASIK. Ophthalmology. 2003;110(2):267-75.
16. Padmanabhan P, Reddi SR, Sivakumar PD. Topographic, tomographic, and aberrometric characteristics of post-LASIK ectasia. Optom Vis Sci. 2016;93(11):1364-70.
17. Duffey RJ, Leaming D. US trends in refractive surgery: 2004 ISRS/AAO survey. J Refract Surg. 2005;21(6):742-8.
18. Kerautret J, Colin J, Touboul D, et al. Biomechanical characteristics of the ectatic cornea. J Cataract Refract Surg. 2008;34(3):510-3.
19. Andreassen TT, Simonsen AH, Oxlund H. Biomechanical properties of keratoconus and normal corneas. Exp Eye Res. 1980;31(4):435-41.
20. Barraquer JI. Queratomileusis y Queratofakia. Bogota: Instituto Barraquer de America. 1980;405-6.
21. Amoils SP, Deist MB, Gous P, et al. Iatrogenic keratectasia after laser in situ keratomileusis for less than –4 to –7 diopters of myopia. J Cataract Refract Surg. 2000;26(7):967-77.

22. Condon PI, O'Keefe M, Binder PS. Long-term results of laser in situ keratomileusis for high myopia: risk for ectasia. J Cataract Refract Surg. 2007;33(4):583-90.
23. Santhiago M, Smadja D, Gomes B, et al. Association between the percent tissue altered and post-laser in situ keratomileusis ectasia in eyes with normal preoperative topography. Am J Ophthalmol. 2014;158(1):87-95.
24. Santhiago M, Smadja D, Wilson S, et al. Role of percent tissue altered on ectasia after LASIK in eyes with suspicious topography. J Refract Surg. 2015;31(4):258-65.
25. Brenner LF, Alió JL, Vega-Estrada A, et al. Clinical grading of post-LASIK ectasia related to visual limitation and predictive factors for vision loss. J Cataract Refract Surg. 2012;38(10):1817-26.
26. Huang X, He X, Tan X. [Research of corneal ectasia following laser in situ keratomileusis in rabbits]. Yan Ke Xue Bao. 2002;18(2):119-22.
27. Tatar MG, Kantarci FA, Yildirim A, et al. Risk factors in post-LASIK corneal ectasia. J Ophthalmol. 2014;2014:204191.
28. Dawson DG, Grossniklaus HE, McCarey BE, et al. Biomechanical and wound healing characteristics of corneas after excimer laser keratorefractive surgery: is there a difference between advanced surface ablation and sub-Bowman's keratomileusis? J Refract Surg. 2008;24(1):S90-6.
29. Randleman JB. Post-laser in-situ keratomileusis ectasia: current understanding and future directions. Curr Opin Ophthalmol. 2006;17(4):406-12.
30. Giri P, Azar DT. Risk profiles of ectasia after keratorefractive surgery. Curr Opin Ophthalmol. 2017;28(4):337-42.
31. Padmanabhan P, Aiswaryah R, Abinaya PV. Post-LASIK keratectasia triggered by eye rubbing and treated with topography-guided ablation and collagen cross-linking—a case report. Cornea. 2012;31(5):575-80.
32. Padmanabhan P, Radhakrishnan A, Natarajan R. Pregnancy-triggered iatrogenic (post-laser in situ keratomileusis) corneal ectasia—a case report. Cornea. 2010;29(5):569-72.
33. Belin M, Ambrósio R. The Belin/Ambrósio enhanced extasia display. [online] Available from http://aspx.apacrs.org/apacrs-publication/Default2.aspx?id=656.
34. Binder PS. Analysis of ectasia after laser in situ keratomileusis: risk factors. J Cataract Refract Surg. 2007;33(9):1530-8.
35. Vahdati A, Seven I, Mysore N, et al. Computational biomechanical analysis of asymmetric ectasia risk in unilateral post-LASIK ectasia. J Refract Surg. 2016;32(12):811-20.
36. Harissi-Dagher M, Frimmel SA, Melki S. High myopia as a risk factor for post-LASIK ectasia: a case report. Digit J Ophthalmol. 2009;15(1):9-13.
37. Binder PS. Ectasia after laser in situ keratomileusis. J Cataract Refract Surg. 2003;29(12):2419-29.
38. Santhiago MR, Giacomin NT, Smadja D, et al. Ectasia risk factors in refractive surgery. Clinical Ophthalmology. 2016;10:713-20.
39. Dawson DG, Randleman JB, Grossniklaus HE, et al. Corneal ectasia after excimer laser keratorefractive surgery: histopathology, ultrastructure, and pathophysiology. Ophthalmology. 2008;115(12):2181-91.
40. Ali Javadi M, Kanavi MR, Mahdavi M, et al. Comparison of keratocyte density between keratoconus, post-laser in situ keratomileusis keratectasia, and uncomplicated post-laser in situ keratomileusis cases. A confocal scan study. Cornea. 2009;28(7):774-9.

41. Akhtar S, Alkatan H, Kirat O, et al. Ultrastructural and three-dimensional study of post-LASIK ectasia cornea. Microsc Res Tech. 2014;77(1):91-8.
42. Liu Y, Konstantopoulos A, Riau AK, et al. Repeatability and reproducibility of corneal biometric measurements using the visante omni and a rabbit experimental model of post-surgical corneal ectasia. Transl Vis Sci Technol. 2015;4(2):16.
43. Maguen E, Maguen B, Regev L, et al. Immunohistochemical evaluation of two corneal buttons with post-LASIK keratectasia. Cornea. 2007;26(8):983-91.
44. Meghpara B, Nakamura H, Macsai M, et al. Keratectasia after laser in situ keratomileusis: a histopathologic and immunohistochemical study. Arch Ophthalmol. 2008;126(12):1655-63.
45. Pahuja NK, Shetty R, Deshmukh R, et al. In vivo confocal microscopy and tear cytokine analysis in post-LASIK ectasia. Br J Ophthalmol. 2017;101(12):1604-10.
46. Elmohamady MN, Abdelghaffar W, Salem TI. Tear matrix metalloproteinase-9 and tissue inhibitor of metalloproteinase-1 in post-LASIK ectasia. Int Ophthalmol. 2018.
47. Guirao A. Theoretical elastic response of the cornea to refractive surgery: risk factors for keratectasia. J Refract Surg. 2005;21(2):176-85.
48. Hiatt JA, Wachler BS, Grant C. Reversal of laser in situ keratomileusis induced ectasia with intraocular pressure reduction. J Cataract Refract Surg. 2005;31(8):1652-5.
49. Kramer EG, Boshnick EL. Scleral lenses in the treatment of post-LASIK ectasia and superficial neovascularization of intrastromal corneal ring segments. Cont Lens Anterior Eye. 2015;38(4):298-303.
50. Mahadevan R, Jagadeesh D, Rajan R, et al. Unique hard scleral lens post-LASIK ectasia fitting. Optom Vis Sci. 2014;91(4 Suppl 1):S30-3.
51. Wollensak G, Spoerl E, Seiler T. Riboflavin/ultraviolet-a-induced collagen crosslinking for the treatment of keratoconus. Amer J Ophthalmol. 2003;135(5):620-7.
52. Greenstein SA, Fry KL, Hersh PS. Corneal topography indices after corneal collagen crosslinking for keratoconus and corneal ectasia: one-year results. J Cataract Refract Surg. 2011;37(7):1282-90.
53. Poli M, Cornut PL, Balmitgere T, et al. Prospective study of corneal collagen cross-linking efficacy and tolerance in the treatment of keratoconus and corneal ectasia: 3-year results. Cornea. 2013;32(5):583-90.
54. Kymionis GD, Diakonis VF, Kalyvianaki M, et al. One-year follow-up of corneal confocal microscopy after corneal cross-linking in patients with post laser in situ keratomileusis ectasia and keratoconus. Am J Ophthalmol. 2009;147(5):774-8.
55. Hersh PS, Greenstein SA, Fry KL. Corneal collagen crosslinking for keratoconus and corneal ectasia: one-year results. J Cataract Refract Surg. 2011;37(1):149-60.
56. Wan Q, Wang D, Ye H, et al. A review and meta-analysis of corneal cross-linking for post-laser vision correction ectasia. J Curr Ophthalmol. 2017;29(3):145-53.
57. Wallerstein A, Adiguzel E, Gauvin M, et al. Under-flap stromal bed CXL for early post-LASIK ectasia: a novel treatment technique. Clin Ophthalmol. 2017;11:1-8.
58. Kanellopoulos AJ, Binder PS. Management of corneal ectasia after LASIK with combined, same-day, topography-guided partial transepithelial PRK and collagen cross-linking: the Athens protocol. J Refract Surg. 2011;27(5):323-31.
59. Tamayo GE, Castell C, Vargas P, et al. High-resolution wavefront-guided surface ablation with corneal cross-linking in ectatic corneas: a pilot study. Clin Ophthalmol. 2017;11:1777-83.
60. Zhu W, Han Y, Cui C, et al. Corneal collagen crosslinking combined with phototherapeutic keratectomy and photorefractive keratectomy for corneal ectasia after laser in situ keratomileusis. Ophthalmic Res. 2018;59(3):135-41.

61. Carrasquillo KG, Rand J, Talamo JH. Intacs for keratoconus and post-LASIK ectasia: mechanical versus femtosecond laser-assisted channel creation. Cornea. 2007;26(8):956-62.
62. Jiang Y, Li Y, Yang S, et al. Tuck-in Lamellar keratoplasty with a lenticule obtained by small incision lenticule extraction for treatment of Post-LASIK ectasia. Sci Rep. 2017;7(1):17806.
63. Tunc Z, Helvacioglu F, Sencan S. Evaluation of intrastromal corneal ring segments for treatment of post-LASIK ectasia patients with a mechanical implantation technique. Indian J Ophthalmol. 2011;59(6):437-43.
64. Hashemi H, Gholaminejad A, Amanzadeh K, et al. Single-segment and double-segment Intacs for post-LASIK ectasia. Acta Med Iran. 2014;52(9):681-6.
65. Yildirim A, Uslu H, Kara N, et al. Same-day intrastromal corneal ring segment and collagen cross-linking for ectasia after laser in situ keratomileusis: long-term results. Amer J Ophthalmol. 2014;157(5):1070-6.
66. Kymionis GD, Bouzoukis DI, Portaliou DM, et al. New INTACS SK implantation in patients with post-laser in situ keratomileusis corneal ectasia. Cornea. 2010;29(2):214-6.
67. McAllum PJ, Segev F, Herzig S, et al. Deep anterior lamellar keratoplasty for post-LASIK ectasia. Cornea. 2007;26(4):507-11.
68. Salouti R, Nowroozzadeh MH, Makateb P, et al. Deep anterior lamellar keratoplasty for keratectasia after laser in situ keratomileusis. J Cataract Refract Surg. 2014;40(12):2011-8.
69. Javadi MA, Feizi S. Deep anterior lamellar keratoplasty using the big-bubble technique for keratectasia after laser in situ keratomileusis. J Cataract Refract Surg. 2010;36(7):1156-60.
70. Tan BU, Purcell TL, Torres LF, et al. New surgical approaches to the management of keratoconus and post-LASIK ectasia. Trans Am Ophthalmol Soc. 2006;104:212-20.
71. Titiyal JS, Agarwal T, Jhanji V, et al. Flap replacement surgery for management of post-LASIK ectasia. Br J Ophthalmol. 2010;94(12):1690-2.
72. Binder PS, Trattler WB. Evaluation of a risk factor scoring system for corneal ectasia after LASIK in eyes with normal topography. J Refract Surg. 2010;26(4):241-50.
73. Miraftab M, Fotouhi A, Hashemi H, et al. A modified risk assessment scoring system for post laser in situ keratomileusis ectasia in topographically normal patients. J Ophthalmic Vis Res. 2014;9(4):434-8.
74. Tomita M, Yoshida Y, Yamamoto Y, et al. In vivo confocal laser microscopy of morphologic changes after simultaneous LASIK and accelerated collagen cross-linking for myopia: one-year results. J Cataract Refract Surg. 2014;40(6):981-90.
75. Nguyen MK, Chuck RS. Corneal collagen cross-linking in the stabilization of PRK, LASIK, thermal keratoplasty, and orthokeratology. Curr Opin Ophthalmol. 2013;24(4):291-5.
76. Aslanides IM, Mukherjee AN. Adjuvant corneal crosslinking to prevent hyperopic LASIK regression. Clin Ophthalmol. 2013;7:637-41.
77. Kanellopoulos AJ, Asimellis G. Epithelial remodeling after femtosecond laser-assisted high myopic LASIK: comparison of stand-alone with LASIK combined with prophylactic high-fluence cross-linking. Cornea. 2014;33(5):463-9.
78. Kymionis GD, Grentzelos MA, Portaliou DM, et al. Corneal collagen cross-linking (CXL) combined with refractive procedures for the treatment of corneal ectatic disorders: CXL plus. J Refract Surg. 2014;30(8):566-76.
79. Moshirfar M, Albarracin JC, Desautels JD, et al. Ectasia following small-incision lenticule extraction (SMILE): a review of the literature. Clin Ophthalmol. 2017:11:1683-8.

CHAPTER
2

Recent Advances in Lamellar Keratoplasty

Casey J Randleman, Soosan Jacob

■ INTRODUCTION

Though penetrating keratoplasty (PK) is known to have a high success rate and is technically easy, it does carry disadvantages such as a higher risk of intraoperative complications such as expulsive hemorrhage and vitreous loss secondary to being an open sky procedure. It is also associated with postoperative complications such as prolonged visual rehabilitation, unpredictability, induced refractive error including irregular astigmatism, higher risk of rejection as well as increased surface issues, and a neurotrophic cornea. It also has the weakest wound, thereby being prone to a higher risk of traumatic graft dehiscence. For these reasons, of late, lamellar keratoplasty (LK) has replaced PK for many indications. Endothelial keratoplasty (EK) in the form of Descemet's stripping automated endothelial keratoplasty (DSAEK), Descemet's membrane endothelial keratoplasty (DMEK), and pre-Descemet's endothelial keratoplasty (PDEK) are a better option for diseases that selectively involve the endothelium where there is no stromal scarring. Similarly, in cases with healthy endothelium and purely stromal pathology, stromal replacement in the form of a deep anterior lamellar keratoplasty (DALK), superficial anterior lamellar keratoplasty (SALK) or tucked-in lamellar keratoplasty (TILK) are better and offer advantages of retention of healthy host endothelium, decreased risk of rejection and secondary failure.

■ RECENT ADVANCES IN ENDOTHELIAL KERATOPLASTY

Descemet's Membrane Endothelial Keratoplasty

Unlike DSAEK, where some stroma is also transferred together with Descemet's membrane (DM) and endothelium, in DMEK, only the DM with endothelium is replaced. This avoids the disadvantages that DSAEK has of additional thickness added to host cornea, induced hyperopia, interface haze, etc. It also has a lesser risk of rejection. However, it is more complex to perform and has a longer learning curve. It also has higher chances of detachment in complex cases such as when DMEK is combined with tubes, aphakia, secondary intraocular lens (IOL) fixation, vitrectomy, etc.

Pre-Descemet's Endothelial Keratoplasty

Description of the pre-Descemet's layer (PDL) in 2013 by Harminder Dua enabled a new kind of EK which also included transplantation of the PDL along with endothelium and DM. Injection of air into a donor corneoscleral graft can result in a type 1, type 2 or a type 3 big bubble (BB) (Figs. 1A to C). A type 1 BB refers to cleavage of a plane between the donor stroma on one side and the PDL, DM, and endothelium on the other side, thus giving a PDEK graft. This type of bubble is formed more commonly in younger donor corneas. A type 2 BB refers to cleavage between the DM and endothelium on one side and the PDL and donor stroma on the other side, thus forming a DMEK graft and this is more commonly formed in older donor corneas. A type 3 BB is when both types of BB are formed simultaneously, i.e. a combination of both in the same donor cornea.[1]

Pre-Descemet's endothelial keratoplasty as described by Amar Agarwal and Harminder Dua grafts have advantages over DMEK grafts in the ability to use young donors,[2] thus giving a more substantial quantum of endothelial cell transfer. The PDL also acts as a splint for the PDEK graft, thus making it a stronger and sturdier graft that is less likely to tear as opposed to the DMEK graft, which is very flimsy and can tear easily. The resilience of the PDEK graft also makes it amenable to easier unfolding and handling within the anterior chamber (AC), thus making surgery easier and faster while still giving comparable results.

Three techniques which have helped make PDEK as well as DMEK surgery easier are—(1) the endoilluminator-assisted PDEK or DMEK (E-PDEK/E-DMEK), (2) the air pump assisted PDEK and (3) the host Descemetic scaffolding techniques, which were described by one of the authors (SJ).

E-PDEK or E-DMEK

As DM is elastic, both DMEK and PDEK grafts scroll toward the DM with endothelium on the outside. It is therefore, essential to have the graft placed in a scrolls-up position before unscrolling and floating it up against the overlying stroma. This is to ensure that the endothelium is transplanted in the right orientation facing the AC. However, the thin nature of DMEK and PDEK grafts, as compared to DSAEK grafts, makes it challenging to identify orientation under the microscope light. This difficulty is compounded by the flimsy nature of the graft, AC currents that easily cause the graft to move and poor visualization in eyes with severe corneal edema. Microscope light that falls perpendicular to the cornea does not provide the ability to distinguish between the layers of the graft's folds, presenting a seemingly two-dimensional image. The use of a vitreoretinal light pipe called an endoilluminator assists with identifying the location and orientation of the graft after injection into the eye. By holding the endoilluminator at an oblique angle, the projected light shines into the AC and onto the graft, providing a three-dimensional view. Reflections bounced off the folds in the graft helps easily identify graft orientation (Figs. 2A and B; Video 1*). The adaptable nature of this technique lets the surgeon check orientation before loading into the cartridge as well

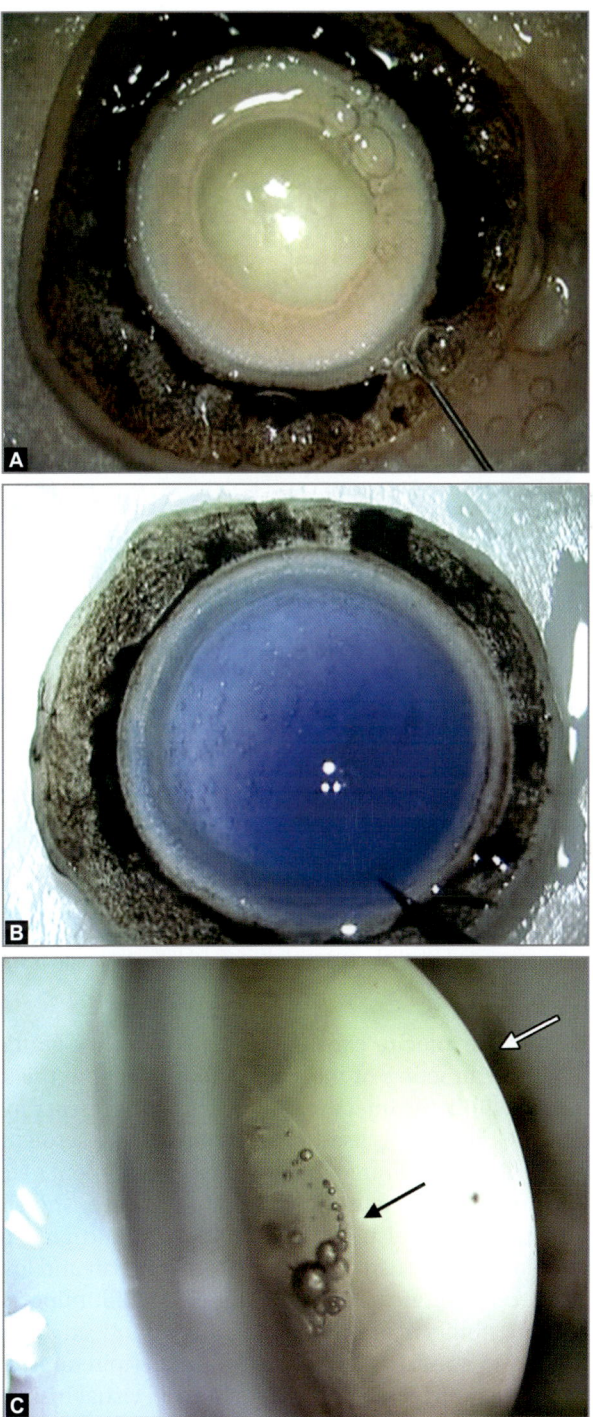

Figs. 1A to C: (A) Type 1 big bubble; (B) Type 2 big bubble; (C) Type 3 big bubble.

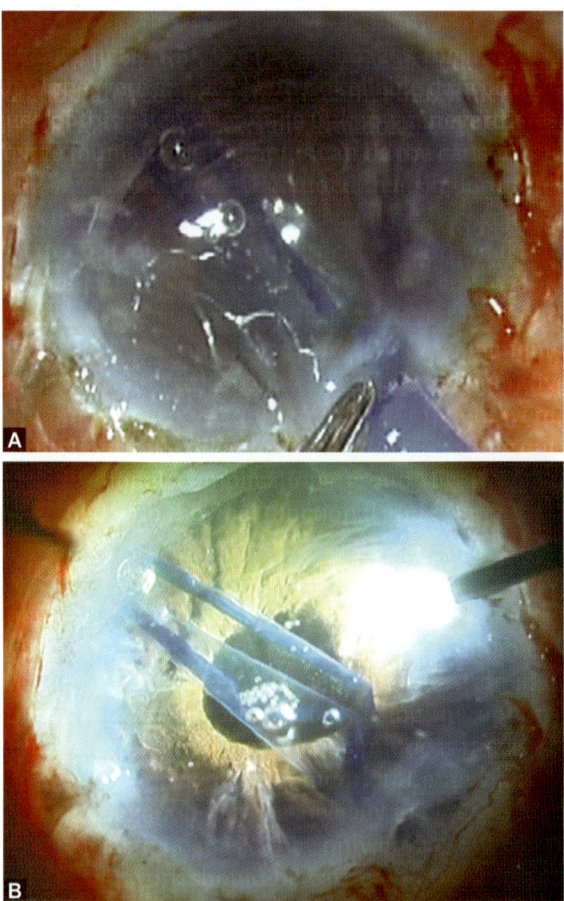

Figs. 2A and B: (A) View with microscope light; (B) View with the endoilluminator-assisted Descemet's membrane endothelial keratoplasty (E-DMEK) technique showing better visualization and depth perception.

as while still within the injector cartridge and also once the graft is inside the AC. By checking the direction of the graft before injection, the surgeon can correct placement within the injector and prevent unnecessary manipulation of the graft in the AC. The light is used to place the graft in a scrolls-up position, which ensures the PDL is stationed flush against the recipient's stroma. It also allows the surgeon to appreciate the entire graft at once, showing both the fold and orientation while also showing the length and graft dimensions. This leads to a faster surgery with more control of the graft and lower chances of damage. Graft unfolding can be done under endoilluminator light, thus eliminating any possibility of graft rotation going unnoticed. Used internally, it can also be used to confirm the patency of the peripheral iridectomy (PI) and is particularly beneficial in cases with a blurred visual inside the AC due to a cloudy cornea. Having the microscope light off during these steps makes three-dimensional perception even better.[3-5]

There are other techniques that are used to help determine the orientation of thinner grafts in the AC. While some of these techniques do allow the surgeon to determine graft orientation prefloatation, each of these techniques also presents challenges not seen with the use of the endoilluminator. The hand held slit lamp may be used once the graft has been injected into the eye. While this does allow prefloatation assessment, it only displays parts of the graft at a time, removing the ability to appreciate the graft in its entirety. It has a lower magnification as compared to the operating microscope and does not allow surgical maneuvers to be performed while using the technique, both because of lack of dexterity and less magnification. It is also a less sterile option with a higher risk of contamination and must be handled using additional sterile methods.

Techniques that do not utilize light have also been described using either a physical marking on the graft itself or an additional object within the AC. The Moutsouris sign[6] is a technique that involves inserting a cannula into the eye, under the graft to determine if it is inverted. If the scroll of the graft falls on top of the cannula, then the graft is determined to be in the correct orientation. The disadvantages of this method include the potential for AC shallowing, induction of AC currents and consequent undesired graft movement due to the insertion of an additional object into the intraocular space, as well as potential damage to the graft secondary to intra-ocular manipulation. The S-stamp approach uses an irreversible sign applied on the graft before injection. After the graft is harvested the surgeon marks an "S" on the Descemetic side which can be used to determine an inverted graft by the direction of the "S" after injection.[7] While this method allows for higher confidence in graft orientation, it has the disadvantage of physical manipulation of the graft outside of the AC. To mark the graft, it must first be folded in half, the donor cornea punched, the graft laid back again and the "S" marked from the epithelial side. This can increases the potential for damage to the endothelial cells, together with potential damage from the marking ink. It also does not allow easy prefloatation determination of the graft orientation as the S may be within the folds and therefore, present a confusing view.

In our experience, the E-PDEK or E-DMEK technique provides accurate determination with few disadvantages. It decreases the need for intraocular manipulation of the graft or physical alterations, increases visibility to allow a full graft appreciation with depth dimensions and allows better visibility through even severe corneal edema.

Air Pump Assisted PDEK

Identification of the orientation of the graft is only one step of EK procedure and is followed by unfolding and placing the graft within the recipient's eye. Though young grafts are ideal in these procedures due their higher endothelial cell counts; however, they are also more elastic, which combined with their thin nature leads to fast and tight scrolling within the AC. The tighter scroll leads to difficulties when approaching centration and unscrolling of a PDEK graft.[8-10]

The air pump assisted PDEK technique utilizes continuous pressurized air infusion delivered via an AC maintainer (ACM) placed through a limbal paracentesis to help certain surgical maneuvers. Air injection can be performed using either a fluid exchange system from a vitrectomy machine or a pressurized air infusion from certain phaco machines. Though using a single air bubble or low-pressure infusion has been described previously for stripping the DM, the air pump assisted technique helps in many other key steps during surgery. The AC is filled with air in the beginning of surgery and the provided pressure acts to tamponade bleeding within the AC that may occur during synechiolysis or PI. The maintained air pressure prevents and stops bleeding and thus prevents a fibrinous sticky atmosphere from forming within the AC, thus avoiding intraoperative difficulty in unscrolling the graft as well as postoperative inflammation and interface blood or fibrin. It also prevents blood from oozing into the AC from peripheral corneal neovascularization. Performing the Descemetorhexis under air after the PI helps give time for bleeding to clot by the time the rhexis is completed. The air also helps make a continuous Descemetorhexis easier to perform while giving greater control over sizing and centration. The ACM is then removed and air replaced with balanced salt solution (BSS) and the graft injected. The orientation of the graft is checked, the graft is unfolded to a large extent and air injected through a cannula placed below the graft to float it against the recipient stroma. This is unlike DMEK or traditional surgery where it is essential to unfold the graft completely from edge to edge as well as make sure of centration before floating the graft up. The ACM is then reinserted and pressurized air infusion started after making sure that the ACM is placed below the graft. The interior pressure provides resistance against the graft from the inside, which creates a firm surface on the cornea through which the surgeon may center the graft. Once the interior pressure is controlled, it only needs increasing when an instrument is moved in or out of the AC. Using a reverse Sinskey hook, the surgeon may then center the graft on the cornea and unfold the edges, which are made more visible against the air. While the graft is held in place by air, adjustments are more controlled, and any creases or folds present in the graft are also addressed, resulting in a smooth placement. Continuous air pressure decreases chances of the graft becoming detached or moving while also maintaining space within the AC for easier graft manipulation. Adequate operating space in the AC helps ensure graft safety, with a lower risk of damage. This technique makes surgery easier and faster and decreases the learning curve. All manipulations to the graft are kept to a minimum and only to the peripheral edge of the graft to prevent cell loss. The continuous air pressure also helps the graft to adhere better and faster and decreases risk of postoperative detachment (Figs. 3 and 4; Video 2**).

Disadvantages include air bubbles escaping from the incisions which may interfere with visualization. This can be solved by placing a cotton wick at the incision which directs the escaping air bubbles away. Conjunctival emphysema can be prevented by putting a nick on the conjunctiva allowing

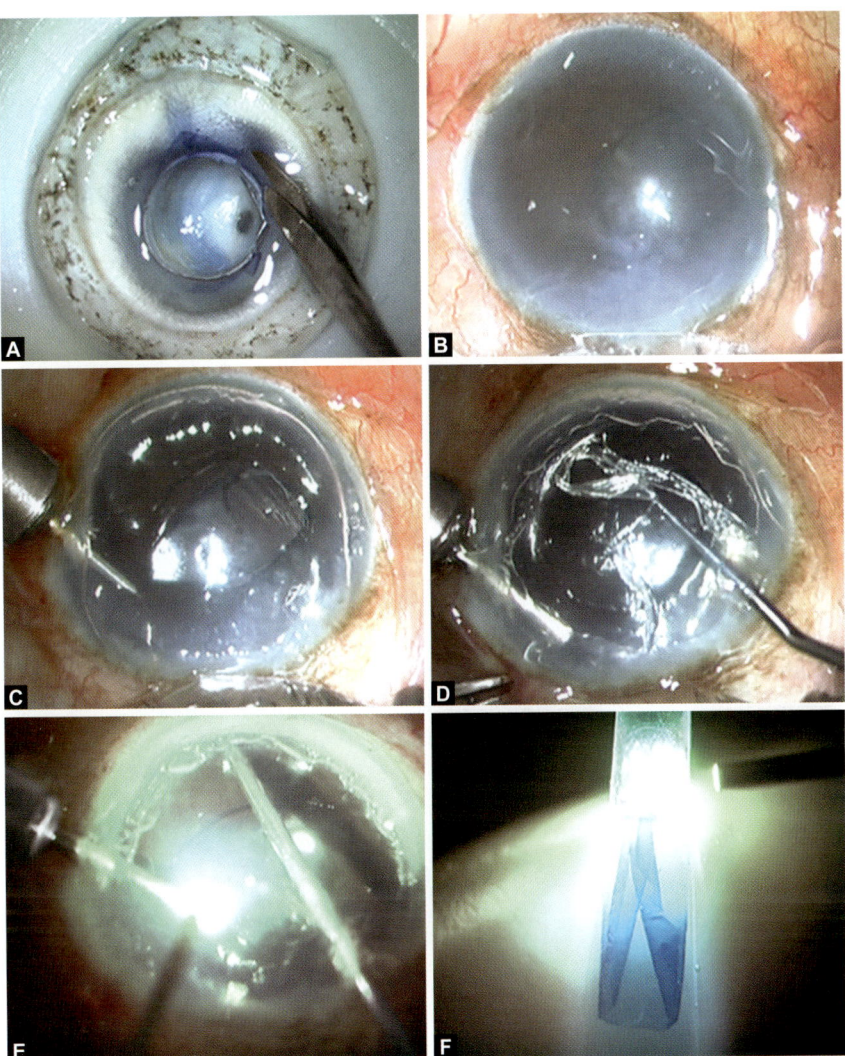

Figs. 3A to F: Air pump assisted pre-Descemet's endothelial keratoplasty. (A) Type 1 big bubble created and PDEK graft dissected; (B) Preoperative view showing endothelial decompensation; (C) Continuous pressurized air infused through an anterior chamber maintainer; (D) Descemetorhexis done with air pump assisted technique; (E) Peripheral iridectomy done with air pump assisted technique; (F) PDEK graft orientation within the cartridge confirmed with the E-PDEK technique.

air to escape. Any cell loss secondary to graft edge unfolding is offset by the absence of repeated attempts at unfolding and centering the graft completely before floatation. It should be remembered that the pressure within the AC is lower than that set on the machine because of continuous leakage of air from the incisions. The estimated pressure should not be allowed to rise to very high levels.

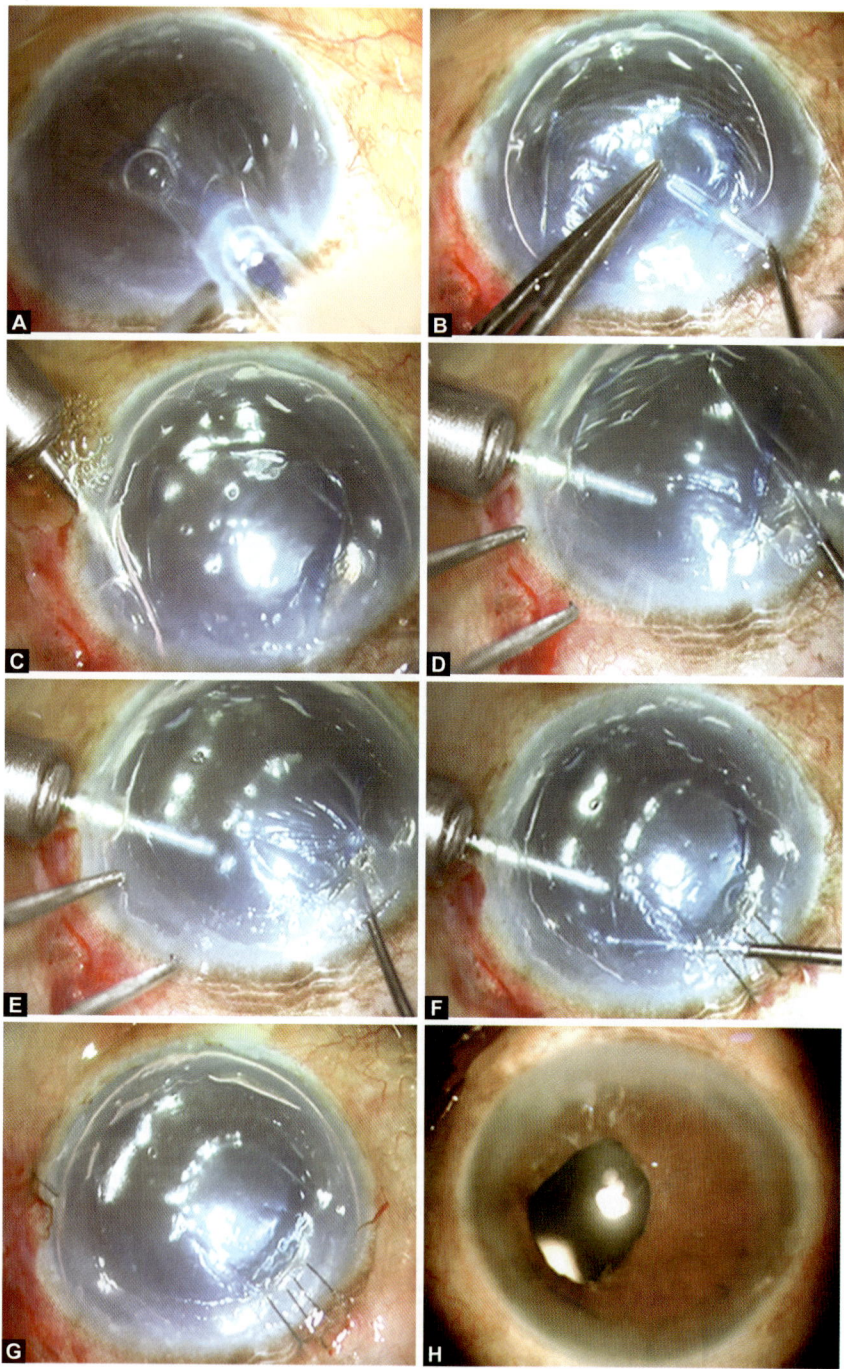

Figs. 4A to H: (A) Graft injected into anterior chamber after removing air; (B) Graft orientation confirmed and then unrolled and floated up with air; (C) Anterior chamber maintainer connected and continuous pressurized air infusion restarted; (D to F) Graft centered and edges unrolled using the air pump assisted technique; (G) Well centered and apposed graft seen at the end of surgery; (H) Postoperative appearance showing a well attached graft and a clear cornea.

Host Descemetic Scaffolding

One of the problems with both PDEK and DMEK is that it has a higher rate of graft detachment in complex cases such as aphakic eyes, vitrectomized eyes, when combined with secondary IOL fixation, or with glaucoma drainage devices or large incision surgeries such as small incision cataract surgery (SICS).[11]

Traditionally, the area of host descemetorhexis is kept larger than the graft size in order to avoid the possibility of the graft overlapping host DM which could be the cause for a graft detachment. The Host Descemetic scaffolding instead uses an area of DM stripping that is smaller than the graft. The host Descemet is then used as a scaffold below the graft to support the graft and prevent graft detachment (Figs. 5 to 7). This is done by sandwiching the graft edge between the host DM and stroma. This can be done as a two-sided or multipoint host DM scaffolding, near total scaffolding or by using a combination of one point scaffolding with wound scaffolding (Figs. 8A to C).

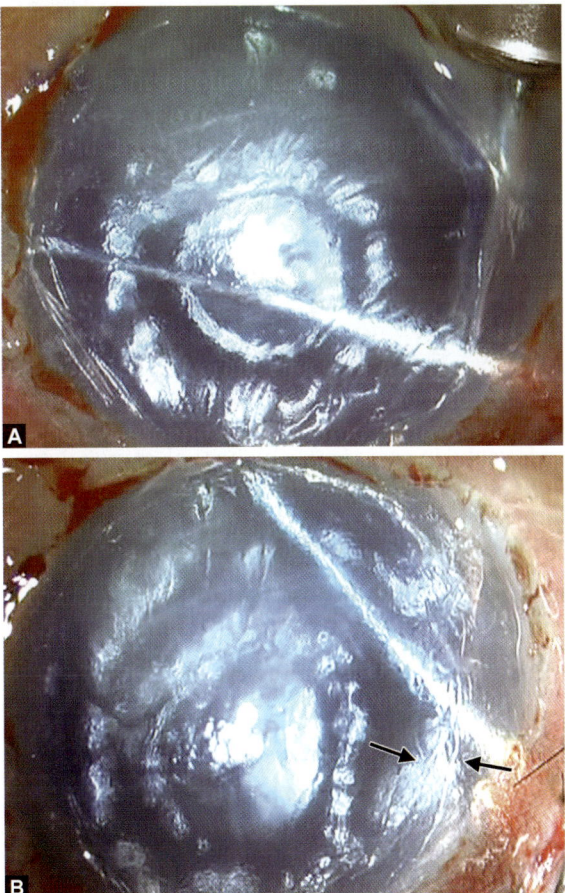

Figs. 5A and B: Host Descemetic scaffolding seen being done for the pre-Descemet's endothelial keratoplasty graft.

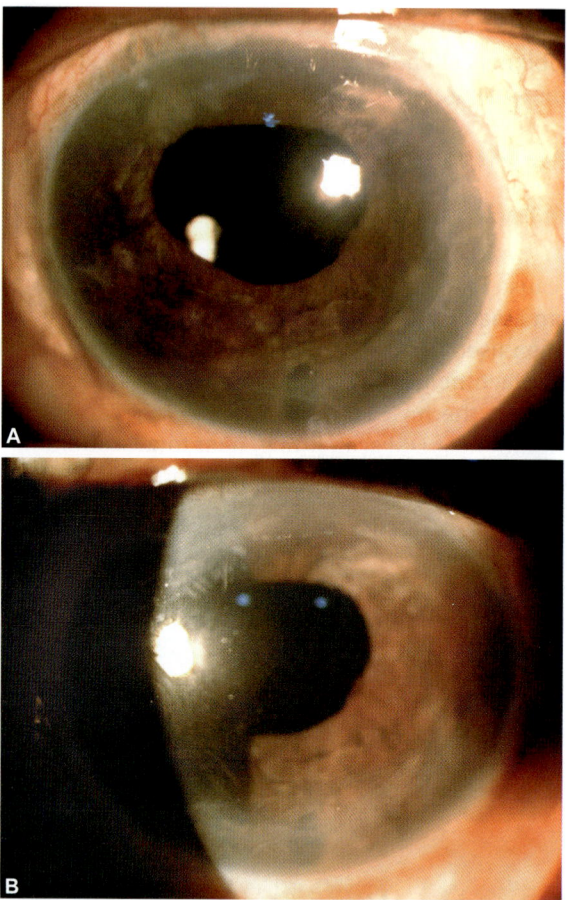

Figs. 6A and B: Postoperative picture showing host Descemetic scaffolding.

This technique is useful in cases with a higher risk of graft detachment. It may also be useful in routine cases as well as during the learning curve.

■ RECENT ADVANCES IN ANTERIOR LAMELLAR KERATOPLASTY

Modified Primary Pre-Descemetic DALK for Acute Hydrops (Jacob Technique)

In cases with cornea pathology anterior to the endothelium, a DALK may be performed. One of the most common indications is keratoconus. Advanced cases of keratoconus may suffer from a rupture of the DM leading to pain, redness, hydration of the cornea, edema, intrastromal fluid clefts, etc.[12,13] This condition referred to as acute corneal hydrops (CH) is typically approached with a two-part treatment plan, initially with injection of intracameral gas to close the break followed later by a keratoplasty procedure to correct the pathology. This could be either a PK or a DALK depending on the location of the ensuing scar. Traditional conservative treatment in the acute stage is with observation, injection of long-acting gas within the AC,[14-16] compression

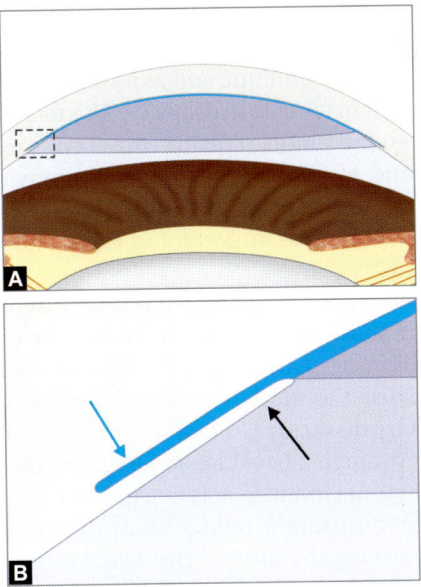

Figs. 7A and B: Host Descemetic scaffolding. Blue arrow shows pre-Descemet's endothelial keratoplasty graft being scaffolded by the host Descemet's membrane (black arrow).

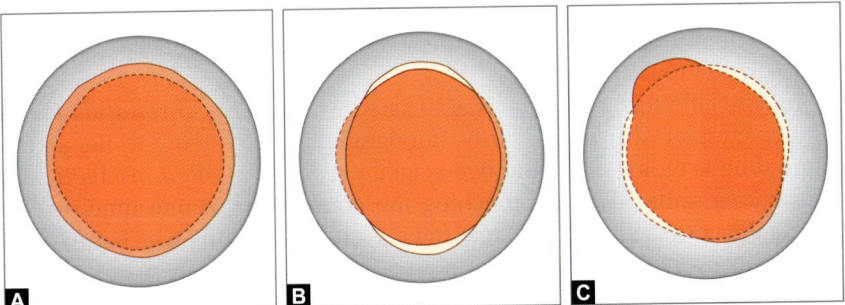

Figs. 8A to C: (A) Total to near total Host Descemetic scaffolding; (B) Two point Host Descemetic scaffolding; (C) Single point Host Descemetic scaffolding with wound scaffolding.

sutures,[17] etc. However, resolution takes time and occurs with scarring. Though scarring may result in some flattening of the cornea and improved contact lens tolerance, the basic pathology remains untreated—the eye still continuing to have all the disadvantages of severe keratoconus—ectasia, poor uncorrected and best spectacle corrected visual acuity, high irregular astigmatism and aberrations, poor corneal topography, thin cornea and the need for contact lens and consequent problems such as limited time of wear, contact lens related scarring, infections, etc. Many patients therefore, need a secondary procedure in the form of a pre-Descemetic DALK. In addition, if post-hydrops scar is over the visual axis, it results in the need for an optical PK, thus exposing the patient to a higher risk of rejection secondary to loss of native endothelium.

One of the authors (SJ) has described a modified technique of safely and effectively performing a pre-Descemetic DALK at the time of acute hydrops as a primary management technique and as a substitute for the conventional conservative management of acute hydrops.[18,19] This technique has advantages of retaining host endothelium, closing the DM break, simultaneously restoring anatomy and treating the pathology, improving uncorrected and best corrected visual acuity, decreasing irregular astigmatism, correction of ectasia and thinning, and most important of all resolution without scarring (Figs. 9A to F; Video 3***).

In the modified technique, the cornea is partially trephined using manual trephine, suction trephine or femtosecond laser. In cases with extensive edema or severe thinning with minimal retained stroma above the tear, an inked trephine is used to mark the corneal surface and a groove is then deepened using a sharp dissector. Graded emphysema is induced by injecting small aliquots of air through a bevel up 30-gauge needle directed away from the break. The emphysema induced acts as a guide to the depth of dissection. Manual deep dissection using a mildly blunt dissector is then done in a centripetal fashion leaving the area of DM tear for the last. The superficial lamellar keratoplasty performed to remove the anterior aspects of the cornea must proceed slowly and carefully, dissecting as close to the tear as possible while maintaining a thin layer of stroma above to support the AC. Minimal stroma is retained above the tear in order to avoid entering the AC. The donor corneoscleral graft is sutured and the DM tear is tamponaded with air in the AC (Figs. 10A to D).

To conclude this technique is associated with success in restoring visual acuity, corneal structure, clarity, topography, pachymetry while at the same time avoiding a lengthy two-staged process that often results in two procedures rather than approaching the entire issue at one time. It also allows the cornea and the DM tear to heal without scarring which is a major advantage over conventional treatment of acute hydrops.

The alternative approaches to repairing CH damage such as pneumodescemetopexy, compressive sutures, and cyanoacrylate glue take significantly longer and often lead to corneal scarring, resulting in decreased visual success. These procedures often occur in two stages over a longer time frame, preventing visual rehabilitation for more time and leading to increased costs and morbidity. Though a more immediate approach such as a PK corrects both CH damage and keratoconus at the same time, it includes removal of the entire recipient cornea, which results in a higher risk of graft failure due to the removal of the patient's endothelium. The modified pre-Descemetic DALK procedure shows the most significant visual rehabilitation with a decreased treatment time. The more direct approach to treatment allows for treatment of

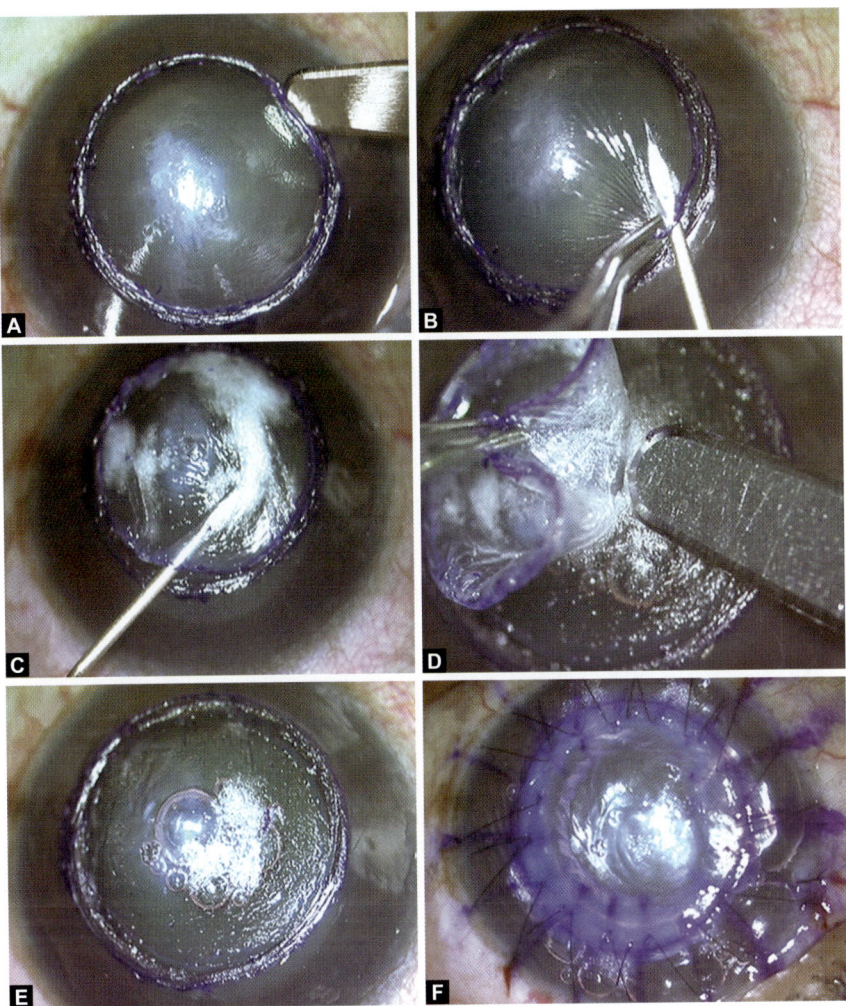

Figs. 9A to F: Modified technique for pre-Descemetic dissection for acute hydrops. (A) Inked trephine mark is deepened manually using a sharp dissector; (B) A 26-gauge needle with bevel bent upward and mounted on a 1 mL syringe is inserted tangentially directed away from the ruptured Descemet's membrane; (C) Surrounding cornea is made emphysematous using small aliquots of air directed away from the break; (D) The overlying stroma is dissected using the emphysematous stroma as a guide for the dissection plane. Melles technique of optical recognition may be used for deeper dissection; (E) Minimal pre-Descemetic stroma is retained to prevent entering the anterior chamber. The anterior chamber is well maintained with no escape of air; (F) Donor graft is sutured into place after removing Descemet's membrane and the DM break is tamponaded with air.

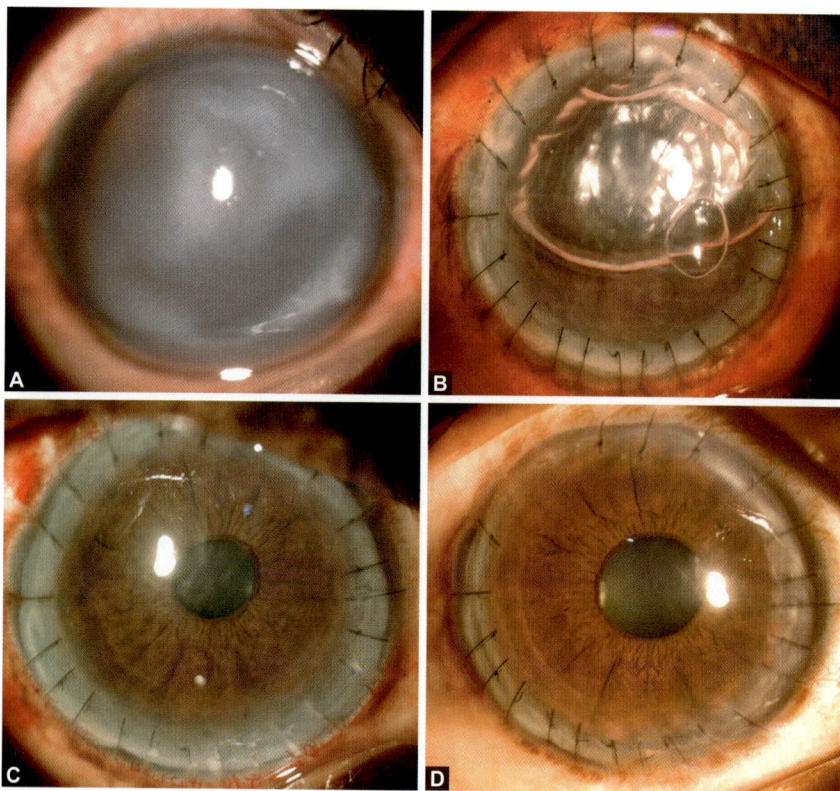

Figs. 10A to D: Resolution of edema seen following the Jacob technique for primary pre-Descemetic deep anterior lamellar keratoplasty for acute hydrops. (A) Preoperatively with acute hydrops; (B) At first postoperative day; (C) At 2 weeks postoperative; (D) At 5 months postoperative follow-up.

the whole issue, rather than only one problem at a time. The DALK procedure also resulted in fewer complications when performed correctly, both through a complete assessment of the issue, while also removing the need for a second surgery and thereby removing the risk associated with increased surgical measures.

REFERENCES

1. Agarwal A, Dua HS, Narang P, et al. Pre-Descemet's endothelial keratoplasty (PDEK). Br J Ophthalmol. 2014;98(9):1181-5.
2. Agarwal A, Agarwal A, Narang P, et al. Pre-Descemet endothelial keratoplasty with infant donor corneas: a prospective analysis. Cornea. 2015;34(8):859-65.
3. Jacob S, Agarwal A, Agarwal A, et al. Endoilluminator-assisted transcorneal illumination for Descemet membrane endothelial keratoplasty: enhanced intraoperative visualization of the graft in corneal decompensation secondary to pseudophakic bullous keratopathy. J Cataract Refract Surg. 2014;40(8):1332-6.
4. Jacob S, Agarwal A, Kumar DA. Endoilluminator-assisted Descemet membrane endothelial keratoplasty and endoilluminator-assisted pre-Descemet endothelial keratoplasty. Clin Ophthalmol. 2015;9:2123-5.

5. Jacob S. E DMEK and E PDEK with audio Soosan Jacob 2 min. [online] Available from https://www.youtube.com/watch?v=4ktkfnOAKmc. [Accessed July, 2018].
6. Dapena I, Moutsouris K, Droutsas K, et al. Standardized "no-touch" technique for Descemet's membrane endothelial keratoplasty. Arch Ophthalmol. 2011;129(1):88-94.
7. Veldman PB, Dye PK, Holiman JD, et al. Stamping an S on DMEK donor tissue to prevent upside-down grafts: laboratory validation and detailed preparation technique description. Cornea. 2015;34(9):1175-8.
8. Jacob S, Narasimhan S, Agarwal A, et al. Air pump-assisted graft centration, graft edge unfolding, and graft uncreasing in young donor graft pre-Descemet endothelial keratoplasty. Cornea. 2017;36(8):1009-13.
9. Jacob S. Use of pressurized air infusion for pre-Descemet's endothelial keratoplasty (PDEK)—the air pump assisted PDEK technique. Open Ophthalmol J. 2018;12:175-80.
10. Jacob S. Air pump assisted PDEK Soosan Jacob 6 2 min with audio final. [online]. Available from https://www.youtube.com/watch?v=onK1R0DG-ow. [Accessed July, 2018).
11. Jacob S. Host Descemetic Scaffold for Pre-Descemet and Descemet Membrane Endothelial Keratoplasty. Best Paper of Session (free paper presentation). ASCRS. 2018 (Washington).
12. Tuft SJ, Gregory WM, Buckley RJ. Acute corneal hydrops in keratoconus. Ophthalmology. 1994;101(10):1738-44.
13. Sharma N, Maharana PK, Jhanji V, et al. Management of acute corneal hydrops in ectatic corneal disorders. Curr Opin Ophthalmol. 2012;23(4):317-23.
14. Ting DS, Srinivasan S. Pneumodescemetopexy with perfluoroethane (C2F6) for the treatment of acute hydrops secondary to keratoconus. Eye (Lond). 2014;28(7):847-51.
15. Basu S, Vaddavalli PK, Ramappa M, et al. Intracameral perfluoropropane gas in the treatment of acute corneal hydrops. Ophthalmology. 2011;118(5):934-9.
16. Poyales-Galán F, Fernández-Aitor-García A, Garzón-Jiménez N, et al. Management of Descemet's membrane rupture by intracameral injection of SF6 in acute hydrops. Arch Soc Esp Oftalmol. 2009;84(10):533-6.
17. Rajaraman R, Singh S, Raghavan A, et al. Efficacy and safety of intracameral perfluoropropane (C3F8) tamponade and compression sutures for the management of acute corneal hydrops. Cornea. 2009;28(3):317-20.
18. Jacob S, Narasimhan S, Agarwal A, et al. Primary modified predescemetic deep anterior lamellar keratoplasty in acute corneal hydrops. Cornea. 2018;37(10):1328-33.
19. Jacob S. Primary pre descemetic DALK for acute hydrops. Soosan Jacob with audio [online] Available from https://www.youtube.com/watch?v=5ZeAXOmVDJw. [Accessed July, 2018].

Useful Links for Videos

(Video 1) *E-DMEK or E-PDEK - https://youtu.be/4ktkfnOAKmc

(Video 2) **Air Pump Assisted PDEK - https://youtu.be/lcIHrzdbDd4

(Video 3) ***Modified Primary Pre-Descemetic DALK for Acute Hydrops (Jacob Technique) -   https://youtu.be/5ZeAXOmVDJw

CHAPTER

3

Keratopigmentation: An Innovative Surgical Option for Therapeutic and Cosmetic Purposes

Olena Al-Shymali, Alejandra E Rodriguez, Maria A Amesty, Jorge L Alió

■ INTRODUCTION

The practice of keratopigmentation (KTP) was practiced in a very rudimentary way in ancient times and it was only sporadically used in the past to treat corneal opacities due to complications and unstable outcomes.[1-3] The clinical and experimental studies of our research group of Alicante from 2002 till present have further developed different types of KTP procedures that have significantly improved the outcomes and perspectives of this innovative surgical technique.

There are a significant number of patients with cosmetically or functionally disfigured eyes that cannot benefit from available treatments. The management of leukomatous corneas is very challenging as they are pathological and constantly are intolerant to contact lenses or external prosthesis due to fitting problems, discomfort sensations, or irregular corneal surface.[4,5] KTP offers an excellent alternative for such patients.[6-8]

The therapeutic effect of KTP has been also demonstrated in sighted eyes with symptomatic glare associated with iris loss, atrophy or trauma;[9-14] in cases of disabling light scattering[15] and photophobia in traumatic aniridia, iris coloboma, or a fixed-dilated pupil;[11,14-16] and even in the treatment of incapacitating diplopia.[13,17] For the purpose of KTP, special pigments and instruments should be available. Pigments had an important evolution coming from vegetable pigments, totally abundant now, till the emerging of the micronized mineral pigments used nowadays. The tolerance and biocompatibility of the latter were tested in different experimental studies with very good results from histopathological and immunological perspectives.[18-20]

No specific instruments existed for the purpose of KTP which animated our team to develop new instruments and implement modern technologies in KTP. Indeed, there is enough evidence of the excellent outcomes provided by KTP to achieve good cosmetic results and high patients' satisfaction, avoiding extensive and mutilating reconstructive surgery like evisceration and enucleation.

■ INSTRUMENTS, PIGMENTS, AND TECHNOLOGIES INVOLVED IN KERATOPIGMENTATION

Instruments

The continuous evolution of KTP fetched the creation of new instruments especially designed for KTP surgery. Depending on the technique, superficial or intrastromal KTP, different instruments and devices are developed. A new automated punctural device Vissum Eye MP System, Madrid, Spain (Apl. No. 2.949.539), provided by Blue Green Medical, Spain (Figs. 1A to D) was designed for superficial KTP. Intrastromal KTP is done using several intrastromal corneal dissectors designed and manufactured by Katena, New York, USA (Figs. 2A to D).

Technologies

After the elaboration of the femtosecond laser and the widening of its indications, intrastromal KTP became much simpler. The femtosecond laser cut is precise and can be created at any level in the stroma, which makes the intrastromal tunnels more homogenous and easier to dissect.

Pigment Selection

According to several studies, pigments should be mineral in origin, indelible, easily sterilizable, nonirritating to the cornea, opaque to luminous rays, and miscible in water but not soluble. Mineral colors are more permanent than vegetable colors when applied to human tissues. However, irritating

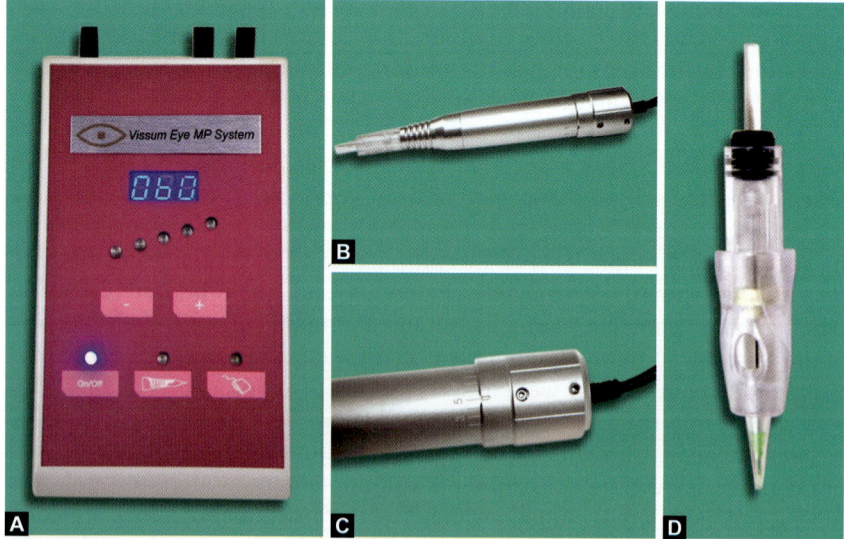

Figs. 1A to D: (A) Device for superficial automated keratopigmentation; (B) Handpiece; (C) Regulated trundle located in the distal part of the handpiece; (D) Disposable tip.

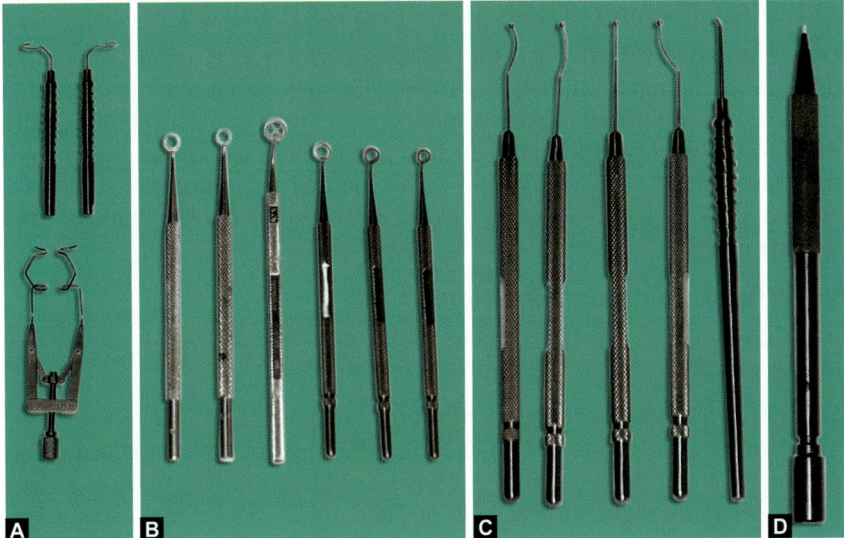

Figs. 2A to D: Intrastromal keratopigmentation instruments. (A) Helicoidal intrastromal corneal dissectors and blefarostate; (B) Pupil optic zone markers of different sizes; (C) Intrastromal corneal dissectors; (D) diamond calibrated knife.

pigments, like the chromes, cadmium, cobalt, and gamboge, should not be employed.[20-22]

During the learning curve and the evolution of KTP, our team has used three different consecutive generations of pigments. The first-generation of pigments were originally used for dermopigmentation. The second-generation were selected pigments that showed good results in the previous stage and were adapted to be used in eyes. Eventually the previous generations were replaced by the third-generation CE (Conformité Européene) mark certificated micronized mineral pigments specially developed for corneal use (Blue Green Company, Spain). In accordance with the Ministry of Health and the Annex IV of European Regulation of Cosmetics the CE mark pigments are composed of different amounts of lactic acid, propanediol, and micronized mineral pigments [color index (CI): 77007, 77491, 77499, 77492, 77288, and 77891].

Micronized mineral pigments have an additional advantage over other natural mineral pigments, because their particle size is reduced by processes of micronization. Therefore, the chance of developing foreign body reactions, against the pigment introduced into the corneal stroma, is much lower than with bigger particles. The particles normally have a diameter of 2.5 microns or smaller.[12-14,19]

Another important advantage of micronized mineral pigments is the wide range of colors available. This is very convenient in KTP because the main objective is to accurately mimic the color of the patient's eye to get a better cosmetic result. The combination of different pigments to achieve the desired color is possible by previously mixing and preparing these micronized mineral pigments in sterile conditions.[12-14,19]

KERATOPIGMENTATION SURGICAL TECHNIQUES

Different methods have been suggested to perform KTP depending on the different pathologies the patients come with such as corneal opacities that can be deep, superficial or both, and other functional visual disabilities. With the development of automated devices, the manual techniques were gradually substituted. However, in rare cases manual techniques are still used. Nowadays, KTP techniques are divided into superficial, intrastromal, and mixed ones.

Superficial Keratopigmentation

It includes superficial manual KTP (SMK) and superficial automated KTP (SAK).

Superficial Manual Keratopigmentation

The center of the cornea is marked with a caliper and the pupil size determined by an optic zone marker (Katena, New York, USA). Then a drop of the adequate pigment is placed on the corneal surface and using a 25G needle micropunctures are performed down to the superficial layers of the stroma. The maneuver is repeated, until the adequate amount of pigment is introduced into the superficial cornea to achieve an acceptable cosmetic appearance.

Superficial Automated Keratopigmentation

This procedure is performed using a special punctural device Vissum Eye MP System, Madrid, Spain (Apl. No. 2.949.539), provided by Blue Green Medical, Spain (Figs. 3A to D).[21] The pupil size and the diameter of the pupil are marked. Automatic micropunctures of the superficial layers of the stroma are performed to an approximate depth of 120 microns from the corneal surface. The penetration depth of the needles previously loaded with pigments is regulated by a trundle located in the distal part of the handpiece. Disposable tips with different number of needles are used depending on the area of the cornea to be pigmented. For example, limbus and pupil simulation is done using the tip with only one needle (Nº1), (Blue Green Medical, Spain). However, for iris simulation we use a tip with several needles (Nº3 or Nº5), from the same company.

Intrastromal Keratopigmentation

It is divided into manual intrastromal KTP (MIK) and femtosecond laser-assisted intrastromal KTP (FIK).

Manual Intrastromal Keratopigmentation

After marking the center of the cornea and the pupil, two to four freehand incisions are performed from the limbus to the border of the marked pupil. From this radial incision the cornea is dissected intralamellarly and circumferentially parallel to the limbus using a microcrescent blade and helicoidal intrastromal corneal dissectors. The dissection is made until reaching the nearest incision on both sides, finally achieving a dissection of the whole

Keratopigmentation: An Innovative Surgical Option for Therapeutic and Cosmetic Purposes

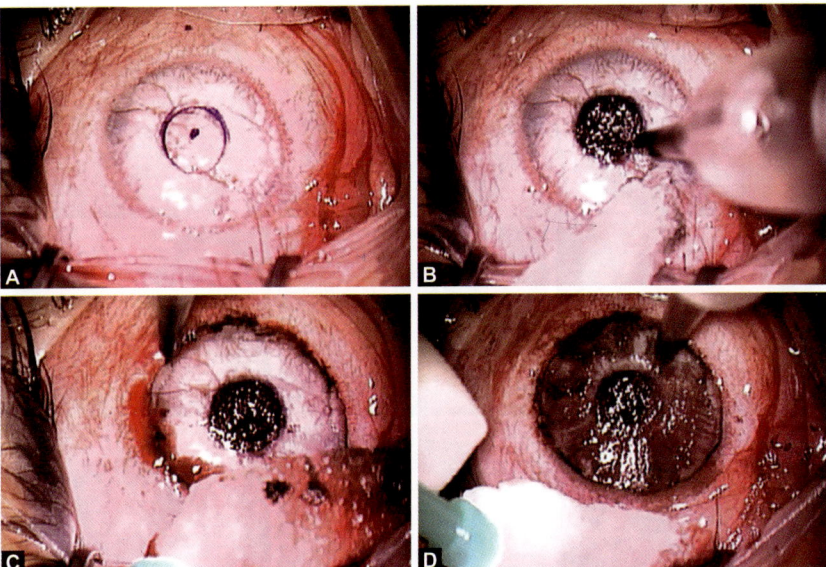

Figs. 3A to D: Superficial automated keratopigmentation technique. (A) Marks in the center of the cornea of the size of the pupil; (B) Simulation of the pupil with black pigment and tip with needle N°1; (C) Limbus pigmentation with black pigment and tip with needle N°1; and (D) Simulation of the iris with dark brown pigment and tip with needle N°3.

cornea from the periphery to the corneal pupil. Afterwards, the adequate pigment previously prepared and loaded into a 1 mL syringe is injected with a 27G flat cannula into the dissected corneal tunnel. When pupil simulation is necessary, an intrastromal corneal dissection is performed within the marked pupil edges (see Fig. 2).

Femtosecond Laser-Assisted Intrastromal Keratopigmentation

Two types of surgeries can be performed, creating just one stromal tunnel (single tunnel technique) or two stromal tunnels (double tunnel technique).[14]

In the single tunnel technique (Figs. 4A to I), femtosecond laser is used to create the circular tunnel of 9.5 mm external and 5.3 mm internal diameters and one superior 90° radial 4 mm incision, at 50% depth of the thinnest cornea. The tunnel is opened to the periphery of the cornea until reaching the limbus with a helicoidal intrastromal corneal dissector followed by the injection of the desired color through the superior incision using a 27G flat cannula.

In the double tunnel technique two tunnels are constructed, one at approximately 400 microns depth and the other at 200 microns depth from the corneal surface. This helps mimic the anatomy of the iris, where the light-colored pigment is applied to the superficial tunnel and the dark-colored pigment is applied to the deep tunnel.

Mixed Keratopigmentation

During this KTP one can combine any of the above-mentioned techniques together. This is used in some cases where only one technique would not offer

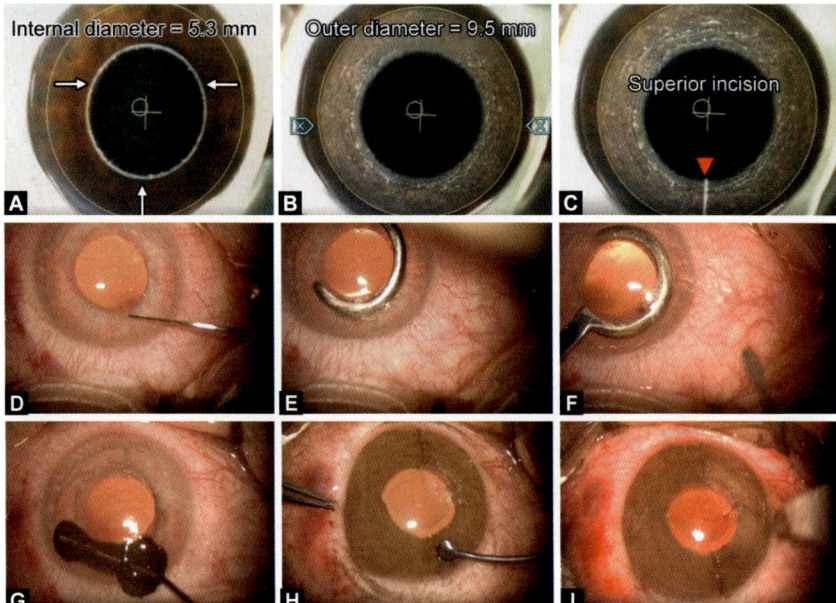

Figs. 4A to I: Femtosecond laser-assisted intrastromal keratopigmentation technique. (A and B) Femtosecond laser cut of the intrastromal tunnel; (C) Radial superior incision; (D) Opening the incision; (E and F) Opening of the intrastromal tunnel using right and left helicoidal dissectors; (G) Pigment injection into the corneal tunnel; (H) Final touch-ups with the curved spoon intrastromal dissector to obtain a nice rounded pupil; (I) Final result.

us the satisfactory results surgeon is aiming to. For example, in a cornea with mild to moderate deep and superficial opacities, the intrastromal technique would mask the deep opacities, yet needing the superficial KTP in order to mask the superficial ones.

Retouches following Keratopigmentation

A retouch is a KTP reoperation that may be needed in order to enhance the color, the ocular function, patient's or investigator's satisfaction. The retouch can be done in any of the four KTP techniques described above, depending on each case and each indication. If a cornea operated with any of the intrastromal techniques needs a retouch, no new tunnels are made. The tunnel made in the primary surgery (either manually or by using femtosecond laser) is opened and the pigments, previously prepared and loaded into a 1 mL syringe, are injected into the tunnel using a 27G flat cannula. If a retouch is needed in eyes formerly operated using any of the superficial techniques, the procedure is repeated exactly as the primary surgery.

In all of the above-mentioned techniques, the pupil diameter of the affected eyes is matched to the mesopic pupil size of the fellow healthy eye when applicable. The same is applied to the pigment choice where the color is customized depending on the color of the fellow eye. The selection of a correct technique depends on the indications and objectives of the KTP to be done. In general, the deepest the introduction of the pigments into the corneal stroma, the better the outcomes and are less prone to complications. Therefore, intrastromal KTP is recommended. However, some corneal conditions like scars and leukomas might not be amenable using this technique and might require more superficial methods.

Postoperative protocol should include the use of antibiotic, anti-inflammatory and analgesic drops to achieve good results and prevent infections, as in any surgical technique. Slit lamp examination and photo documentation is recommended 1 day, 1 week, 1 month, 3 months, 6 months and then annually after the surgery to detect possible complications.

■ INDICATIONS

In general, KTP can be indicated as therapeutic cosmetic or therapeutic functional procedure depending on the patient's ocular pathology.

Therapeutic Cosmetic Keratopigmentation

This technique is done with cosmetic purposes in pathological corneas because of various morbidities (Figs. 5A and B), such as:
- Total or partial corneal leukomas with or without corneal neovascularization due to different reasons such as traumas, infections, opacification of the donor-recipient borders in eyes with previous keratoplasties.
- Chronic corneal edema after several unsuccessful keratoplasties, cataract or phakic intraocular lenses (IOLs) surgeries, congenital glaucoma, ocular infections, or Fuchs' dystrophy.
- Corneal calcification [in addition to KTP, it is treated by 2% ethylenediaminetetraacetic acid (EDTA)].

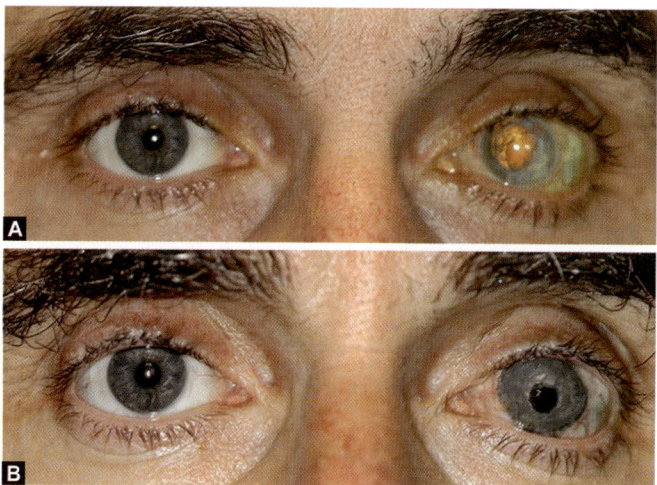

Figs. 5A and B: Therapeutic cosmetic keratopigmentation case. (A) Preoperative aspect of the eyes of a patient after suffering a trauma in his left eye when he was a child; (B) Postoperative appearance of the eyes after superficial automated keratopigmentation in the left eye. Gray and black pigments were used and the color was adjusted to the iris color of the fellow eye. After 2 months a keratopigmentation (KTP) retouch was applied. The patient is satisfied with the final cosmetic appearance of his eye.

- Phthisis bulbi.
- Sclerocornea.
- Leukocoria secondary to cataract in a blind eye; if cataract surgery is not recommended.

Therapeutic Functional Keratopigmentation

It was studied since 1872, when Wecker emphasized the importance of performing corneal pigmentation or tattooing for optical purposes. Corneal opacities are optically translucent and this characteristic can cause blurriness. To resolve this problem, Wecker conducted an experiment in which he created a pinhole pupil slightly downward and inward, and he covered the rest of the central cornea with an opaque black pigment, achieving excellent results.[22-24] These studies and some others have shown beneficial results after corneal tattooing for optical reasons (Figs. 6A and B).[12-14]

Among the indications for therapeutic functional purposes are the following:
- Albinism (translucent iris)
- Aniridia, total or partial
- Iris coloboma
- Iridodialysis
- Irido-corneal-endothelial syndrome
- Progressive iris cysts
- Diffuse corneal opacity and related glare
- Essential iris atrophy
- Urrets-Zavalia syndrome.

Other Applications: Purely Cosmetic Keratopigmentation

Keratopigmentation was described and applied as a purely cosmetic procedure. It is done in adequately selected patients who wish to change the color of their eyes to acquire a desired cosmetic appearance.[25] All purely cosmetic KTP are done using the femtosecond laser-assisted intrastromal technique, and in advance customized pigments that are agreed with the patient (Figs. 7A and B). As this is a permanent procedure, the patient should be properly informed to take an adequate decision in order to choose the adequate apparent color of the eye that will be created by the procedure.

■ OPHTHALMOLOGICAL ASSESSMENT

A complete ophthalmological examination should be performed in every case, including:
- Uncorrected and corrected visual acuity measured under cycloplegic conditions.
- Biomicroscopy.
- Ocular surface check-up for dry eye.
- Fundus evaluation, if possible, to rule out any underlying ophthalmic pathology that could potentially limit the degree of visual acuity after the procedure.

Keratopigmentation: An Innovative Surgical Option for Therapeutic and Cosmetic Purposes

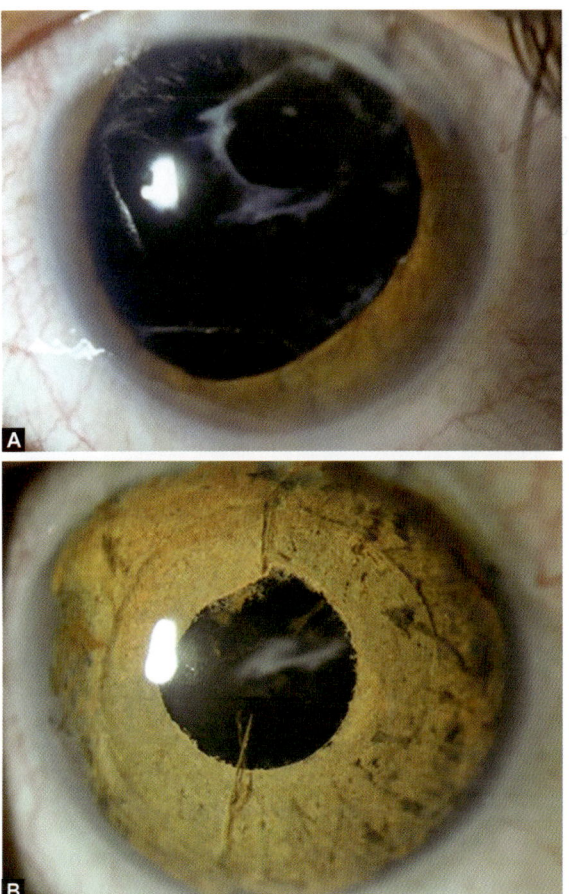

Figs. 6A and B: Functional therapeutic keratopigmentation. (A) 46-year-old man with aniridia of the left eye with a mild central corneal scar and strabismus after a trauma with a metallic wire. The BCVA was CD2; (B) The eye was treated with femtosecond laser-assisted intrastromal keratopigmentation technique in combination with strabismus surgery. After 2 months a retouch was applied. Finally, the patient was satisfied and the BCVA remained CD2.

- Corneal pachymetry.
- Corneal topography.
- Anterior segment optical coherence tomography (OCT) to assess depth and length of corneal opacities.
- Photo documentation of the cornea.
- Assessment of the patient's satisfaction after the procedure.

CONTRAINDICATIONS TO KERATOPIGMENTATION

Patients with any of the following conditions should be excluded from undergoing KTP for either therapeutic functional or cosmetic purposes:
- Any active ocular inflammation.
- Chronic corneal epithelial defects and ulcers.

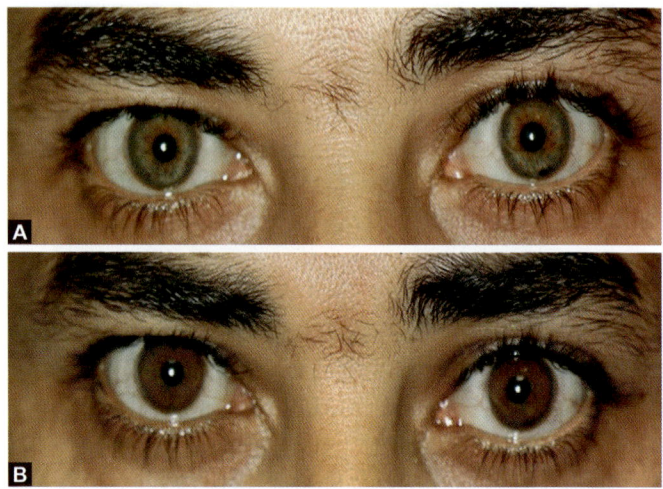

Figs. 7A and B: Cosmetic outcome of a pure cosmetic keratopigmentation case. (A) Preoperative hazel greenish color of the iris; (B) Postoperative medium brown color of the eyes after femtosecond laser-assisted intrastromal technique.

- History of herpetic keratitis.
- Corneal dellen.
- Ocular surface chronic inflammation.
- Severe dry eye.
- Corneal thickness less than 300 μm.

OUTCOMES

During the active years of practicing KTP, our team had very good and satisfactory outcomes, beginning from our experimental studies and ending with everyday practice.

The tolerance, biocompatibility and safety of the micronized mineral pigments were studied in animal models, where the pigments showed good and adequate behavior when introduced both intrastromally and superficially.[18,19,21] They presented good cosmetic results with no adverse effects. This encouraged us to go on with further development of the techniques.

From the year 2002 till 2018, we had operated around 280 eyes of 240 patients. The total number of procedures including the primary surgeries and all the retouches is 390 procedures.

In 2010, Alio et al. described and compared severely impaired eyes operated using superficial and intrastromal techniques.[8] Both techniques presented satisfactory results, however, the intrastromal one showed to be more advantageous as it provided a more homogenous aspect of the pigmented area. The surgery was faster, the patient showed a faster and less symptomatic postoperative recovery, the corneal surface was untouched and the staining was not exposed to tear film, what theoretically makes the pigments more stable and less prone to be washed out.

In a recent study, Al-Shymali et al.[26] reviewed all the patients that underwent superficial KTP, where almost 55% of the patients were operated only once, not needing more intervention, and 45% had one or more retouches. We assessed patients' satisfaction using a grading system of excellent or very happy, good or happy and poor or unhappy. Most of our patients (around 98%) were satisfied and declared they are very happy or happy. Thus, KTP can be a solution for many patients with cosmetic or functional ocular deformities, especially if alternatives like cosmetics lenses, keratoplasties, evisceration, enucleation or implants are not suitable procedures.

As many of our patients have pathological eyes, we frequently do mixed KTP in order to reach the perfect outcomes that will satisfy both the surgeon and the patient. Additionally, many of our patients who seek for KTP have blind decompensated eyes that show other pathologies like strabismus, ptosis, terminal glaucoma, aniridias, nystagmus. Therefore, we perform other surgeries before, after or even the same day with KTP, such as strabismus corrections, transscleral diode laser cyclophotocoagulation, ptosis repair, nystagmus surgeries, and pupiloplasties.

As mentioned previously, we used KTP[8,13,14,17,27] in patients with functionally impaired eyes that complained of photophobia, glare and photic phenomena due to several reasons such as fixed dilated pupil (Urrets-Zavalia syndrome), traumatic aniridia (partial or total), iris coloboma, intractable diplopia, very large peripheral iridotomies, iris atrophy, translucent iris in albinism, and progressive iris cysts. In most of the patients the visual complains disappeared or decreased significantly after KTP.

Regardless of the technique used, the visual acuity of the patients changed insignificantly and sometimes increased especially in the therapeutic functional groups. However, we observed that the intraocular pressure decreased significantly in patients pigmented with superficial techniques. This feature remains unexplained; however, we suggest that the procedure changes the corneal resistance and induces corneal irregularities and consequently the intraocular pressure measures lower but the actual intraocular pressure probably does not.

COMPLICATIONS

As any surgical procedure, KTP is faced with some complications. In our recent report of KTP complications, we studied and divided the complications encountered into organic and functional ones.[28]

Organic complications were described as change in color, color fading, and neovascularization. Functional complications included light sensitivity, visual field limitations, and magnetic resonance imaging (MRI) alterations. The percentage of complications in that series was 12.8%, of which 55% were functional and 45% were organic complications. Light sensitivity occupied 49% of the complications, followed by color fading and change in color (19% each), neovascularization 7%, visual field limitations 4% and MRI alterations 2%.

Concerning the MRI, one of our patients pigmented with SAK suffered severe pain during a head MRI. In the MRI images, the intraocular structures and the ocular globe were smeared and no reliable data could be taken from them. The cause of this phenomenon is unknown, nevertheless we propose that the iron oxide found in the pigments can be the cause.

Based on our observations, we concluded that single-tunnel technique is more preferable than the double-tunnel technique as well as deep corneal tunnels offer better outcomes than superficial intrastromal tunnels. In order to avoid visual field limitations, the internal diameter of the intrastromal tunnel (artificial pupil) created manually or using femtosecond laser should be minimally 5.3 mm. In our opinion, washing out the pigments at the end of the operation decreases the risk of light sensitivity postoperatively.

Despite the complications encountered, most of them were overcome by repeated pigmentation in the organic group and by washing out the pigments in some of the functional complications group. Eventually, most of our patients were satisfied with the final functional and cosmetic results.

CONCLUSION

Keratopigmentation is a modern surgery that provides an excellent solution for patients where other treatment options are not suitable. Femtosecond laser technology allows the surgeon to perform intrastromal dissections for pigmenting different types of corneal areas using the options provided by the software. The corneal tunnel creation technique is precise, safe, and easy to perform. However, with the development of the new automated device, superficial KTP is gaining popularity especially in cases where corneal opacities are too superficial to be masked by only intrastromal techniques. Still, more investigation and work should be carried out in order to decrease the postoperative complications.

REFERENCES

1. Holth S. Revival of Galen's corneal staining with copper sulfate and tannine should be abandoned. Am J Ophthalmol. 1931;14:378-9.
2. Mannis MJ, Eghbali K, Schwab IR. Keratopigmentation : a review of corneal tattooing. Cornea. 1999;18(6):633-7.
3. Van der Velden/Samderubun EM, Kok JH. Dermatography as a modern treatment for colouring leukoma corneae. Cornea. 1994;13(4):349-53.
4. Yildirim N, Basmak H, Sahin A. Prosthetic contact lenses : adventure or miracle. Eye Contact Lens. 2006;32(2):102-3.
5. Masoudi S, Stapleton F, Willcox M. Contact lens-induced discomfort and protein changes in tears. Optom Vis Sci. 2016;93(8):955-62.
6. Pitz S, Jahn R, Frisch L, et al. Corneal tattooing. An alternative treatment for disfiguring corneal scars. Br J Ophthalmol. 2002;86(4):397-9.
7. Kim C, Kim KH, Han YK, et al. Five-year results of corneal tattooing for cosmetic repair in disfigured eyes. Cornea. 2011;30(10):1135-9.

8. Alio JL, Sirerol B, Walewska A, et al. Corneal tattooing (keratopigmentation) with new mineral micronised pigments to restore cosmetic appearance in severely impaired eyes. Br J Ophthalmol. 2010;94(2):245-9.
9. Reed J. Corneal tattooing to reduce glare in cases of traumatic iris loss. Cornea. 1994;13(5):401-5.
10. Remky A, Redbrake C, Wenzel M. Intrastromal corneal tattooing for iris defects (letter). J Cataract Refract Surg. 1998;24(10):1285-7.
11. Beekhuis WH, Drost BHIM, van der Velden/ Samderubun EM. A new treatment for photophobia in posttraumatic aniridia: a case report. Cornea. 1998;17(3):338-41.
12. Alio J, Rodriguez A, Toffaha B, et al. Femtosecond-assisted keratopigmentation for functional and cosmetic restoration in essential iris atrophy. J Cataract Refract Surg. 2011;37(10):1744-7.
13. Alio JL, Rodriguez AE, Toffaha BT. Keratopigmentation (corneal tattooing) for the management of visual disabilities of the eye related to iris defects. Br J Ophthalmol. 2011;95(10):1397-401.
14. Alio JL, Rodriguez AE, Toffaha BT, et al. Femtosecond-assisted keratopigmentation double tunnel technique in the management of a case of Urrets-Zavalia syndrome. Cornea. 2012;31(9):1071-4.
15. Sekundo W, Seifert P, Seitz B, et al. Long-term ultrastructural changes in human corneas after tattooing with non-metallic substances. Br J Ophthalmol. 1999;83:219-24.
16. Burris T, Holmes-Higgin D, Silvestrini T. Lamellar intrastromal corneal tattoo for treating iris defects (artificial iris). Cornea. 1998;17:169-73.
17. Laria C, Alio J, Pinero D. Intrastromal corneal tattooing as treatment in a case of intractable strabismic diplopia (double binocular vision). Binocul Vis Strabismus Q. 2010;25(4):238-42.
18. Amesty MA, Rodriguez AE, Hernández E, et al. Tolerance of micronized mineral pigments for intrastromal keratopigmentation : a histopathology and immunopathology experimental study. Cornea. 2016;35(9):1199-205.
19. Sirerol B, Walewska-Szafran A, Alio J, et al. Tolerance and biocompatibility of micronized black pigment for keratopigmentation simulated pupil reconstruction. Cornea. 2011;30(3):344-50.
20. Amesty MA, Alio JL, Rodriguez AE. Corneal tolerance to micronised mineral pigments for keratopigmentation. Br J Ophthalmol. 2014;98(12):1756-60.
21. Rodriguez AE, Amesty MA, El Bahrawy M, et al. Superficial automated keratopigmentation for iris and pupil simulation using micronized mineral pigments and a new puncturing device: an experimental study. Cornea. 2017;36(9):1069-75.
22. Ziegler S. Multicolor tattooing of the cornea. Trans Am Ophthalmol Soc. 1922;20:71-87.
23. Alio J, Agdeppa M, Uceda-Montanes A. Femtosecond laser-assisted superficial keratectomy for the treatment of superficial corneal leukomas. Cornea. 2011;30(3):301-7.
24. Von Wecker L. Tatouage de la cornee. Union Med. 1870;27:41.
25. Alio J, Rodriguez A, El Bahrawy M, et al. Keratopigmentation to change the apparent color of the human eye: a novel indication for corneal tattooing. Cornea. 2016;35(4):431-7.

26. Al-Shymali O, Rodriguez AE, Amesty MA, et al. Superficial keratopigmentation: an alternative solution for patients with cosmetically or functionally impaired eyes. Cornea. 2019;38(1):54-61.
27. Rodriguez AE, Toffaha BT, Alio JL, et al. Femtosecond-assisted keratopigmentation for functional and cosmetic restoration in essential iris atrophy. J Cataract Refract Surg. 2011;37(10):1744-7.
28. Alio J, Al-Shymali O, Amesty MA, et al. Keratopigmentation with micronised mineral pigments: complications and outcomes in a series of 234 eyes. Br J Ophthalmol. 2018;102(6):742-7.

CHAPTER
4

Ocular Blood Flow in Glaucoma

Murali Ariga, Pratheeba Nivean, Malarchelvi Palani, Maithri Arun Kumar

INTRODUCTION

Blood supply to the eye is mainly by the ophthalmic artery (a branch of internal carotid artery). The posterior ciliary artery is the main source of blood supply to the optic nerve head, the choroid up to the equator, the retinal pigment epithelium, the outer 130 μ of retina and the medial and lateral segments of the ciliary body and iris while the central retinal blood vessels supplies the retina.[1] Whenever there are changes in blood pressure, ocular perfusion pressure and intraocular pressure (IOP) an internal autoregulatory mechanism functions.[2] Ocular hemodynamics though complex, can be assessed to an extent. The quantification of blood flow in these vessels can give information about the pathological processes underlying retinal and optic nerve head diseases such as glaucoma and vessel occlusions.

Changes in IOP can influence the blood flow within intraocular structures due to the arteriovenous pressure differences. Optic nerve head ischemia may have a role to play in the causation and progression of glaucoma. Similarly, vascular impairment is also seen in diseases such as age-related macular degeneration (AMD), arterial and vein occlusions as well as diabetic retinopathy.

ASSESSMENT OF OCULAR BLOOD FLOW

In the last few decades, from the highly invasive and experimental technique of using radioactive tracers to the latest noninvasive optical coherence tomography (OCT) angiography, assessment of ocular blood flow has come a long way. These techniques can be simply classified into two groups: invasive and noninvasive.
1. **Invasive methods:** Scanning laser ophthalmoscopic angiography (SLOA) with fluorescein and/or indocyanine green (ICG).
2. **Noninvasive methods:** Color Doppler imaging (CDI), laser Doppler velocimetry (LDV), laser speckle technique, laser Doppler flowmetry, retinal vessel analyzer (RVA), retinal oximetry, Doppler OCT, and the latest OCT angiography (OCTA; Table 1).

Table 1: Comparison of various techniques for measuring ocular blood flow.

Techniques	Vascular bed	Measurements	Main limitations
Color Doppler imaging	Retrobulbar blood vessels	Velocity	Measures velocity not flow
Laser Doppler flowmetry	Optic nerve head and choroidal capillaries	Flow in arbitrary units	• No absolute flow measurements • Comparison between subjects difficult.
Scanning laser ophthalmoscopic angiography	Retina and choroid (dye dependent)	Velocity	Measures velocity and filling time not flow
Pulsatile ocular blood flow	Mainly choroid	Pulse amplitude, pulsatile ocular blood flow (POBF)	No direct measurement is made. Relation to flow is unclear
Confocal scanning laser Doppler flowmetry	Optic nerve and retinal capillaries	Flow in arbitrary units	• Flow measured in arbitrary units. • Comparison between subjects difficult.
Interferometry	Choroid	Fundus pulsation amplitude	Doubtful relationship between fundus pulsation amplitude and ocular blood flow
Laser speckle flowgraphy	Optic nerve head and subfoveal choroid	Tissue blood velocity	Measurement is not clearly understood
Retinal vessel analyzer	Large retinal vessels	Retinal vessel diameter	No flow or velocity information. Retinal vessel diameter in arbitrary units
Bidirectional laser Doppler velocimetry (CLBF) model	Large retinal vessels	Velocity, diameter and calculated flow	Good fixation and clear media required
Retinal oximetry	Retinal vessels	Oxygen saturation in arteries and veins	Not fully validated

(CLBF: Canon Laser Blood Flowmeter)

SCANNING LASER OPHTHALMOSCOPIC ANGIOGRAPHY

Scanning laser ophthalmoscopic angiography is a set of techniques that quantify various aspects of blood filling the retinal and choroidal vasculature. It consists of a scanning laser which illuminates the retina in a faster scan pattern and the intensities are used to construct a video signal which can be displayed on the monitor and stored.

Using the principle of fluorescein angiography, either fluorescein dye or ICN dye is injected in a vein and the vasculature of interest is observed as the video signal is constructed. The mean dye velocity, arteriovenous passage time (AVP) and the mean transit time are calculated. Prolonged AVP time has been noticed in some glaucomatous eyes.[3]

Advantages

The AVP is very sensitive to hemodynamic changes and allows visualizing even mild changes in blood flow. SLOA with ICG is the only method available now to assess the choroidal vasculature.

Limitations

It is invasive and requires highly skilled operators to utilize the processing software which is laborious and not commercially available.

■ COLOR DOPPLER IMAGING

Based on principles of ultrasound, CDI uses pulse-Doppler measurements or Doppler-shifted frequencies with B-scan grayscale images (Fig. 1). CDI is done for the ophthalmic artery, central retinal artery and short posterior ciliary arteries. Doppler measurements of the peak and trough waveforms of the three arteries are taken. The peak systolic velocity (PSV), end-diastolic volume (EDV) and resistivity index (RI) are calculated. CDI is known to be especially useful in glaucomatous optic neuropathy wherein, studies have demonstrated low PSV and EDV levels in these vessels.[4]

A normal wave pattern in a Doppler imaging is biphasic with a peak and trough (Fig. 2). However, this normal biphasic pattern is lost in vascular occlusions and glaucoma patients particularly in normal tension glaucoma (NTG) subjects (Figs. 3 and 4). A biphasic peak may also be observed in

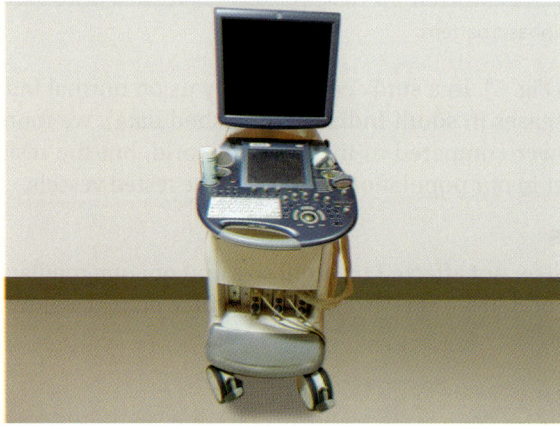

Fig. 1: Color Doppler imaging machine.

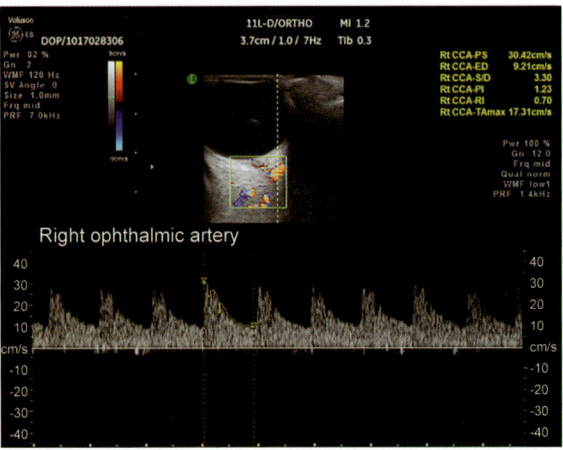

Fig. 2: Biphasic normal pattern.
Source: Prof Venkatasai Bharat Scans.

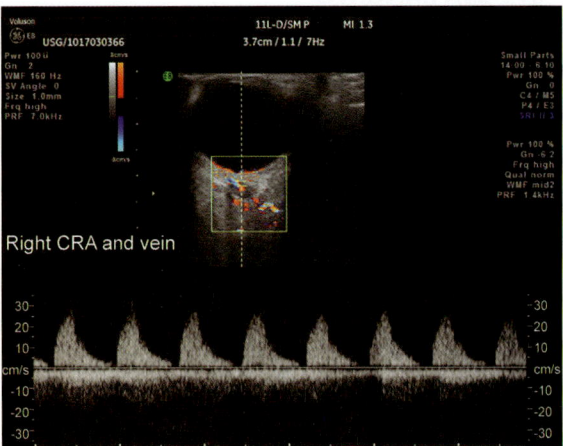

Fig. 3: Loss of biphasic pattern.

certain eyes (Fig. 5). In a study conducted by us on normal individuals with no ocular diseases in south India (unpublished data), we found the PSV to be slightly lower compared to the western world, but the resistive index is slightly higher in our population in all the three tested vessels.

Advantages

It is noninvasive; not affected by pupil size and opaque media; reproducible and capable of detecting resistance to vascular beds distal to the points of measurement.[5]

Limitations

Color Doppler imaging is an expensive test and requires an expert certified technician to give reproducible results. It measures blood flow velocities and not net flow as diameter of the vessels cannot be assessed.

Ocular Blood Flow in Glaucoma

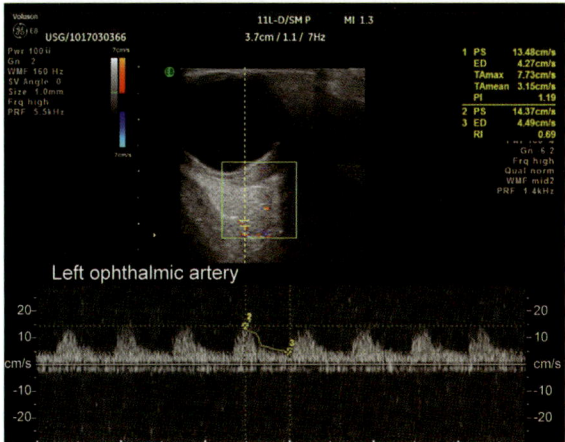

Fig. 4: Loss of biphasic pattern with decreased peak systolic velocity.

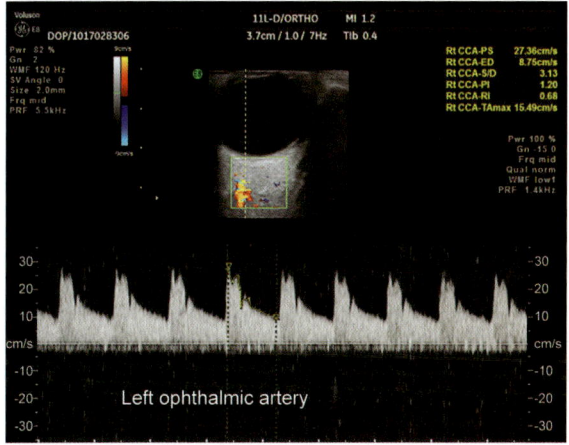

Fig. 5: Biphasic peak systole.

It may be difficult to locate the small vessel posterior ciliary artery signals in certain patients.

LASER DOPPLER VELOCIMETRY

Bidirectional laser doppler velocimetry (LDV) can be used to quantify blood velocity in the large retinal vessels. The blood velocity and vessel diameter are calculated and retinal blood flow is obtained.[6] It has been used to investigate vascular diseases of the retina such as vein occlusions and diabetic retinopathy. Changes in blood flow have also been documented following the use of pharmacological agents.

Advantages

Laser Doppler velocimetry with diameter measurements helps to determine blood flow in absolute units.

Limitations

Only a single segment of the vessel can be measured. Clear optical media and pupil dilatation are required. The machine, into which this technique is incorporated, is no longer commercially available.

LASER DOPPLER FLOWMETRY

It is a Doppler device that consists of a modified fundus camera and computer system. It provides noninvasive confocal scanning laser Doppler flowmetry of retinal capillary blood flow. It is a confocal system with a plane thickness of 400 microns and tends to concentrate on surface vasculature. Another method of laser Doppler flowmetry utilizes manual pixel-by-pixel analysis and displays them as histograms with percentile flow values. Retinal capillary blood flow seems to be reduced within the neuroretinal rim and peripapillary area in glaucoma and have also been found to correspond to visual field defects.[7]

Advantages

Measures volumetric retinal capillary blood flow and is sensitive to small changes in blood flow.

Limitations

Measurements are in arbitrary values and clear optical media and good fixation are required.

RETINAL VESSEL ANALYZER

The retinal vessel analyzer (RVA) has a camera, a real time monitor and a computer with vessel diameter analysis software. The vessel diameters are assessed in real time and consecutive fundus images are digitized. This is based on the principle that the blood vessel has a transmittance profile due to the absorbing properties of hemoglobin. Adaptive algorithms are used based on these profiles to measure the diameters. It is known to be especially useful in evaluating prognosis in diabetic retinopathy where it improves after panretinal photocoagulation.[8]

Advantages

The RVA enables continuous monitoring of vessel diameter, and different segments of different vessels can be evaluated simultaneously. Fundus images can be stored and recovered at any time.

Limitations

A major limitation is that it is a method to estimate the diameter of the vessel and not the actual blood flow. It requires clear optical media, good fixation and a dilated pupil.

RETINAL OXIMETRY

It is a noninvasive technique of measuring hemoglobin oxygen saturation in retinal structures by digital imaging. Images of vessels are recorded at oxygen sensitive and insensitive wavelengths through narrow band-pass filters specific for different wavelengths.

Retinal oximetry can give us information regarding the metabolic activity of the retina. The possible presence of hypoxia and its effects in various diseases can be studied. In a pilot study, eyes with NTG showed significantly decreased arteriolar oxygen saturation than primary open-angle glaucoma (POAG).[9]

Advantages
It is noninvasive procedure that provides the metabolic link in glaucoma pathology.

Limitations
Clear optical media are required. However, new tests are not sufficiently validated.

DOPPLER OPTICAL COHERENCE TOMOGRAPHY

Doppler optical coherence tomography is based on the principle that red blood cells induces an interference pattern when a light is scattered and the phase difference between sequential B-scans can be recorded as an image. Doppler OCT can be used to measure blood velocity and volumetric flow rate in retinal branch vessels. Both the peak and average velocity can be analyzed along the cardiac cycle. Vessel diameter can also be measured directly.

Eyes with glaucoma, diabetic retinopathy, retinal vein occlusions (RVOs), and anterior ischemic optic neuropathy were had reduced retinal blood flow. The reduction in retinal blood flow correlated with visual field changes in glaucomatous eyes.[10]

Advantages
Blood flow is measured in absolute units of μL/min and vessel dimensions are also directly measured.

Limitations
Quantitative measurements are limited to major vessels and capillary flow cannot be demonstrated. Error in vessel orientation occurs due to eye movement and scan time required is more.

OPTICAL COHERENCE TOMOGRAPHY ANGIOGRAPHY

Optical coherence tomography angiography is a more recent noncontact imaging technique that allows for visualization of the retinal and choroidal vasculature (Fig. 6). OCTA detects the motion of red blood cells as intrinsic contrast. Some of the features that can be detected on OCTA are (Figs. 7 and 8):
- Vascular density;
- Flow index;
- Vascular density in the peripapillary retina; and
- Vascular density in the macula.

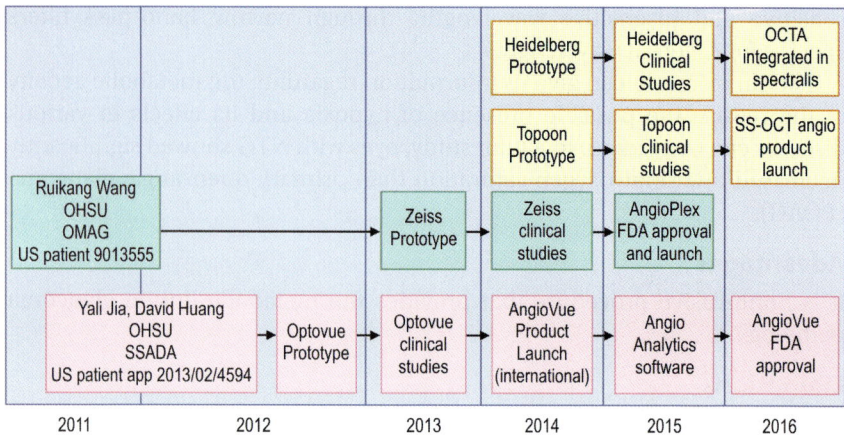

Fig. 6: Ophthalmic OCTA development timeline.
(FDA: Food and Drug Administration; OCTA: optical coherence tomography angiography; OHSU: Oregon Health and Science University; OMAG: optical microangiography; SSADA: split-spectrum amplitude-decorrelation angiography; SS-OCT: swept-source OCT.)
Source: Makita S, Hong Y, Yamanari M, et al. Optical coherence angiography. Opt Express. 2006;14(17): 7821-40.

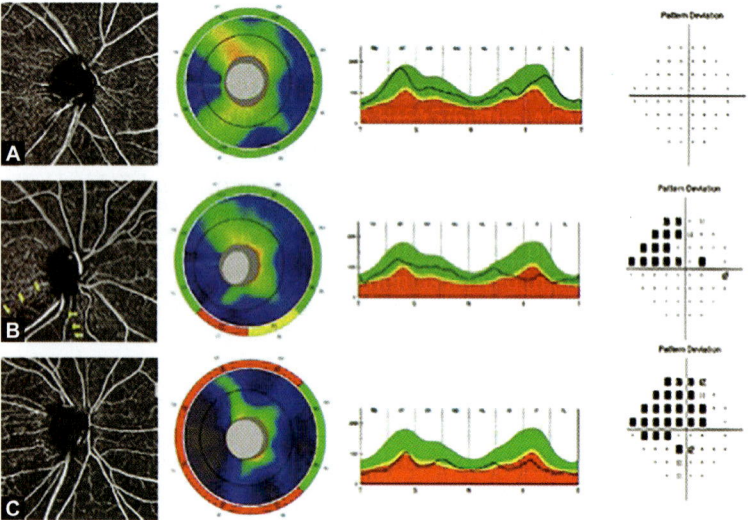

Figs. 7A to C: Correlating optical coherence tomography angiography with retinal nerve fiber layer and fields.

In glaucoma (including glaucoma suspect and preperimetric glaucoma) significant reduction of blood flow, capillary diameter, and vascular density was noticed proportional to the severity of glaucoma damage. Figures 9 and 10 show a glaucoma patient with inferior notch in neural rim and retinal nerve fiber layer (RNFL) defect. This is also seen in OCTA with decreased capillary density in the area of the RNFL loss. This also correlates with a corresponding

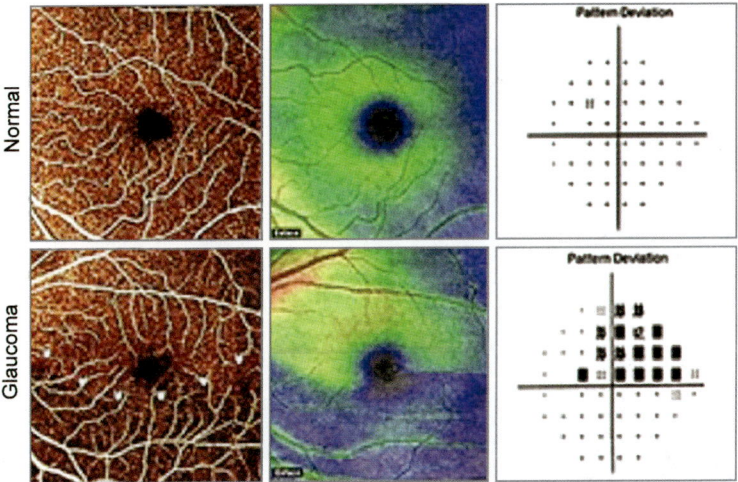

Fig. 8: Optical coherence tomography angiography correlation with ganglion cell complex and fields.

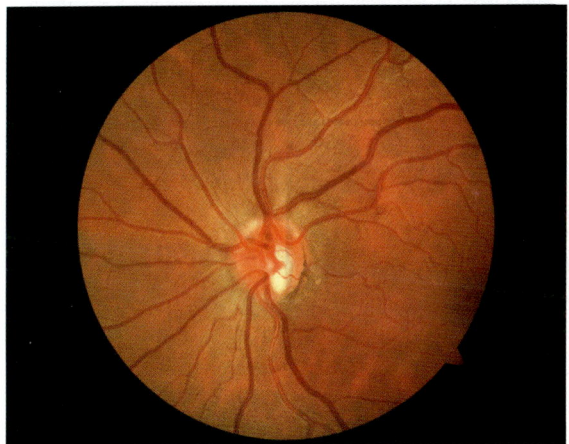

Fig. 9: Optic disk showing inferior glaucomatous notch and retinal nerve fiber layer defect.

visual field loss and loss of inferior RNFL or ganglion cell complex (GCC) in this example (Figs. 11 and 12). Some studies have suggested a higher correlation between vascular indices and functional (visual field) data compared to thickness.

Optical coherence tomography angiography has been shown to be useful in the evaluation of retinal vascular occlusive disease to define areas of nonperfusion in ischemic RVOs. It is useful in detecting occult neovascular AMD which is difficult to do so with conventional fluorescein angiography. Microvascular changes and enlargement of foveal avascular zone in diabetic retinopathy is easily picked up in an OCTA. It is also a useful tool for evaluating optic disk perfusion.[11]

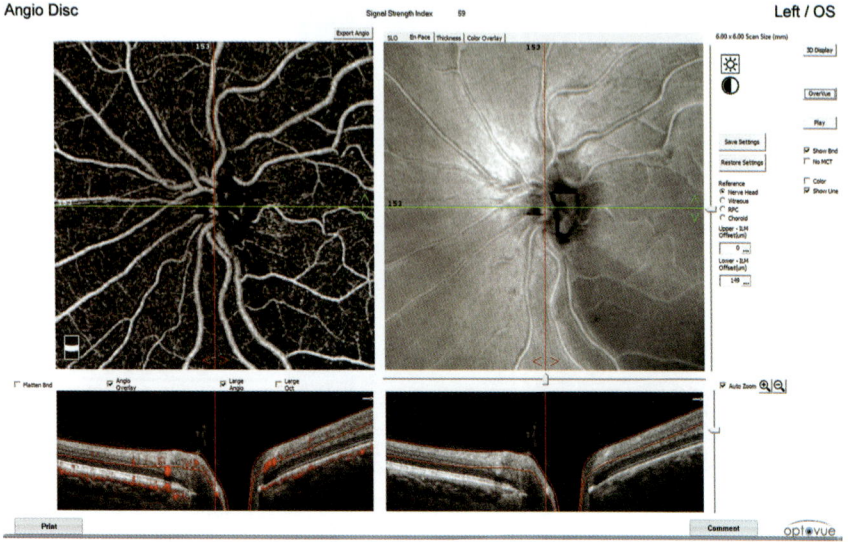

Fig. 10: OCT angio of optic disc showing decreased capillary density in the region of the RNFL defect.
Courtesy: Dr Arulmozhi Varman, Uma Eye Clinic.

Advantages

It is noninvasive and can assess both retinal and choroidal blood flow. It gives quantitative and qualitative data and is superior to fluorescein angiography and conventional OCT.

Limitations

The major limitations of OCTA are the artifacts produced by eye movement, attenuation artifact (due to loss of signal with depth), segmentation artifact (due to difficulties in selecting consistent boundaries for the *en face* slabs), and projection artefact (due to decorrelation tails from more superficial vessels). OCTA is a recent development and has yet to be validated for routine clinical use.

■ FACTORS THAT AFFECT OCULAR BLOOD FLOW

Physiologic Factors

Age

A reduction of ocular circulation has been observed with increasing age in the ophthalmic and central retinal artery. Capillary flow in the retina, neuro-retinal rim, and lamina cribrosa reduces in the elderly (over 60 years).[12]

Posture

When position is changed from sitting to supine, ocular perfusion pressure is usually increased. CDI demonstrated autoregulatory response in ophthalmic and central retinal artery in normal subjects on change of position while the same was not seen in glaucoma subjects, suggesting that there could by faulty autoregulation of retinal circulation in glaucoma.[13]

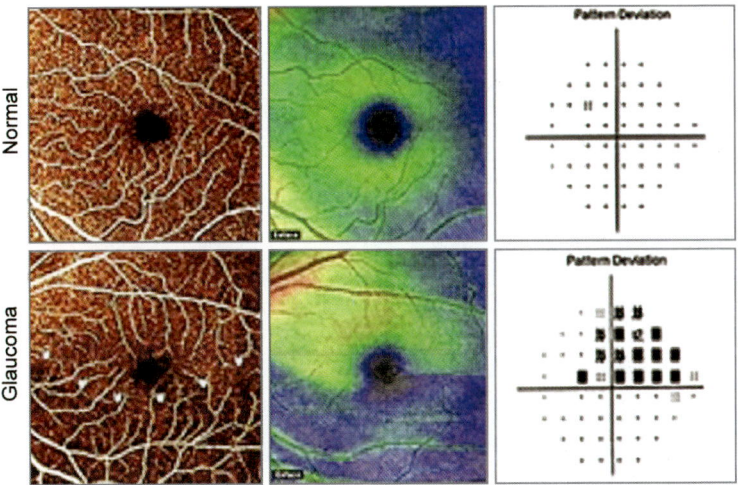

Fig. 8: Optical coherence tomography angiography correlation with ganglion cell complex and fields.

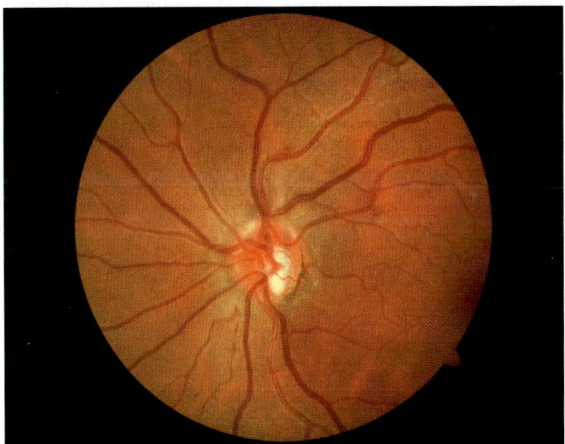

Fig. 9: Optic disk showing inferior glaucomatous notch and retinal nerve fiber layer defect.

visual field loss and loss of inferior RNFL or ganglion cell complex (GCC) in this example (Figs. 11 and 12). Some studies have suggested a higher correlation between vascular indices and functional (visual field) data compared to thickness.

Optical coherence tomography angiography has been shown to be useful in the evaluation of retinal vascular occlusive disease to define areas of nonperfusion in ischemic RVOs. It is useful in detecting occult neovascular AMD which is difficult to do so with conventional fluorescein angiography. Microvascular changes and enlargement of foveal avascular zone in diabetic retinopathy is easily picked up in an OCTA. It is also a useful tool for evaluating optic disk perfusion.[11]

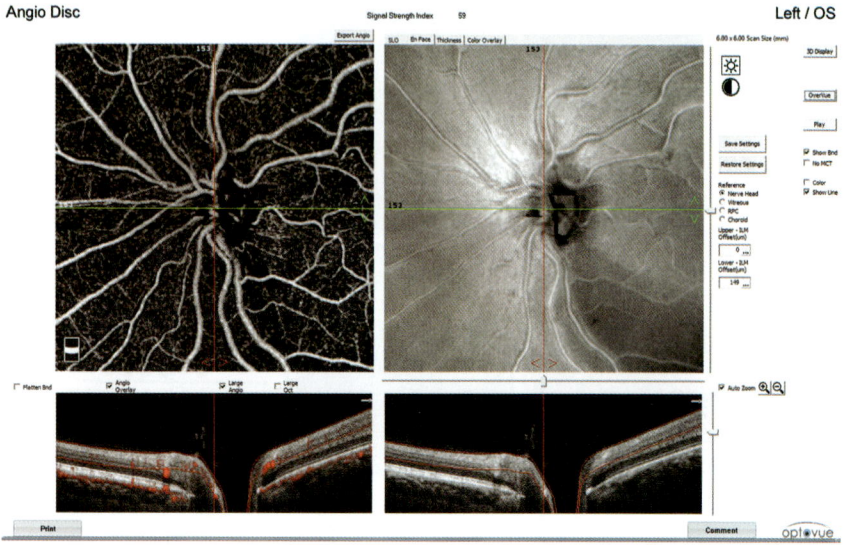

Fig. 10: OCT angio of optic disc showing decreased capillary density in the region of the RNFL defect.
Courtesy: Dr Arulmozhi Varman, Uma Eye Clinic.

Advantages

It is noninvasive and can assess both retinal and choroidal blood flow. It gives quantitative and qualitative data and is superior to fluorescein angiography and conventional OCT.

Limitations

The major limitations of OCTA are the artifacts produced by eye movement, attenuation artifact (due to loss of signal with depth), segmentation artifact (due to difficulties in selecting consistent boundaries for the *en face* slabs), and projection artefact (due to decorrelation tails from more superficial vessels). OCTA is a recent development and has yet to be validated for routine clinical use.

■ FACTORS THAT AFFECT OCULAR BLOOD FLOW

Physiologic Factors

Age

A reduction of ocular circulation has been observed with increasing age in the ophthalmic and central retinal artery. Capillary flow in the retina, neuro-retinal rim, and lamina cribrosa reduces in the elderly (over 60 years).[12]

Posture

When position is changed from sitting to supine, ocular perfusion pressure is usually increased. CDI demonstrated autoregulatory response in ophthalmic and central retinal artery in normal subjects on change of position while the same was not seen in glaucoma subjects, suggesting that there could by faulty autoregulation of retinal circulation in glaucoma.[13]

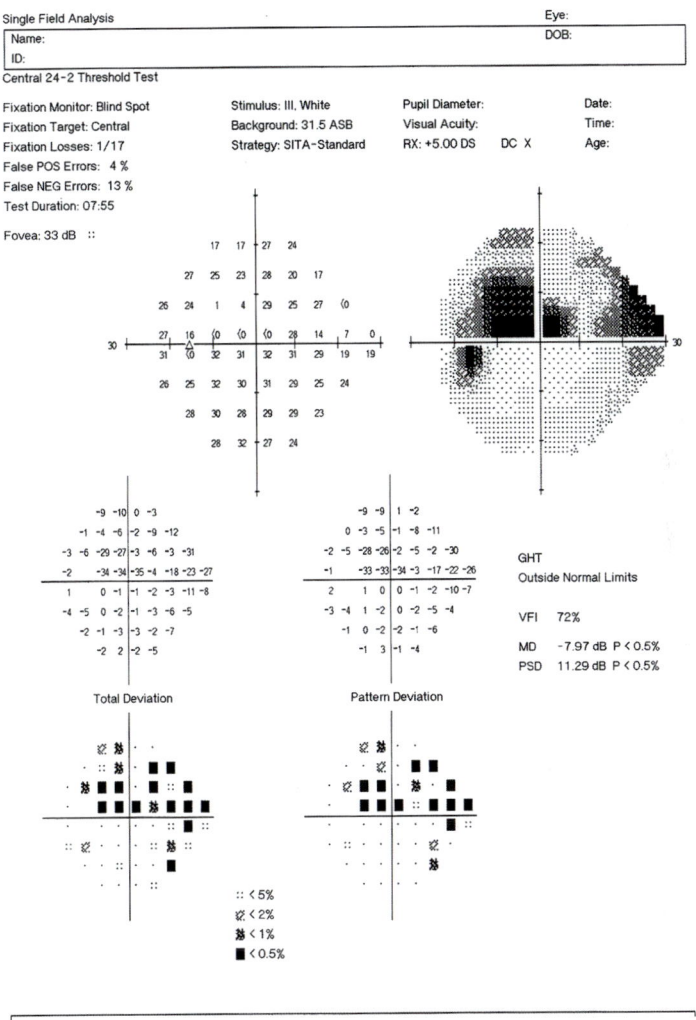

Fig. 11: Field left eye.

Circadian Rhythm

A nocturnal dip in blood pressure and an increase in IOP at night is well-known. Using CDI, nocturnal decrease in blood velocity was seen in short posterior ciliary artery but not significant in the ophthalmic artery. There was no difference noted between normal and glaucomatous eyes.[14]

Systemic Disease

Ocular vascular dysregulation can occur in any disease that involves the vascular system. Vasospasm, migraine, rheological factors such as platelet hyperaggregability, diabetes, arteriosclerosis, and atherosclerosis caused by systemic hypertension, systemic hypotension, sleep apnea, and atrial fibrillation can cause changes in ocular perfusion and blood flow. Endothelial

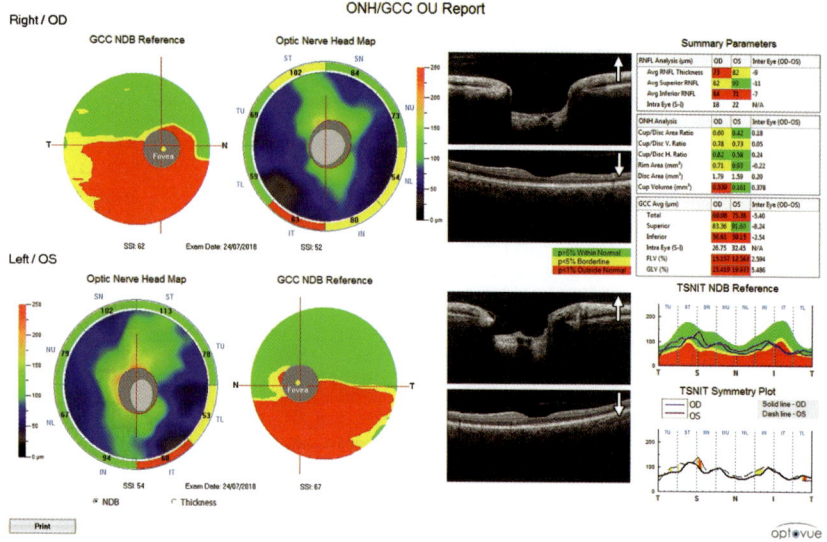

Fig. 12: Optical coherence tomography showing the inferior retinal nerve fiber layer loss.
Source: Dr Arulmozhi Varman.

dysfunction may be the link between systemic and ocular dysregulation in glaucoma.[15]

Pharmacological Factors

Intraocular Pressure Lowering Drugs

Treatment with timolol in POAG and ocular hypertension (OHT) patients for 6 months showed no significant effect in optic nerve head blood flow (HRF) while topical carbonic anhydrase inhibitors such as dorzolamide showed significant increase in the optic nerve head circulation.[16] In normal subjects, a single instillation of dorzolamide or timolol showed no effect on blood flow. Topical prostaglandin analogues such as latanoprost failed to show any effect on retrobulbar hemodynamics in POAG, NTG, or OHT patients.

Systemic Drugs

Calcium channel blockers such as nifedipine showed no significant change in ocular blood flow while instillation of topical verapamil was reported to increase optic nerve head circulation.[17] Little effects on choroidal flow was reported with the use of losartan, a renin-angiotensin inhibitor.[18] Intravenous administration of dopamine was found to increase blood flow velocity in major retinal vessels.

■ CONCLUSION

Technology through decade has brought us to this golden era of imaging where we can visualize and understand the subtle physiological and pathological processes that lead to the diseases we treat. There is insufficient data comparing blood flow and retinal diseases and progression of glaucoma.

Further studies with better study designs are required to validate its use with respect to treatment and prognosis. In the future, with newer methods of estimation of ocular blood flow, we can evaluate and characterize ocular circulation and this may become an integral part of our clinical practice.

ACKNOWLEDGMENTS

Professor Venkatsai has taken the ocular blood flow scans, Dr Arulmozhi Varman has contributed pictures and Professor Alon Harris has trained us in ocular blood flow.

REFERENCES

1. Investigative ophthalmology and visual science. 2004;45:749-57.
2. Bill A, Sperber GO. Control of retinal and choroidal blood flow. Eye (Lond). 1990;4(Pt 2):319-25.
3. Wolf S, Arend O, Haase A, et al. Retinal hemodynamics in patients with chronic open-angle glaucoma. Ger J Ophthalmol 1995;4(5):279-82.
4. Plange N, Kaup M, Weber A, et al. Performance of colour Doppler imaging discriminating normal tension glaucoma from healthy eyes. Eye (Lond). 2009;23(1):164-70.
5. Halpern EJ, Merton DA, Forsberg F. Effect of distal resistance on Doppler US flow patterns. Radiology. 1998;206(3):761-6.
6. Feke GT, Goger DG, Tagawa H, et al. Laser Doppler technique for absolute measurement of blood speed in retinal vessels. IEEE Trans Biomed Eng. 1987;34(9):673-80.
7. Sato EA, Ohtake Y, Shinoda K, et al. Decreased blood flow of neuroretinal rim of optic nerve head corresponds with visual field deficit in eyes with normal tension glaucoma. Graefes Arch Clin Exp Ophthalmol. 2006;244(7):795-801.
8. Seifert BU, Vilser W. Retinal Vessel Analyser (RVA)—design and function. Biomed Tech (Berl). 2002;47(Supp l Pt 2):678-81.
9. Michelson G, Scibor M. Intravascular oxygen saturation in retinal vessels in normal subjects and open-angle glaucoma subjects. Acta Ophthalmol Scand. 2006;84(3):289-95.
10. Wang Y, Tan O, Huang D. Investigation of retinal blood flow in normal and glaucoma subjects by Doppler Fourier-domain optical coherence tomography. Proc SPIE; 2009. p. 7168.
11. Maram J, Srinivas S, Sadda SR. Evaluating ocular blood flow. Indian J Ophthalmol. 2017;65(5):337-46.
12. Embleton SJ, Hosking SL, Roff Hilton EJ, et al. Effect of senescence on ocular blood fow in the retina, neuroretinal rim and lamina cribrosa, using scanning lase Doppler flowmetry. Eye. 2002;16(2):156-62.
13. Evans DW, Harris A, Garrett M, et al. Glaucoma patients demonstrate faulty autoregulation of ocular blood flow during posture change. Br J Ophthalmol. 1999;83(7):809-13.
14. Harris A, Evans D, Martin B, et al. Nocturnal blood pressure reduction: effect on retrobulbar hemodynamics in glaucoma. Graefes Arch Clin Exp Ophthalmol. 2002;240(10):372-78.
15. Resch H, Garhofer G, Fuchjager-Mayrl G, et al. Endothelial dysfunction in glaucoma. Acta Ophthalmol. 2009;87(1):4-12.

16. Fuchsjager-Mayrl G, Wally B, Rainer G, et al. Effect of dorzolamide and timolol on ocular blood flow in patients with primary open angle glaucoma and ocular hypertension. Br J Ophthalmol. 2005;89(10):1293-7.
17. Netland P, Feke G, Konno S, et al. Optic nerve head circulation after topical calcium channel blocker. J Glaucoma. 1996;5(3):200-6.
18. Spicher T, Orgul S, Gugleta K, et al. The effect of losartan potassium on choroidal hemodynamics in healthy subjects. J Glaucoma. 2002;11(3):177-82.

CHAPTER 5

Selective Laser Trabeculoplasty

Purvi R Bhagat, Shivani Dixit, Nikunj Tank

■ INTRODUCTION

The management of glaucoma aims to lower the intraocular pressure (IOP) either by improving the aqueous outflow or by decreasing the aqueous humor production. The options for lowering the IOP include drug therapy, laser treatment or surgical management. Laser iridotomy has a definitive role for primary angle closure disease, while laser trabeculoplasty increases the outflow from the trabecular meshwork (TM).

■ HISTORY AND CONCEPT

The role of lasers in glaucoma was described in 1970s, when investigators reported that argon laser can create holes in localized areas of the TM.[1] In 1979, Wise and Witter introduced the use of argon laser trabeculoplasty (ALT) to treat open-angle glaucoma.[2] Since ALT causes thermal coagulative damage and subsequent scarring of the uveoscleral part of the TM, alternative technology was looked into, to reduce the energy delivery on the TM, consequently minimizing the side effects without losing the efficacy of the procedure.[3]

Anderson and Parish discovered that selectively absorbed radiation could damage pigmented structures.[4] These inherent properties of a tissue determining its destruction, in other words, selective photothermolysis became the principle of selective laser trabeculoplasty (SLT). Working on this concept, Latina and Park[5] used Q-switched 532 nm Neodymium:Yttrium Aluminum Garnet (Nd:YAG) laser to irradiate a mixed cell population of pigmented and nonpigmented cells. They developed a technique that could selectively target pigmented meshwork cells. A 3 ns SLT pulse, combined with a 1 μs thermal relaxation time of melanin, minimizes the thermal dissipation to surrounding tissues.

■ MECHANISM OF ACTION

It has been shown by histopathological studies that ALT treated eyes showed coagulative damage to TM while the ones treated with SLT did not.[6]

The mechanism of action of SLT is proposed by various theories:
- **Mechanical theory:** It proposes that SLT causes stretching of the TM beams and thereby increases aqueous humor outflow.
- **Biological theory:** It states that injury to the pigmented TM cells releases chemoattractants which invite monocytes which are then transformed into macrophages. These macrophages clear pigment granules from the TM and finally exit through the Schlemm's canal.[7]
- **Cell division theory:** This states that laser applications stimulate cell division in the anterior TM, providing pluripotent cells for the repopulation of treated sites. Loss of endothelial cells over the trabecular beams causes the peripheral corneal endothelial cells to divide and slide over the treated areas. These cells produce different extracellular matrix, enhancing the aqueous outflow.

Indications
- Ocular hypertension.
- *Primary open angle glaucoma:* When IOP is uncontrolled despite maximally tolerated medical therapy or patient is noncompliant to medications or is intolerant to the drugs or when the surgery cannot be done due to patient's local or systemic condition or patient is unwilling for surgery. One such important condition is glaucoma in pregnancy.
- *Secondary open-angle glaucoma* like pseudoexfoliation, pigmentary and steroid induced.
- Combined mechanism glaucoma, with a patent iridotomy with adequate visualization of the TM.

Contraindications
- Inadequate visualization of the TM.
- Hazy media.
- Uveitic glaucoma.
- Neovascular glaucoma.
- Traumatic glaucoma.
- Heavily pigmented TM, especially with a previous history of ALT. This may be a relative contraindication considering an increased risk for IOP spikes after SLT.[8]

Advantages
- Noninvasive procedure.
- Fewer complications compared to ALT and various glaucoma surgeries.
- Can be repeated, if and when necessary.

Disadvantages
- Cost of the equipment.
- Effect is not long lasting.
- Cooperation of the patient at slit lamp is essential.

Technique

Patient Preparation
- Complete baseline evaluation for glaucoma.
- In gonioscopic evaluation of the angle, one should confirm adequate visibility of TM. The presence of synechiae should be ruled out as these are contraindications to the procedure.
- The patient should be explained about the laser procedure and written informed consent should be taken.
- Some surgeons prefer to instill alpha 2 agonists, either apraclonidine or brimonidine, prior to the laser to counteract the risk of a post-procedure IOP rise.
- Topical anesthetic like proparacaine (0.5%) eye drop is applied just prior to the procedure.

Procedure
- Selective laser trabeculoplasty uses frequency-doubled Q-switched Nd:YAG laser (532 nm).
- The laser is attached with a slit lamp system.
- A low-power helium-neon laser beam provides aiming of the treatment area.
- The patient is seated comfortably at the laser slit lamp system. A Goldmann three-mirror goniolens, Latina SLT lens or a Ritch trabeculoplasty lens is inserted into the eye using a coupling agent (Fig. 1).
- The spot size is 400 micron with a pulse duration of 0.3 ns (in ALT, the argon green laser is set to a spot size of 50 micron with 0.1 second duration. A larger spot size covers most of the angle structures including the iris root (Fig. 2).

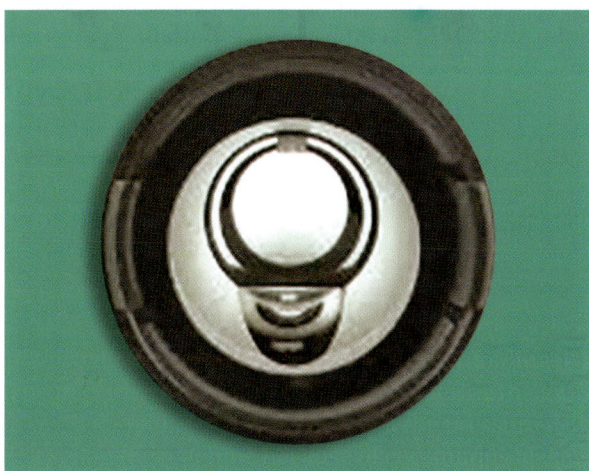

Fig. 1: Trabeculoplasty lens, with single gonioscopy mirror.

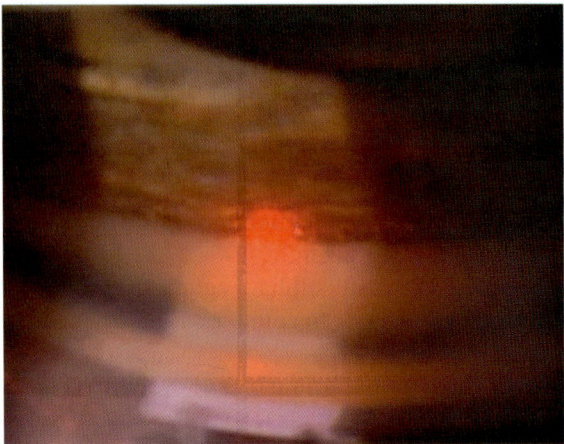

Fig. 2: Selective laser trabeculoplasty (SLT) laser spot focused at the pigmented part of the trabecular meshwork.

- The power is usually set to 0.8 megajoule (MJ) but can be adjusted within a range of 0.2–1.7 MJ depending on the extent of TM pigmentation. More the TM pigmentation, lesser is the energy required. The end point of SLT pulse energy is identified by the production of tiny "champagne" type bubbles (Fig. 3).
- The energy is increased or decreased in intervals of 0.1 MJ till minimal bubble formation is detected. Treatment is then continued through single-pulse mode.
- The extent of treatment of the TM is controversial. The standard treatment protocol uses 50 spots delivered at 0.6–1 MJ applied over 180° of meshwork.
- Eyes treated 360° show a greater IOP reduction but there is also a higher rate of adverse effects in this group. Patient discomfort, anterior chamber inflammation and IOP spikes have been reported.[9]

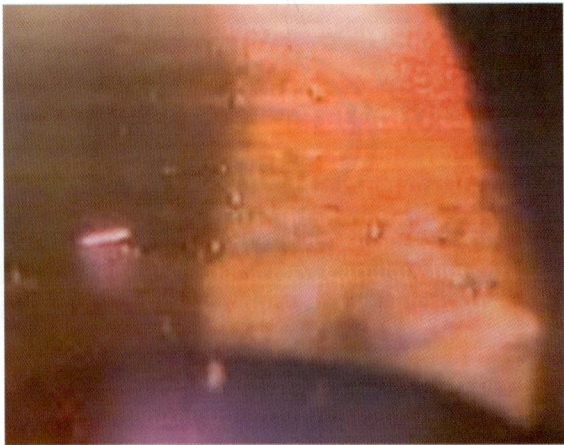

Fig. 3: Champagne bubbles, suggesting adequate energy delivery.

Postprocedure Management
- Use of a topical steroid or a nonsteroidal anti-inflammatory drug in the postoperative week is controversial for concern of the neutralization effect of these drugs on the desired inflammation.
- Intraocular pressure is checked approximately 1 hour after the procedure. IOP-lowering drugs are prescribed if there is significant IOP elevation.
- If patients are on antiglaucoma medications prior to the laser, they may continue the same for a week.
- Depending on the IOP response after 6–8 weeks, further decision either to discontinue the drops or to perform a repeat SLT can be made.

Complications
Most studies report fewer complications with SLT, which is mainly due to the lesser energy delivery compared to that in ALT.
- *Post-laser IOP spike*: This is usually associated with use of higher energy levels, treatment through 360° of TM, posterior placement of the laser shots, heavy pigmentation in the angle, and a significantly compromised preoperative outflow facility.[10] The IOP spikes are usually transient, occurring within the first hour of treatment and most often resolve with medications.
- *Uveitis*: Mild uveitis has been reported in majority of patients treated with SLT.[11,12] However, such sequelae usually resolve in 24 hours.
- Although SLT is quite a safe procedure, hyphema and bleeding are also known to occur.

Outcomes
Selective laser trabeculoplasty may require several weeks or months to achieve its complete IOP-lowering effect. In a study on 67 patients with uncontrolled primary open-angle glaucoma who had undergone SLT, the mean IOP reduction was found to be 4.4 mm Hg from a mean preoperative IOP of 22.4 mm Hg at 6 months follow-up.[13] The IOP reduction was almost double 5 months later demonstrating that SLT needs time to have its effect completely established and to determine whether a repeat procedure shall be necessary. Studies show that the strongest predictor of SLT success is a high preoperative IOP.[14,15]

Hodge et al. in their study comparing SLT and ALT, collected data on 72 patients treated with SLT and defined successful SLT as an IOP reduction of at least 20% at 1 year.[14] They concluded that age, gender, type of open-angle glaucoma, degree of TM pigmentation, and other glaucomatous risk factors were not predictors of the success of SLT. On the contrary, certain studies do show that increased angle pigmentation correlates with the efficacy of the procedure. In a study done by Wasyluk et al.[16] 63 eyes were subdivided into 3 groups based on their angle pigmentation and all were treated with 270° SLT. The mean IOP reduction noted were 2.06, 2.46, and 4.75 mm Hg in subgroups having low, marked, and high pigmentation, respectively. Although the absolute IOP reduction was found to be lesser in eyes with low pigmentation, such patients may still be considered candidates for SLT.

Another study found that the type of glaucoma and preoperative IOP influenced the success of SLT.[17]

CONCLUSION

Selective laser trabeculoplasty is now established as an effective solution for those patients who have uncontrolled IOP, intolerant to antiglaucoma drugs or noncompliant with medical treatment and poor candidates for surgery. Though the effect of the procedure may last for few months to few years, repeatability of the procedure is a great advantage.

REFERENCES

1. Krasnov MM. Laseropuncture of anterior chamber angle in glaucoma. Am J Ophthalmol. 1973;75(4):674-8.
2. Wise JB, Witter SL. Argon laser therapy for open-angle glaucoma. A pilot study. Arch Ophthalmol. 1979;97(2):319-22.
3. Latina MA, de Leon JM. Selective laser trabeculoplasty. Ophthalmol Clin North Am. 2005;18(3):409-19.
4. Anderson RR, Parish JA. Selective photothermolysis: precise microsurgery by selective absorption of pulsed radiation. Science. 1983;220(4596):524-7.
5. Latina MA, Park C. Selective targeting of TM cells: in vitro studies of pulsed and CW laser interactions. Exp Eye Res. 1995;60(4):359-71.
6. Kramer TR, Noeker RJ. Comparison of the morphologic changes after selective laser trabeculoplasty and argon laser trabeculoplasty in human eye bank eyes. Ophthalmology. 2001;108(4):773-9.
7. Alvarado JA, Murphy CG. Outflow obstruction in pigmentary and primary open angle glaucoma. Arch Ophthalmol. 1992;110(12):1769-78.
8. Harasymowycz PJ, Papamatheakis DG, Latina M, et al. Selective laser trabeculoplasty (SLT) complicated by intraocular pressure elevation in eyes with heavily pigmented trabecular meshworks. Am J Ophthalmol. 2005;139(6):1110-3.
9. Nagar M, Ogunyomade A, O'Brart DP, et al. A randomised, prospective study comparing selective laser trabeculoplasty with latanoprost for the control of intraocular pressure in ocular hypertension and open angle glaucoma. Br J Ophthalmol. 2005;89(11):1413-7.
10. Keightley SJ, Khaw PT, Elkington AR. The prediction of IOP rise following argon laser trabeculoplasty. Eye (Lond). 1987;1(Pt 5):577-80.
11. Latina MA, Gulati V. Selective laser trabeculoplasty: stimulating the meshwork to mend its ways. Int Ophthalmol Clin. 2004;44(1):93-103.
12. Leahy KE, White AJ. Selective laser trabeculoplasty: current perspectives. Clin Ophthalmol. 2015;9:833-41.
13. Kano K, Kuwayama Y, Mizoue S, et al. Clinical results of selective laser trabeculoplasty. Nippon GankaGakkai Zasshi. 1999;103(8):612-6.
14. Hodge WG, Damji KF, Rock W, et al. Baseline IOP predicts selective laser trabeculoplasty success at one year post treatment; results from a randomized clinical trial. Br J Ophthalmol. 2005;89(9):1157-60.
15. Martow E, Hutnik CM, Mao A. SLT and adjunctive medical therapy: a prediction rule analysis. J Glaucoma. 2011;20(4):266-70.

16. Wasyluk JT, Piekarniak-Wozniak A, Grabska-Liberek I. The hypotensive effect of selective laser trabeculoplasty depending on iridocorneal angle pigmentation in primary open angle glaucoma patients. Arch Med Sci. 2014;10(2):306-8.
17. Miki A, Kawashima R, Usui S, et al. Treatment outcomes and prognostic factors of selective laser trabeculoplasty for open-angle glaucoma receiving maximal-tolerable medical therapy. J Glaucoma. 2016;25(10):785-9.

CHAPTER
6

Shunts in the Management of Intractable Glaucoma

Rengaraj Venkatesh, Annamalai Odayappan, MG Pavan Kumar

■ INTRODUCTION

Intractable or refractory glaucoma refers to those types of glaucoma wherein despite conventional medical or surgical treatment, the intraocular pressure (IOP) fails to reduce to the desired levels and usually requires resurgery. Although cyclodestructive procedures are effective in reducing IOP by decreasing aqueous production, vision loss remains a persistent threat. Glaucoma drainage devices (GDD) offer a new treatment option in these conditions. They create a new bypass pathway for the aqueous to drain from the anterior chamber to the subconjunctival space. Introduced in 1969 by Molteno and colleagues,[1-3] the past 50 years has seen improvements in design modifications and surgical technique resulting in higher success rate and lower complications. Other GDDs introduced offer unique design and features adding them to the armamentarium of glaucoma surgeon in tackling these difficult to treat glaucomas.

■ TYPES OF GLAUCOMA DRAINAGE DEVICES

There are three types of GDD as follows:
1. **Setons:** They are solid stents or wicks which allows drainage either by bulk flow by preventing apposition or by means of surface tension along material, e.g. horsehair, silicone, gold tubes, silk, and metal sutures.
2. **Nonvalved or nonrestrictive implants or shunts:** They are open-tubed devices without valves incapable of influencing anterograde or retrograde flow, e.g. Molteno implant, Baerveldt implant, Schocket procedure, Aurolab aqueous drainage implant.
3. **Valved or restrictive implants:** They are open-tubed devices with valves that allow pressure sensitive unidirectional flow, e.g. Krupin valve, Ahmed valve, Joseph valve, White, Optimed.

Functioning of Implants
The basic design of a drainage device usually consists of a tube which extends from the anterior chamber, ciliary sulcus, or in some cases from the vitreous

cavity to a plate, disc, or encircling band placed beneath conjunctiva and Tenon's capsule. The surface area of the plate or disc plays an important role in the fibrous capsule formation and thereby in the amount of aqueous drainage, resistance to outflow, and control of IOP. At the edge of the external plate, where the distal end of the tube gets inserted, a ridge is designed to prevent obstruction of the tube from outside by the developing fibrous capsule. All plates have got fixation holes on their anterior edge for securing the plate to the sclera with sutures. The devices without valve restriction need to have their tubes ligated to prevent early postoperative hypotony since the fibrous capsule around the implant takes a few weeks to months to develop. During this period of the blocked tube, the IOP remains elevated which is termed as the hypertensive phase needing antiglaucoma medications.[4,5]

When to use Glaucoma Drainage Devices?

A drainage device comes into place when conventional trabeculectomy (or repeated attempts) had failed to control IOP or when it is least likely to succeed. The indications for GDD implant includes (Figs. 1A to D):

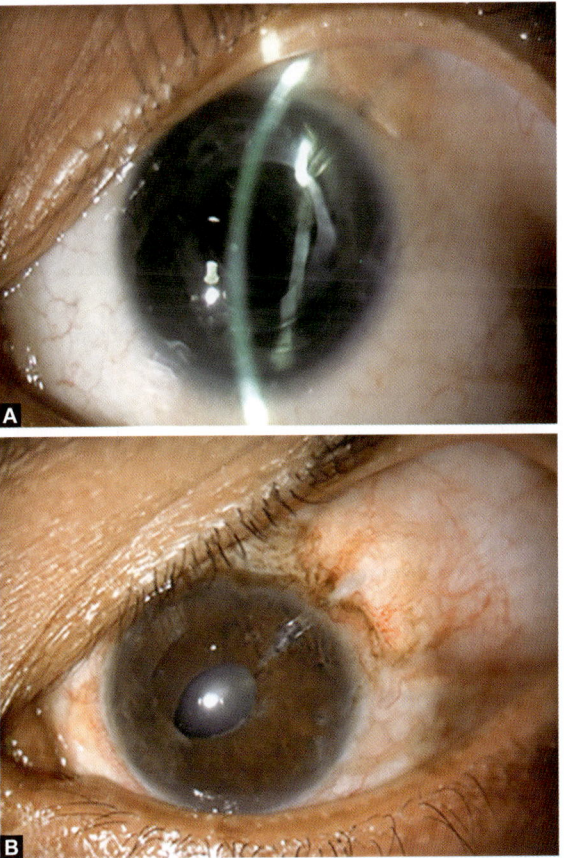

Figs. 1A and B

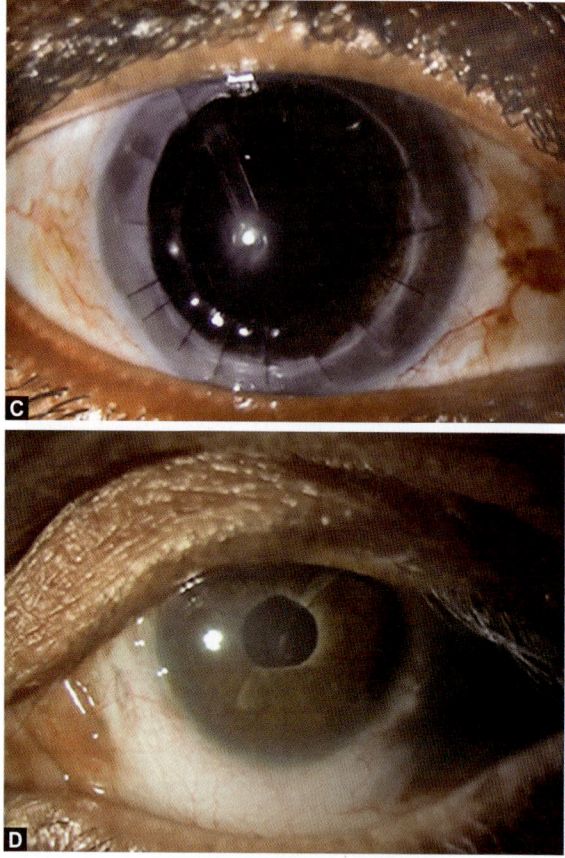

Figs. 1C and D

Figs. 1A to D: Few indications of GDD; (A) Aniridia; (B) ICE syndrome; (C) After penetrating keratoplasty; (D) Pseudoexfoliation glaucoma.
(ICE: iridocorneal endothelial; GDD: glaucoma drainage devices)

- Neovascular glaucoma
- Iridocorneal endothelial (ICE) syndrome
- Uveitic glaucoma
- Traumatic glaucoma
- Excessive conjunctival scarring
  - Multiple surgeries
  - Ocular surface diseases
  - Chemical burns
  - Steven-Johnson syndrome
  - Cicatricial pemphigoid
- Previously failed glaucoma surgery
- Postpenetrating keratoplasty glaucoma
- Glaucoma following retinal detachment surgery
- Pseudophakic and aphakic glaucoma

- Refractory infantile glaucoma
- Aniridia with glaucoma
- Sturge-Weber syndrome
- Epithelial downgrowth
- Primary procedure for uncontrolled primary open-angle glaucoma when there are high chances of complications following trabeculectomy.

CURRENT DRAINAGE DEVICES

Nonvalved Implants

Molteno Implant (Molteno Ophthalmic Limited, Dunedin, New Zealand; IOP, Incorporation, Costa Mesa, CA, USA)

The original design has undergone many modifications. The single plate type implant consists of a 10 mm long silicone tube with a 0.63 mm outer diameter and 0.33 mm inner diameter which connects to a polypropylene plate which has a 13 mm diameter and surface area of 133 mm^2.

To increase the surface area and filtration, the double-plate model was introduced with an addition of another 13 mm second plate to the primary plate through a silicone tube 90° away from the primary intracameral tube. Both left and right eye versions are available. Pediatric plate size of 8 mm is also available. It could be used for eyes with axial length is less than 17 mm.

Third generation Molteno implant comes with larger and thinner flexible endplate with an elliptical subsidiary ridge over the upper surface. It is proposed that this modification which consists of a ridge with the overlying Tenon's tissue growth acts as a biological valve which prevents post-operative hypotony.

All Molteno implants have been described to be magnetic resonance imaging (MRI) safe (Table 1).

Schocket Procedure

A silicone tube, i.e., 30 mm long with a 0.30 mm inner diameter is used to shunt the aqueous from the anterior chamber to an encircling band placed as in retinal detachment surgery.[6,7] First, the tube is sutured within the groove of the silicone band, leaving 15 mm of the tube extending freely. This encircling

Table 1: Various models of the Molteno implant.

Type (Model)	Size
Single plate (S1)	133 mm^2
For pediatric/microphthalmic eyes (P1)	80 mm^2
Double plate L2 (Left) and R2 (Right)	266 mm^2
Molteno 3 SS	185 mm^2
Molteno 3 SL	245 mm^2
Molteno 3 GS	175 mm^2
Molteno 3 GL	230 mm^2

Table 2: Various models of the Baerveldt implant.

Model	Surface area
Model BG-101–350	350 mm²
Pars Plana model BG-102–350	350 mm²
Model BG-103–250	250 mm²

band with the tube is then sutured to the sclera circumferentially, 10–12 mm behind the limbus and under the four recti muscles. The free-end of the tube is finally inserted into the anterior chamber. Providing about 350–450 mm² surface area for drainage, its IOP lowering effect have been comparable to the double plate Molteno implant.

Baerveldt Implant (Advanced Medical Optics, Incorporation, Santa Ana, CA, USA)

Designed by Dr George Baerveldt in 1990, the plate is made of soft silicone material with a silicone tube attached to it. The outer diameter of the tube is 0.63 mm and the inner diameter of the tube is 0.3 mm.[8] It is available in 2 sizes with surface areas of 250 mm² (20 × 13 mm) and 350 mm² (32 × 14 mm).

The smaller implant is suitable for small eyes as in children, in eyes with scleral buckles where the 350 mm² plate is too large to fit and in eyes with uveitic glaucoma where the aqueous production might be limited.

The pars plana implant has a tube which enters the eye at 90° via the Hoffman elbow which is secured over the vitreous base 4 mm from the limbus. It is useful in eyes undergoing vitrectomy or in those after keratoplasty.

It has a patented "bleb control mechanism". The plate has got fenestrations through which the fibrous tissue grows. This secures the plate in situ controlling the height and volume of the bleb and minimizing motility disturbances. The plate is barium impregnated which allows it to be identified in X-ray, computed tomography (CT), and MRI. The various models of the Baerveldt implant are given in Table 2.

Aurolab Aqueous Drainage Implant (AADI) (Aurolab, Madurai, TN, India)

The Baerveldt 350 mm² design is the prototype for the AADI. Professor George Baerveldt authorized its use thereby allowing the device to be manufactured at Aurolab, India in collaboration with the Bascom Palmer Eye Institute, Miami, Florida. It has been commercially available since June 2013 and has recently been reported to be safe and effective as comparable to the Ahmed glaucoma valve and the Baerveldt implant.[9,10]

The plate is made up of silicone and measures 32 mm long with a 13 mm convex radius and a surface area of 350 mm². A 35 mm long silicone tube is connected to it. There are 2 fixation holes in the anterior portion of the plate which are used to suture the plate to the underlying sclera using 8-0 or 9-0 nylon sutures (Figs. 2A and B). The larger surface area of the plate helps to achieve a comparatively lower IOP in the long-term as compared to valved devices. It is the only nonvalved device available in India till date.

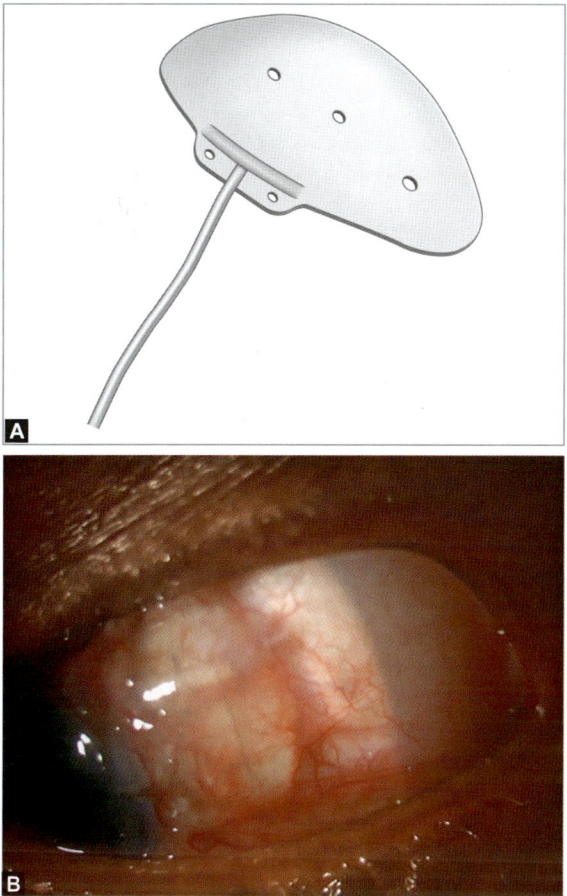

Figs. 2A and B: (A) Aurolab aqueous drainage implant (AADI); (B) Postoperative appearance after the placing AADI.

Valved Implants

The valve in these devices tend to close below a certain pressure level thereby reducing the chances of postoperative hypotony.

Krupin Implants (Benson Hood Laboratories, Pembroke, Massachusetts, USA)

In 1976, Krupin and associates introduced a valved implant that opens at a predetermined IOP level.[11] It has undergone various modifications since its introduction.

It now consists of a silastic tube attached to an oval silastic disc, conforming to the curvature of the globe. It measures 13 × 18 mm. The valve at the tube's distal end is a simple slit and is manometrically calibrated so that it opens when the IOP is over 11 mm Hg and closes at 9 mm Hg thereby avoiding the early postoperative hypotony.

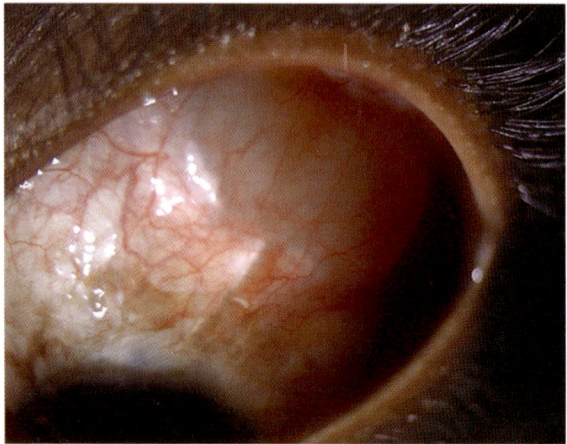

Fig. 3: Postoperative appearance after the placing Ahmed glaucoma valve (AGV).

Table 3: Various models of the Ahmed glaucoma valve (AGV).

Model	Size	Material
AGV-S2	184 mm^2	Polypropylene
AGV-FP7	184 mm^2	Silicone
AGV-FP8	102 mm^2	Silicone

Ahmed Glaucoma Valve (AGV) (New World Medical, Rancho Cucamonga, CA, USA)

It was introduced by Mateen Ahmed in 1993. It is a 184 mm^2 polypropylene or silicone plate with silicone valve. To increase the area of filtration, a second plate can be attached to the first one. The tube is 25.4 mm long, has a 0.63 mm outer diameter and 0.3 mm inner diameter.[8] (Fig. 3) A smaller pediatric version is also available which has a surface area of 102 mm^2.

It has a venturi valve consisting of two thin silicone elastomer membranes which is engineered to open at an IOP of 8 mm Hg. However, if it leaks around the tube at the site where it enters the anterior chamber, it can still result in over-filtration and hypotony. The various models of the AGV are given in Table 3.

A new valve can have adhesions between the silicone elastomer membranes. Therefore, there is a unique maneuver of priming the AGV before placement. It is done by a retrograde injection of saline into the free end of the silicone tube with a 30-gauge cannula. This facilitates the separation of the membranes and thereby priming the valve system within the plate initiating the fluid flow.

■ PREOPERATIVE EVALUATION

The conjunctiva mobility should be assessed to determine the site of placement of the drainage device. Gonioscopy should be performed preoperatively to look for synechiae-free areas for the placement of tube and to identify any neovascularization in angles. In case of neovascular glaucoma, pretreatment with an anti-VEGF agent reduces the risk of intraoperative and postoperative bleeding. In the presence of significant cataract, combining cataract surgery and GDD placement may be a good option. Conditions which lead to thinning of sclera like high myopes, pediatric patients, and collagen vascular disease need special surgical precautions and needles while fixing the device to sclera. Dense arcus and corneal scars might obscure the placement of intracameral tubes and may lead to misdirection. Intracameral tube might cause endothelial decompensation, hence it is wiser to choose pars planar placement of GDD tube in vitrectomized eyes.

■ CHOOSING GLAUCOMA DRAINAGE DEVICES

Choice of an implant depends on multiple factors like the type of disease, patient factors, and surgeon factors. In conditions needing early postoperative control of IOP, or if the patient is poorly compliant with medications and follow-up visits or if the surgeon is a beginner, valved implant is better compared to nonvalved device.

The availability of scar-free conjunctiva determines the size of the implant. Previous studies have showed that the size of implant is an important determinant of postoperative IOP control to a certain extent, however, the influence of size, composition, and shape of the devices needs to be studied further.

■ SURGICAL PROCEDURE

Surgery is usually performed under retrobulbar or peribulbar block. Subtenon's anesthesia is also an option. Intravenous sedation or general anesthesia is reserved for patients who are highly uncooperative, anxious, or claustrophobic.

These devices are ideally placed under a fornix-based conjunctival flap. For a single plate implant, a conjunctival dissection of 90–120° centered between two recti will usually suffice. The tube is checked for patency. In case of valved implants, priming of the valve must be done prior to scleral anchoring. After the peritomy, the corresponding recti muscles are hooked. The drainage plate is then placed under the recti, over the equator of the globe around 8–10 mm behind the limbus. Placing the implant posteriorly adds to the advantage of bypassing the scarred limbal area. The plate is fixed to the underlying sclera by passing sutures through the eyelets on the anterior portion of the plate. In case of a non-valved device, if the surgery is performed as a single stage procedure, usually the tube is closed temporarily with 6-0 Vicryl (Polyglactin 910, Ethicon Incorporation) sutures to avoid excessive filtration and hypotony during the immediate postoperative period. The bleb is, therefore, not exposed to the inflammatory mediators from the anterior chamber until the tube opens up as the suture gets absorbed, which is typically after 4–6 weeks, thereby, having lesser chances of bleb encapsulation. If the IOP was high despite maximal medications or if some filtration is needed in the immediate postoperative period, a suture needle can be passed perpendicularly through and through in the tube at two locations thereby creating four holes just proximal to the external ligature. These fenestrations are described as the 'garden hose sprinkling system,' and it allows for aqueous leakage in the immediate postoperative period thereby reducing the IOP till the ligation suture gets absorbed. The tube is then inserted into the anterior chamber through a track created by a 23-gauge needle starting 2–3 mm behind the limbus parallel to the iris plane. The tube should extend for about 3 mm into the anterior chamber so that it stays away from the cornea and the iris. Excessive length of the tube is trimmed with scissors with a bevel facing the cornea. The tube may or may not be secured with nonabsorbable sutures. To minimize the chances of erosion by the tube through the overlying conjunctiva, the tube is covered by a 6 x 6 mm patch graft using either donor sclera or clear corneal graft which may be of partial thickness (Figs. 4A and B).

Finally, watertight 8-0 Vicryl sutures are used to suture the conjunctival flap to the limbus. Figures 5 and 6 describe the surgical procedures of AADI and AGV, respectively.

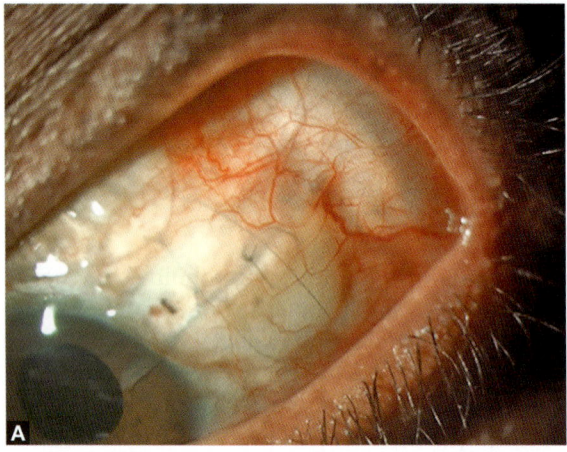

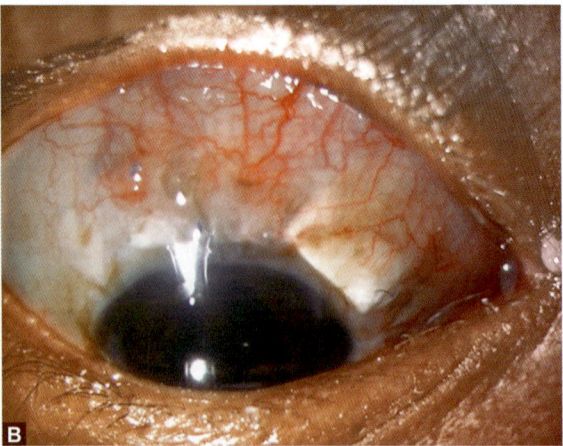

Figs. 4A and B: (A) Tube covered by a corneal patch graft; (B) Tube covered by a scleral patch graft.

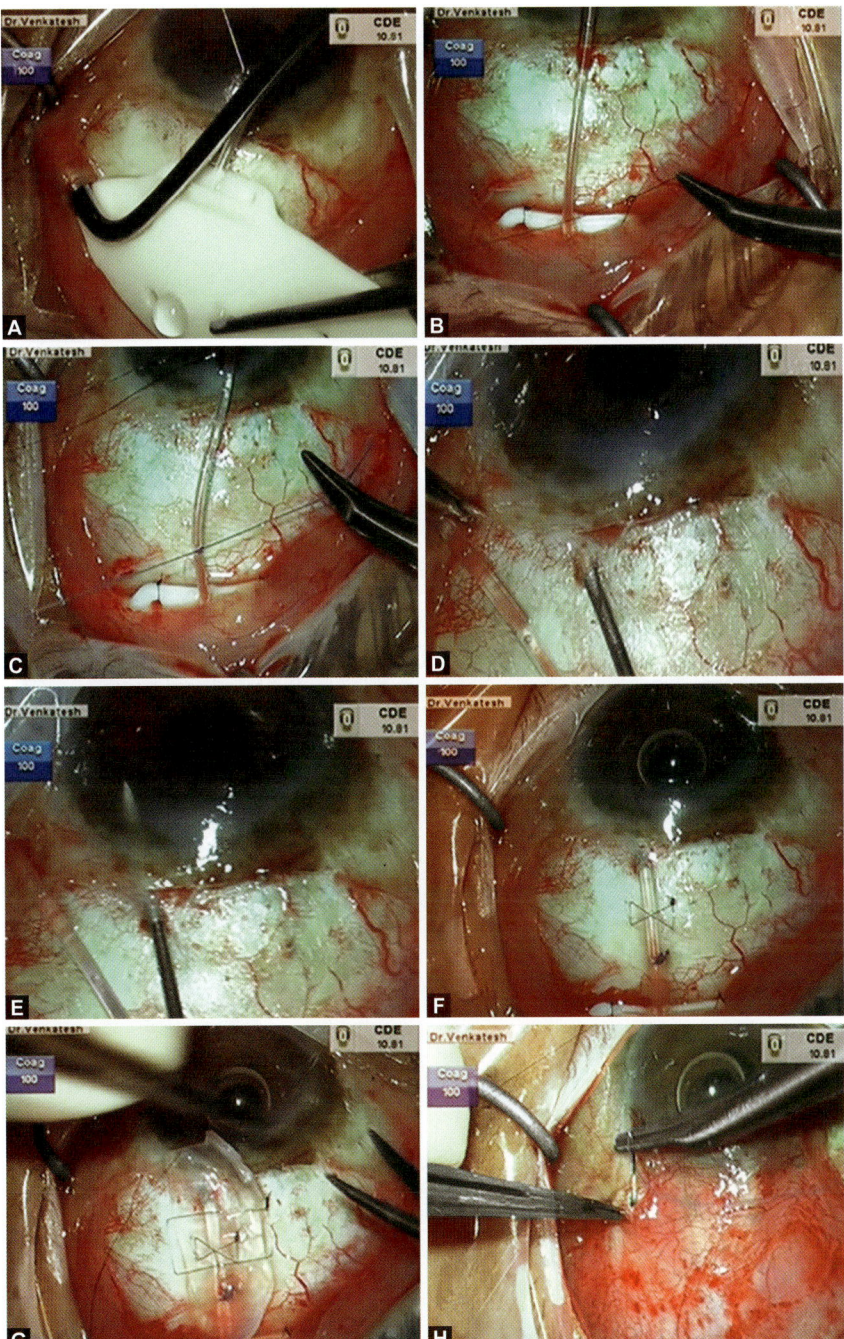

Figs. 5A to H: (A) Placing the Aurolab aqueous drainage implant (AADI) plate under the hooked muscle; (B) Suturing the plate to the sclera with nonabsorbable sutures through the fixation holes; (C) External ligation of the tube; (D and E) Anterior chamber entry with a 23-gauge needle; (F) Tube is secured with nonabsorbable sutures; (G) Tube is covered with patch graft; (H) Fornix based conjunctival flap is sutured with 8-0 Vicryl sutures.

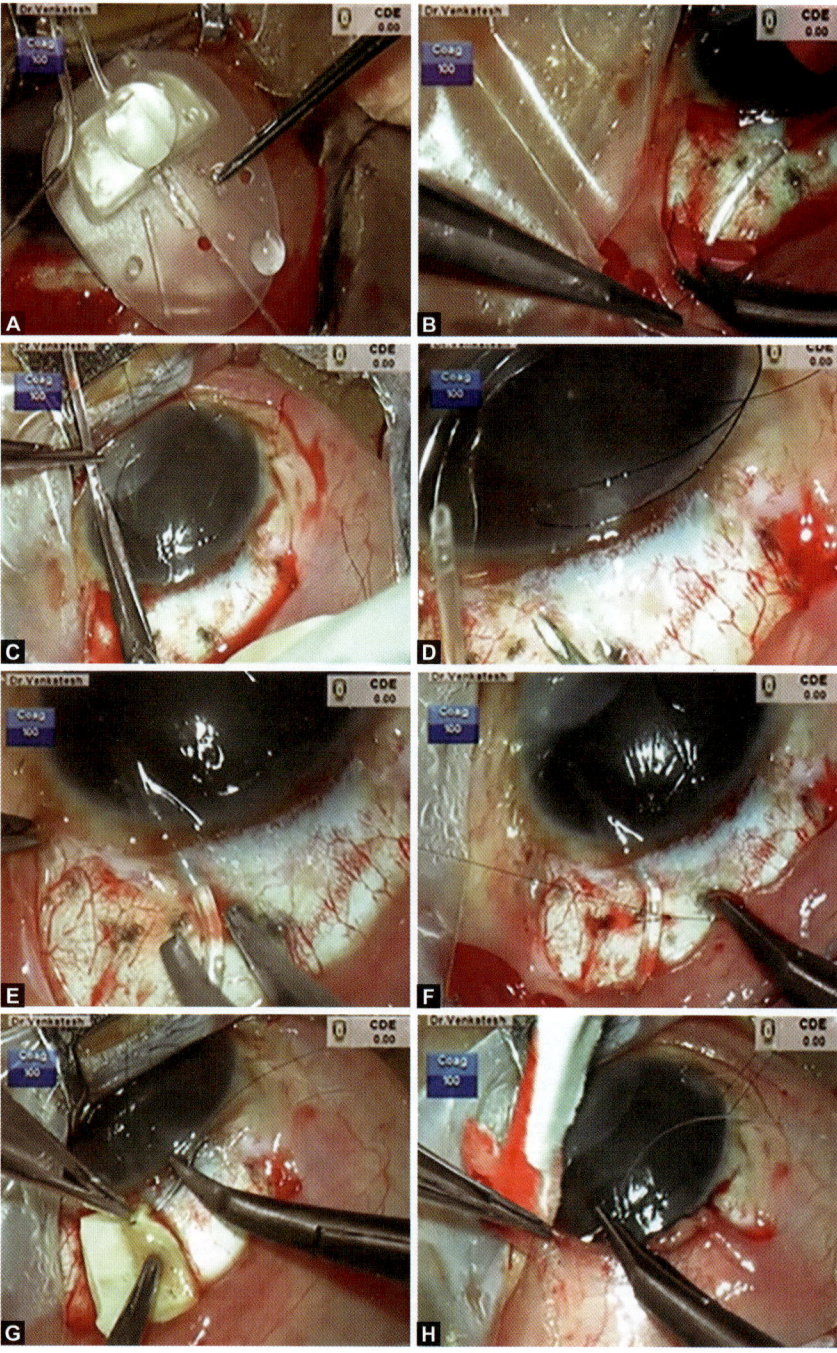

Figs. 6A to H: (A) Priming the Ahmed glaucoma valve (AGV); (B) Placing the AGV plate and suturing it to the sclera with sutures passed through the fixation holes; (C) Trimming the tube; (D) Anterior chamber entry with a 23-gauge needle; (E) Tube insertion into the anterior chamber; (F) Securing of the tube with nonabsorbable sutures; (G) Donor scleral patch graft is being used to cover the tube; (H) Fornix based conjunctival flap sutured with 8-0 Vicryl sutures.

PLACEMENT OF THE TUBE

In most surgeries, the GDD tube is placed in the anterior chamber. However, it may also be positioned in the sulcus in a pseudophakic eye or in the pars plana in which case it requires either a Hoffman elbow (for a Baerveldt implant) or a Pars Plana Clip. Pars plana route is chosen in conditions when there is compromised cornea, corneal scar, after penetrating keratoplasty or vitrectomy (Figs. 7A to C).

SITE OF IMPLANTATION

Most drainage devices are placed in the superotemporal quadrant. This is preferred because there is easy and wide access to implant the plate and is less likely to cause motility disturbances. Superonasal quadrant placement has been associated with Brown's syndrome.[12] In eyes where previous retinal detachment surgery has been performed and has silicone oil inside, the plate is preferably placed in the inferior quadrant to minimize the loss of oil, however, hypertropia and down gaze limitation have been reported.

USE OF ANTIFIBROTICS

Trials have shown that there is no higher success rate with the intraoperative use of Mitomycin-C. So, these antifibrotic agents are rarely being used with drainage devices currently.[13]

COMPLICATIONS

Early Postoperative Complications

- Hypotony or flat anterior chamber may be due to excessive filtration or tube site leak. It can be managed by ligation of the tube or removal and inserting in a new site.
- Choroidal effusion
- Suprachoroidal hemorrhage
- *Hyphema:* It can occur in case of neovascular glaucoma. Adjunctive use of anti-VEGF agent might reduce the chances of hyphema.
- Elevated IOP.

Late Postoperative Complications

- *Uveitis:* It may occur if tube is in contact with iris and may cause raised IOP later (Fig. 8).
- *Motility disturbances and diplopia:* They are seen more commonly with large plate implants. It may need implant removal in certain cases.
- *Cataract:* It can occur due to tube lens touch (Fig. 9).
- *Tube retraction:* It may occur due to slippage of anchoring sutures.
- Tube block by vitreous or debris. Vitreous may block the tube when tube in placed in pars plana with inadequate vitrectomy (Figs. 10 and 11).
- *Tube or plate erosion:* It can be prevented with patch grafts (Figs. 12A and B).
- Tube or plate extrusion can rarely happen.

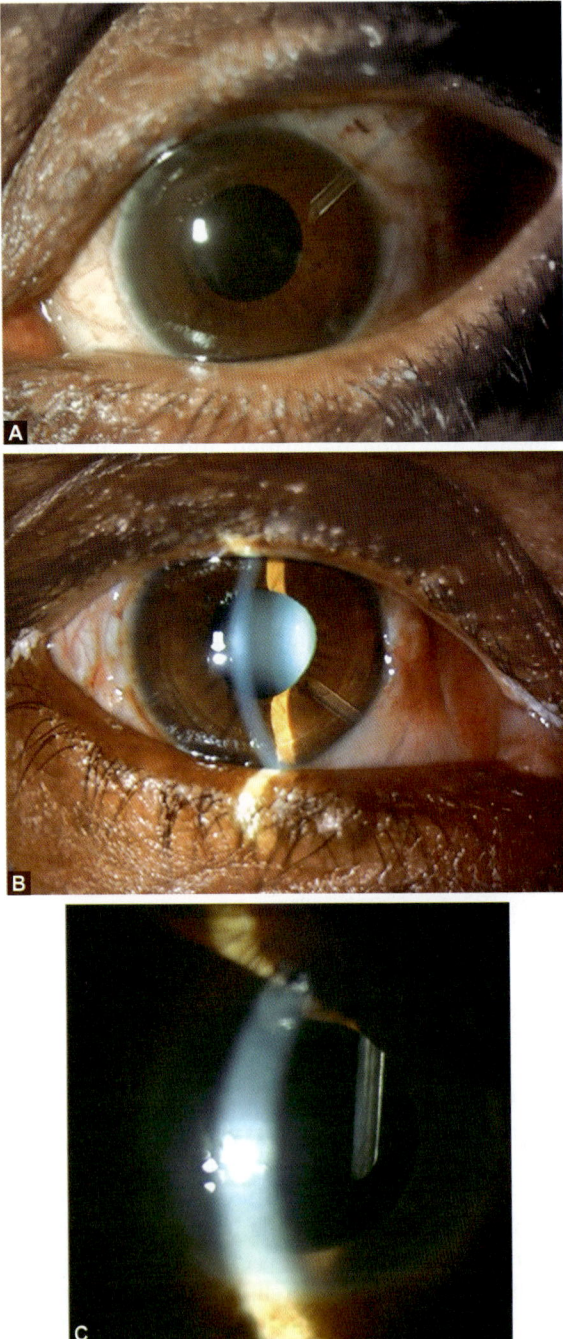

Figs. 7A to C: (A) Tube in anterior chamber with glaucoma drainage devices (GDD) in the superotemporal quadrant; (B) Tube in anterior chamber with GDD in the inferonasal quadrant; (C) Tube inserted through the pars plana.

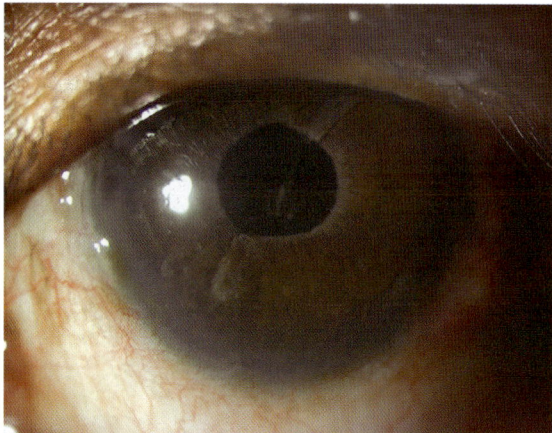

Fig. 8: Fibrinous membrane in a patient with glaucoma drainage devices (GDD).

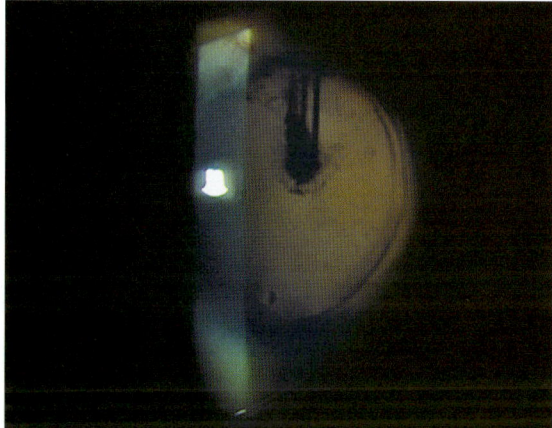

Fig. 9: Lens touch by tube.

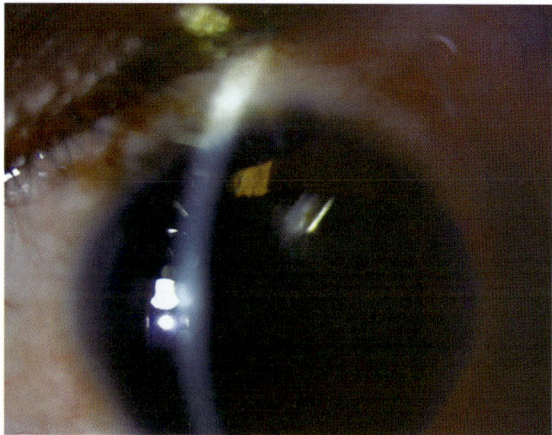

Fig. 10: The tube which is placed through the pars plana of the aphakic eye is blocked by vitreous.

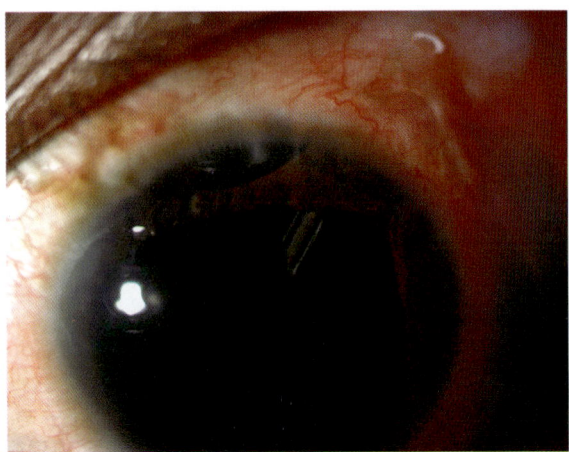

Fig. 11: The tube is blocked by debris.

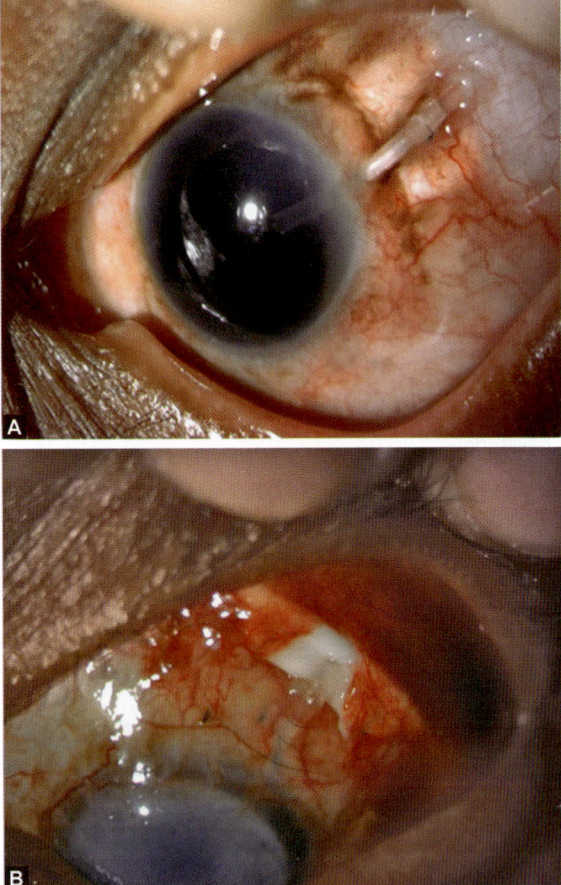

Figs. 12A and B: (A) Tube exposure; (B) Plate edge and tube exposure after erosion through the conjunctiva.

- *Corneal touch and decompensation:* Due to tube endothelial touch. This may need explant removal or penetrating keratoplasty with tube reposition
- Loss of preexisting visual acuity may happen due to hypotony maculopathy, retinal detachment, vitreous hemorrhage, or cystoid macular edema.
- Encapsulated bleb or Tenon's cyst occurs most commonly with Ahmed glaucoma valve implant needs bleb needling or revision surgery.
- Endophthalmitis may rarely occur.

REFERENCES

1. Molteno AC, Straughan JL, Ancker E. Long tube implants in the management of glaucoma. S Afr Med J. 1976;50:1062-6.
2. Molteno ACB. New implant for drainage in glaucoma: clinical trial. Br J Ophthalmol. 1979;53:606-15.
3. Molteno ACB. The optimal design of drainage implants for glaucoma. Trans Ophthal Soc. 1981;33:39-41.
4. Ayyala RS, Zurakowski D, Smith JA, et al. A clinical study of the Ahmed glaucoma valve implant in advanced glaucoma. Ophthalmol. 1998;105:1968-76.
5. Molteno AC, Dempster AG. Methods of Controlling Bleb Fibrosis Around Draining Implants. In: Mills KB (Ed). Glaucoma: Proceedings of the Fourth International Symposium of the Northern Eye Institute, Manchester, UK, 14-16 July 1988. Oxford: Pergamon Press; 1989. pp.192-211.
6. Schocket SS. Investigations of the reasons for success and failure in the anterior shunt-to-the encircling-band procedure in the treatment of refractory glaucoma. Trans Am Ophthalmol Soc. 1986;84:743-98.
7. Schocket SS, Lakhanpal V, Richards RD. Anterior chamber tube shunt to an encircling band in the treatment of neovascular glaucoma. Ophthalmol. 1982;89:1188-94.
8. Lim KS, Allan BD, Lloyd AW, et al. Glaucoma drainage devices; past, present, and future. Br J Ophthalmol. 1998;82:1083-9.
9. Kaushik S, Kataria P, Raj S, et al. Safety and efficacy of a low-cost glaucoma drainage device for refractory childhood glaucoma. Br J Ophthalmol. 2017;101:1623-7.
10. Pathak RV, Rao DP. Surgical outcomes of a new low-cost nonvalved glaucoma drainage device in refractory glaucoma: Results at 1 Year. J Glaucoma. 2018;27:433-9.
11. Krupin T, Podos SM, Becker B, et al. Valve implants in filtering surgery. Am J Ophthalmol. 1976;81:232-5.
12. Ball SF, Ellis GS, Herrington RG, et al. Brown's superior oblique tendon syndrome after Baerveldt implant. Arch Ophthalmol. 1992;110:1368.
13. Costa VP, Azuara-Blanco A, Netland PA, et al. Efficacy and safety of adjunctive mitomycin C during Ahmed glaucoma valve implantation: A prospective randomized clinical trial. Ophthalmol. 2004;111:1071-6.

CHAPTER
7

Recent Advances in Intraocular Lens Power Calculation

Prashob Mohan, Arup Chakrabarti

■ INTRODUCTION

Since, the first intraocular lens (IOL) was implanted in 1949,[1] cataract surgery has advanced quite a lot. The adoption of highly accurate and universally reproducible surgical techniques and instrumentation along with cutting edge IOL technology has made cataract surgery no less than a refractive surgery. Increasing public awareness regarding these advances in technology has also increased the pressure on the ophthalmic surgeon in achieving near perfect outcomes. One of the most important factors that determine the refractive outcome of a cataract surgery is IOL power. In such a scenario, accurate calculation of IOL power becomes a necessity rather than a luxury.

Accurate IOL power calculation hinges on two factors—(1) accurate measurement of parameters such as axial length (AL), keratometry, anterior chamber depth (ACD), lens thickness, horizontal white-to-white (WTW), etc., and accurate predictive formulae which use these parameters to determine IOL power.

■ BIOMETRY

The first ultrasound amplitude scan (A-scan) to measure AL was performed in 1956 by Mundt and Hughes.[2] Applanation A-scan had its fair share of pitfalls such as variable corneal compression. Immersion ultrasound biometry solved the problem of variable corneal compression and had better repeatability.[3,4] For more than 50 years, ultrasound was the only commercially available tool to measure ocular AL. This changed in 1998 with the introduction of optical biometry which used infrared light to determine AL.[5]

The introduction of optical biometry lead to a quantum shift in ophthalmologists practice pattern towards optical biometers from ultrasound biometers and is currently the most preferred method of measuring ocular distances.

Advantages of Optical Biometry

It has several advantages over ultrasound biometry.
- It measures the true axial length of the eye. Ultrasound biometers measure axial length from the anterior surface of the cornea to the internal limiting membrane of the retina whereas optical biometers measure the distance between the tear film and the retinal pigment epithelium.[5] Ultrasound biometers add an arbitrary value of 200 µ to the measured AL to account for retinal thickness, but the thickness of the retina varies in different individuals. This is a source of error in ultrasound biometry.
- Optical biometers measure AL along the visual axis, i.e., to the center of the macula while ultrasound biometers measure AL along the anatomic axis of the eye which is different from the visual axis.[6] It is the distance along the visual axis that is required to obtain accurate refractive results.
- Due to the above property optical biometers can be used to accurately measure ALs in eyes with posterior staphyloma.[6] Ultrasound biometers may erroneously measure axial length up to the pit of a staphyloma where the fovea may not be located.
- In silicone oil-filled eyes and in eyes with aphakia or pseudophakia the AL measured by ultrasound biometers requires adjustments for variation in the velocity of sound in different media while no such adjustment is required for optical biometers.[7,8]
- Optical biometers are noncontact instruments and hence faster and more comfortable for the patient. Furthermore with applanation A-scans, there may be variable corneal compression that can lead to an error in AL calculation, the chance of which is eliminated by noncontact optical biometry.[9]
- The precision of measurement is greater with optical biometers as they use a partially coherent light source with a narrow wavelength as opposed to ultrasound biometers which use a broad beam.[10,11]

Disadvantages of Optical Biometry

- Optical biometers are significantly more expensive than ultrasound biometers.[12]
- AL measurements in dense cataracts and posterior subcapsular cataracts may be difficult.[13] However, these difficulties have been overcome with the arrival of swept source optical coherence tomography (SSOCT) technology.[14]

Optical Biometry

The optical biometers available today make use of three technological principles:
1. Partial coherence interferometry (PCI)
2. Optical low coherence reflectometry (OLCR)
3. SSOCT.

Partial Coherence Interferometry

This technology was developed by Fercher and Roth in 1986. PCI and ultrasound biometry work on similar principles. However, PCI uses infrared light, unlike ultrasound A-scan which uses sound waves. Interfaces between tissues of different refractive indices reflect this light. It is difficult to directly measure the time delay in receiving the echoes as in ultrasound as light travels at too high velocity. Therefore, interferometric techniques have to be used.[15] An interferometer with a dual coaxial beam setup is used with the aim of eliminating the sensitivity of a classical Michelson interferometer to longitudinal eye movements. Two beams of light which have a mutual time delay equal to twice the arm length difference of the interferometer are introduced into the eye. This light gets reflected off tissue interfaces. For axial length measurement the beams reflected at the anterior corneal surface and the retinal pigment epithelium are considered. The interferometer then detects a partial coherence interferometry signal. This instrument enables highly accurate AL measurements.[15]

The devices using this technology are IOLMaster 500 from Carl Zeiss, the AL-scan from Nidek and Pentacam AXL from Oculus.

Optical Low Coherence Reflectometry

The OLCR technique is based on a Michelson interferometer which uses a superluminescent diode producing low coherence infrared light. The light is split into two beams by a coupler. One beam enters the eye and the other is directed towards a scanning reference mirror. Light is reflected at each tissue interface within the eye. The emitted and reflected light travel coaxially. An interference pattern is thus formed which is detected by a detector. The reference beam is scanned, so as to produce an interference signal and thus the exact location from which the light was reflected from within the eye is determined.[16]

The biometers which use this principle are Lenstar LS900 (Haag Streit), Aladdin (Topcon), Galilei G6 (Ziemer).

Swept Source Optical Coherence Tomography

A swift sweeping laser is used as the source instead of a superluminescent diode. The reference mirror does not move in this case. The interference signal captured by the detector then undergoes Fourier transformation.[17,18]

The devices using this technology are the IOLMaster 700 (Carl Zeiss), Argos (Movu), and the Eyestar 900 (Haag Streit).

Optical Biometers

IOLMaster 500

In 1999, the IOLMaster from Carl Zeiss (Fig. 1) became the first optical biometer to be launched. The IOLMaster 500 is a modified Michelson interferometer that uses a 780 nm infrared laser. The principle of PCI is used to measure the true AL of the eye. It was calibrated against an ultra-high resolution 40-MHz Grieshaber Biometric System. The IOLMaster measures AL to within 0.02 mm accuracy as against 0.10–0.12 mm in a standard immersion ultrasound biometer, which represents a five-fold increase in accuracy.[19]

The A-constants for IOLs to be used while performing optical biometry are different from that used for ultrasound biometry. More than 270 lens constants optimized for use with the IOLMaster are provided online on the user group for laser interference biometry (ULIB) website.

The IOLMaster 500 also measures keratometry, ACD, and horizontal WTW distance in addition to AL. These values are important in IOL power calculation using modern formulae. Keratometry is measured using a telecentric method where the image is formed at the focal plane of the cornea and is more accurate than nontelecentric methods of keratometry.[20] ACD is measured optically using a projected slit.

The IOLMaster 500 has onboard Haigis-L and Holladay 2 formulae in addition to SRK II, SRK-T, Haigis, Hoffer Q, and Holladay-1 formulae.

There is also a facility to export data via Universal Serial Bus (USB) to the Callisto (Fig. 2)—a computer-assisted surgery system that can display an

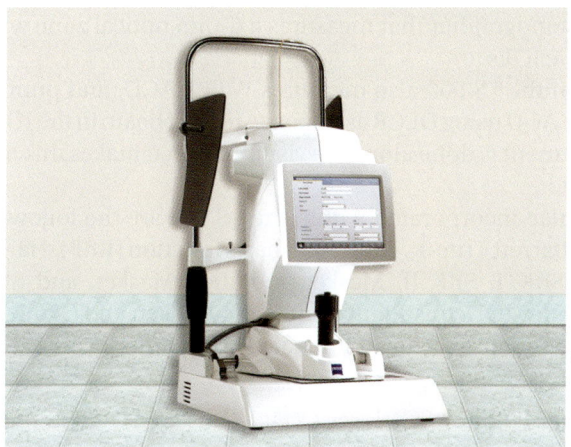

Fig. 1: Intraocular lens Master 500.

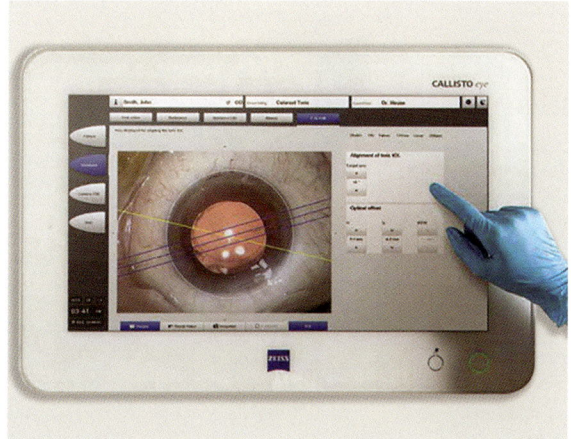

Fig. 2: Callisto.

overlay in the microscope eyepiece during cataract surgery, which is helpful during toric IOL implantation.

A drawback of the IOLMaster was its inability to reliably measure AL in eyes with corneal opacities and dense cataract. This has been addressed to a certain extent by a software upgrade with help of which multiple scans can be averaged resulting in a better ability to obtain accurate biometry in opaque media.[21]

Lenstar LS 900
Launched in 2009, the Lenstar (Fig. 3) was the first device that could measure the lens thickness. It uses a superluminescent diode to produce a low coherent infrared light beam of 820 nm wavelength. The principle of OLCR is employed to accurately calculate AL, ACD, and lens thickness.

For keratometry, it uses a dual-zone keratometry measurement system with 32 closely spaced measurement points. The Pro-version of the Lenstar LS 900 comes with the T-Cone, a double-ring (1.65 and 2.3 mm diameter) placido disk topographer that measures a 6-mm optical zone which helps in planning Toric IOLs.

In addition the LS 900 also measures WTW, ACD, and pupil diameter. It measures the ACD using OLCR as opposed to a slit beam in the IOLMaster 500. This measurement is done along the visual axis that makes this measurement more accurate.

The formulae incorporated within the LS 900 are the following— Barrett Universal II, Barrett True-K, Hill-radial basis function (RBF), Haigis, Hoffer-Q, Holladay 1, SRK/T, SRK II, Masket, modified Masket, and Shammas no-history. Holladay IOL consultant professional, Olsen and Okulix's ray-tracing methods are available via an additional software interface.

IOLMaster 700
The IOLMaster 700 from Carl Zeiss (Fig. 4) uses SSOCT to measure ocular distances. At 2,000 scans per second, the device performs an accurate and

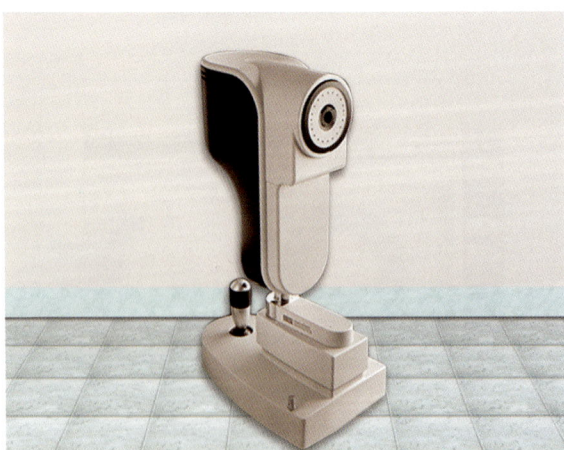

Fig. 3: Lenstar LS 900.

fast imaging of the eye. Anatomical irregularities such as crystalline lens tilt, and to a certain extent macular edema and macular holes can be visualized with the IOLMaster 700. It also uses a telecentric keratometer like the IOLMaster 500.[20] SSOCT technology enables measurement through dense cataracts and media opacities as well. In addition, the machine also allows for a visual verification of fixation. Scans which do not show the pit of the fovea can be discounted.[22,23]

The formulae included are Haigis, Haigis-T for torics, and Haigis-L for postrefractive surgery eyes, Holladay 1 and 2, SRK/T, Hoffer Q, and Barrett Universal II.

For toric IOL implantation, the IOLMaster 700 also captures a reference image of the eye and the surgeon can use blood vessels as landmarks to identify the axis of alignment intraoperatively thereby eliminating the need for external marking. There is also an in-built toric IOL calculator.

Aladdin HW3.0
Topcon's Aladdin HW3.0 (Fig. 5) is a combined OLCR-based optical biometer and placido disk-based corneal topographer. The Aladdin can perform three-zone keratometry at 3, 5, and 7 mm from the central cornea. The topographer uses 24-placido rings to map the cornea. Lens centration and mesopic pupil size can be assessed with the help of dynamic pupillometry. Zernike wavefront analysis evaluates higher-order aberrations and corneal surface anomalies like early-stage keratoconus.

The Aladdin provides the surgeon with a range of popular IOL power calculation formulae including postrefractive surgery formulae and toric IOL calculators.

In terms of AL, anterior chamber depth and mean keratometry values, the Aladdin biometer has demonstrated good agreement with the IOLMaster 500.[24]

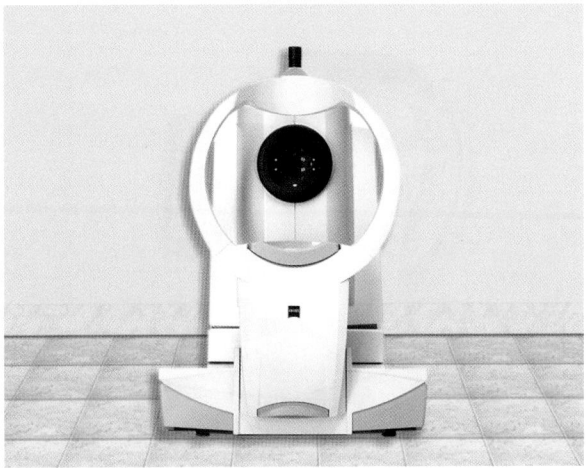

Fig. 4: Intraocular lens Master 700.

Axial Length-scan
Based on the PCI principle, the AL-scan from Nidek (Fig. 6) can measure keratometry, AL, ACD, WTW, pupil size, and central corneal thickness (CCT). The AL-scan incorporates automatic tracking and shooting features for ease of use. CCT and ACD are captured using Scheimpflug imaging. Double mire rings reflected onto the cornea help in performing topography and keratometry. They also aid in evaluating corneal aberrations. Axes may be determined from visible landmarks on the eye which aids in toric IOL positioning. Nidek claims that by adjusting signal-to-noise ratio to amplify the signal, AL-scan can perform biometry in denser cataracts. The device in addition also has an ultrasound A-scan and pachymeter which may be used in very dense cataracts in which AL is not measurable using PCI.[25]

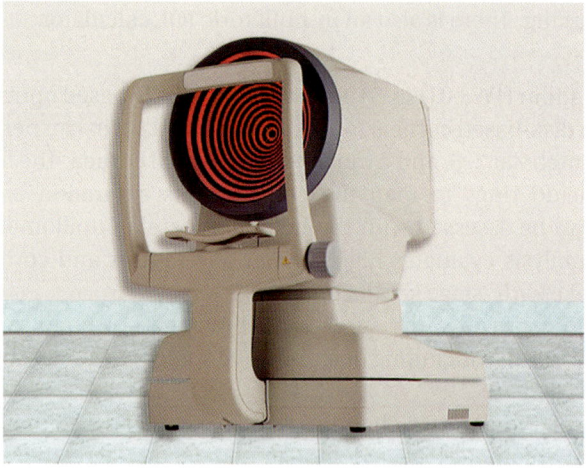

Fig. 5: Aladdin HW 3.0.

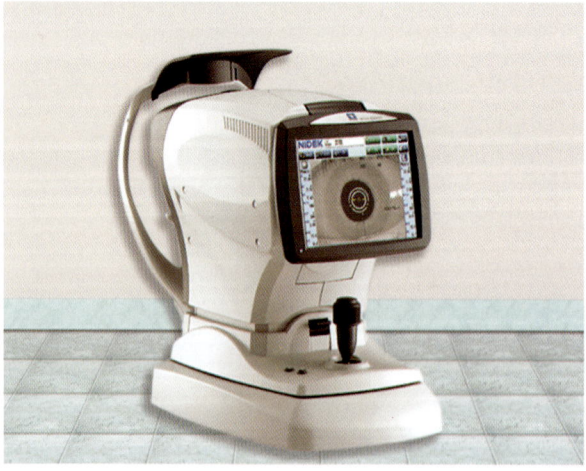

Fig. 6: Axial length-scan.

The incorporated formulae include Camellin-Calossi for postrefractive eyes; SRK/T, Shammas PL; Binkhorst Regression; Regression II; Hoffer Q; Haigis, and Holladay 1.

Argos

Argos from Movu (Fig. 7) is an SSOCT-based biometer that measures AL, CCT, aqueous depth, ACD, lens thickness, pupil size, WTW, and keratometry. Like the IOLMaster 700, the argos is capable of making measurements through dense cataracts. The analyze mode allows technicians to check the plausibility of measurements. The OCT image helps to ensure that the measured parameters do actually align with correct boundaries.

The built-in software includes the Barrett Suite, Hoffer Q, Haigis, Holladay 1, SRK/T, and Shammas no-history formulae. There is also a toric IOL calculator that is incorporated.

Pentacam-AXL

The Pentacam-AXL (Fig. 8) combines Scheimpflug imaging device with a PCI biometer. The Scheimpflug camera helps in capturing corneal tomographic data. The PCI biometer measures the AL. Additionally, the CCT and WTW are also measured. The Pentacam-AXL can estimate true corneal power by accurately determining astigmatism on the anterior and posterior corneal surfaces. The Pentacam AXL's software has the ability to estimate changes in the corneal shape incurred by previous Photo Refractive Keratectomy (PRK) or LASIK, based on its current evaluation of the shape of the cornea. Hence, it can arrive at the approximate pre-LASIK level of myopia or hyperopia. It can also has wavefront analysis capability which helps in premium IOL planning.

The formulae incorporated include Haigis, SRK/T, Holladay, Hoffer Q, Potvin-Shammas-Hill and Potvin-Hill.

Galilei G6

The Galilei G6 from Zeimer (Fig. 9) combines an OLCR biometer with dual Scheimpflug imaging and placido disk topography. Placido disk topography

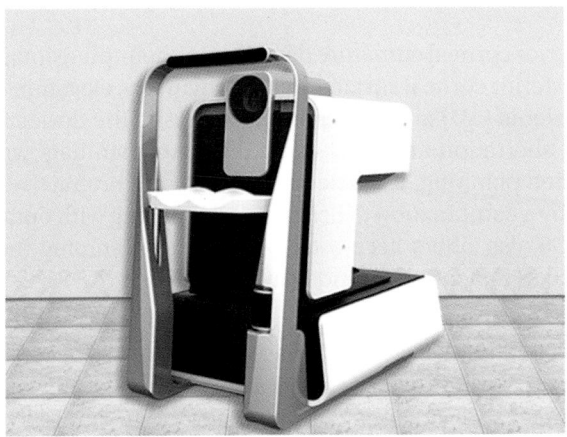

Fig. 7: Argos.

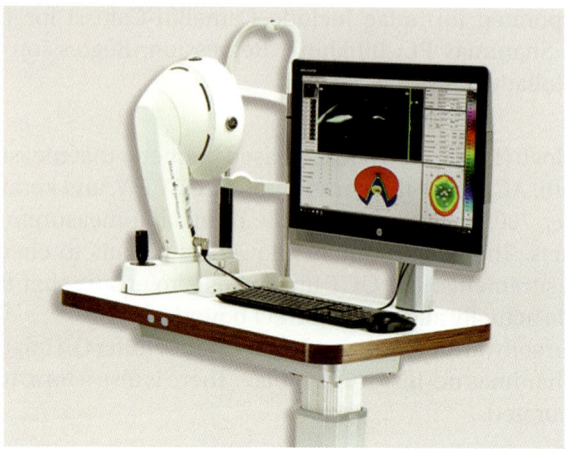

Fig. 8: Pentacam AXL.

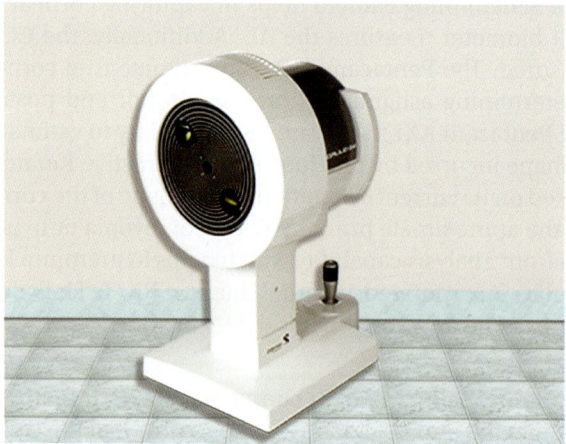

Fig. 9: Galilei G6.

provides anterior corneal curvature data. Dual Scheimpflug imaging provides ray traced posterior corneal surface data, pachymetry, elevation data and also three-dimensional (3D) anterior chamber analysis. The device also provides higher order aberration and total corneal astigmatism data which helps in corneal incision planning. IOL selection in postkeratorefractive surgery eyes is facilitated by a combination of Scheimpflug imaging with optical biometry. The Galilei G6 also offers access to formulae that employ the ray tracing principle such as Phaco Optics and Okulix.

Eyestar 900
The Eyestar 900 (Fig. 10) is a SSOCT-based device from Haag-Streit currently under development. It provides elevation-based topography of anterior and posterior corneal surface along with biometry of the entire eye. The latest-generation IOL calculation formulae such as Hill-RBF, Barrett and Olsen and the Barrett's toric IOL calculator are provided onboard.

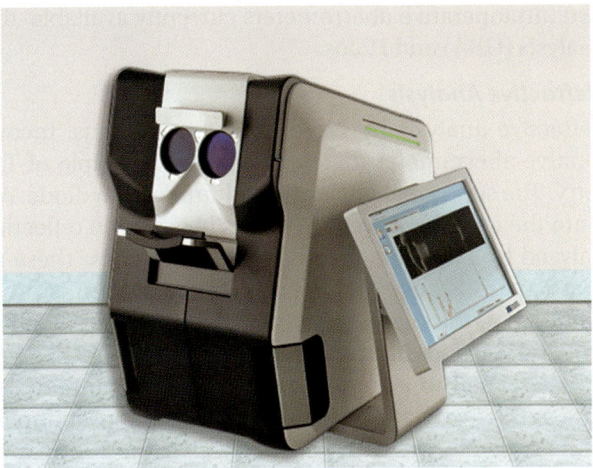

Fig. 10: Eyestar 900.

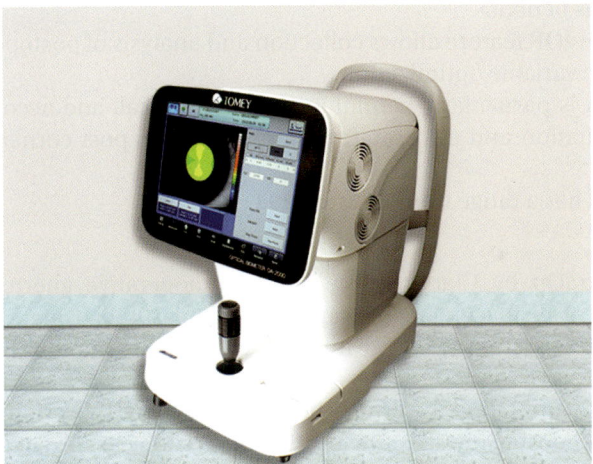

Fig. 11: OA-2000.

OA-2000
The OA 2000 by Tomey (Fig. 11) is an SSOCT based biometer. It also has a placido disk based topographer. It measures CCT, ACD, AL, keratometry, lens thickness, WTW, pupil diameter, and corneal topography 2, 2.5, and 3-mm diameter optical zone. It has the ability to make AL measurements in dense cataracts.

The software package allows access to all the popular IOL calculation formulae including ray tracing formulae.

Intraoperative Aberrometry

Intraoperative aberrometers are instruments that perform wavefront aberrometry during cataract surgery to aid surgeons in taking both aphakic and pseudophakic refractive measurements to avoid refractive surprises.

There are two intraoperative aberrometers currently available–the optiwave refractive analysis (ORA) and Holos.

Optiwave Refractive Analysis

Optiwave refractive analysis by WaveTec Vision Systems, Incorpotation is an intraoperative aberrometer that works on the principle of Talbot moiré interferometry. The source of light is a superluminescent diode. A light beam is directed into the eye. The wavefront of this beam upon reflection from the retina is analyzed by a system consisting of two gratings. These gratings are offset at a particular distance and angle. A fringe pattern is produced light undergoes diffraction through the gratings. The computer then analyzes this fringe pattern and provides information about refraction.

The ORA is attached to a surgical microscope. Continuous information regarding the refractive status of the aphakic and pseudophakic eye is available to the surgeon. The ORA system also has the VerifEye+ technology where by information on axis of placement of a toric IOL, position of limbal relaxing incisions, etc. are displayed real time via the microscope oculars for the surgeons benefit.

The AnalyzOR feature allows collection and analysis of postoperative data for dynamic variable optimization.

The ORA is particularly helpful in toric, multifocal, and accommodative IOL implantation and also cataract surgery in eyes post-corneal refractive surgery.[26,27]

The ORA has a range from –5 D to +20 D

Holos

HOLOS IntraOp by Clarity is the latest intraoperative aberrometer. The magnitude of displacement of wavefront is measured using a microelectromechanical system (MEMS) mirror which rotates rapidly, and a quad detector.

Similar to the ORA, the Holos helps in verifying the pre-planned IOL power and choosing the size and location of incisions to correct astigmatism intraoperatively.

The Holos has a range of measurement from –5D to +16 D. Like the ORA it is attached to the microscope.

IOL POWER CALCULATION FORMULAE

Dr Harold Ridley implanted the first IOL in 1949. Even though this was a landmark event in the history of ophthalmology, the patient had a postoperative refractive error of -21 D![28]

Since then, technology to measure ocular distances has improved by leaps and bounds. But an accurate measurement of AL and keratometry would mean nothing if they are not fed into a formula that can accurately calculate the refractive power of an IOL.

A plethora of IOL power calculation formulae have sprung up since the 1980s when standard power IOL implantation was practiced.

Classification
The various IOL power calculation formulae can be classified as follows[29]
- Historical or refraction-based formulae
- Regression formulae
- Vergence formulae
  - 2 variable formulae
  - 3 variable formulae
  - 5 variable formulae
  - 7 variable formulae
- Artificial intelligence based formulae
- Ray tracing

Historical or Refraction-based Formulae
This represents an obsolete method of adding a fixed power to the patient's cataractous refraction.

Regression Formulae
These formulae rely purely on statistics and analysis of previous data. They do not take into account the optics of the eye. For example, SRK and SRK II which were linear regression formulae.

Vergence Formulae
These formulae are based on Gaussian optics—the basic premise that image vergence = object vergence + lens vergence. Most of these formulae rely on the equation formulated by Fyodorov.

IOLP= [1336/(AL-ELP) − (1336/{1336/[1000/(1000/D PostRx) − V] + K} − ELP)]

Where, K is net corneal power, AL is axial length, IOLP is IOL power, ELP is effective lens position, DPostRx is desired refraction, and V is Vertex distance.

The fundamental weakness of these formulae is their inability to calculate ELP accurately. Hence, calculating an accurate ELP is the primary goal of these formulae. ELP can be calculated using a number of variables. Thus, these formulae also use a certain amount of regression in addition to theoretical optics in order to estimate ELP. According to the number of variables used to calculate ELP, vergence formulae may be further classified into:

2 Variable Formulae
Holladay 1, SRK –T, Hoffer Q

3 Variable Formulae
- *Haigis:* Most IOL formulae have a fixed formula-specific IOL power prediction curve. The present system of IOL constants works by simply moving the position of an IOL power prediction curve for the utilized formula up or down. The Haigis formula developed by Professor Wolfgang Haigis differs from these formulae in that it uses three constants (a0, a1, and a2) to set both the position and the shape of the power prediction curve.

The effective lens position d = a0 + (a1 * ACD) + (a2 * AL)
Where, ACD is the anterior chamber depth and AL is axial length.

The a0, a1, and a2 constants are derived by multi-variable regression analysis from a large sample which includes a wide range ACD and ALs. These constants are surgeon and IOL specific. So, the Haigis formula provides a degree of personalization. Each surgeon can download an excel spreadsheet from https://doctor-hill.com/physicians/download.htm and use it to derive their own sets of a0, a1, and a2.[30]

- *Ladas super formula:* Dr John G Ladas, Dr Albert Jun, Dr Aazim Siddiqui, and Dr Uday Devgan jointly developed a method to represent IOL calculations in three dimensions. Initially, the Hoffer Q, Holladay 1, Holladay 1 with Wang-Koch adjustment, Haigis and SRK-T formulae were included in their study. The points of agreement between these formulae for various ranges of AL and keratometry were delineated and the areas where these formulae disagree with each other were also determined. A super surface was created that included the ideal portions from four of the five formulae to generate the super formula. This formula is not a static formula and is constantly undergoing optimization using inputs from surgeons around the world.[31]

5 Variable Formulae

- **Barrett Universal 2:** The Barrett Universal 2 was developed by Dr Graham D Barrett. Its basis lies in a theoretical model eye in which ACD is related to AL and keratometry.

  The formula is called universal because it can be used without modification in all eyes and all IOL designs irrespective of whether the eye is short, medium or long.

  The effective lens position is calculated based on 5 variables—the AL, keratometry, ACD, lens thickness (optional), and horizontal WTW corneal diameter (optional). In addition, the postoperative desired refraction and the lens factor or A-constant of the particular IOL to be implanted is required.

  The lens factors of a selected number of IOLs can be found on the website https://www.apacrs.org/barrett_universal2/. Alternatively, the SRK-T A-constant for the IOLs listed on the ULIB website may be used. The A-constants used in Barrett Universal 2 formula need not be optimized.

  For obtaining optimum results, it is recommended that data be input from an optical biometer and that appropriate optical A-constants be used.

  One of the key advantages of this formula is its accuracy in predicting IOL power for extremely long eyes in which IOL power may be negative. Even when meniscus lenses are implanted, no modifications in IOL power are necessary.[32-34]

7 Variable Formulae

- *Holladay 2*: Holladay 2 is a vergence formula designed by Dr Jack T Holladay that attempts to estimate the effective lens position using 7 variables, namely, AL, average keratometry, horizontal WTW distance,

Recent Advances in Intraocular Lens Power Calculation

refraction ACD, lens thickness, and age. Of these, after AL and keratometry, the WTW emerged as the next most significant variable that determined effective lens position. Dr Holladay classified eyes into 9 types (Table 1). He also determined that there was no correlation between the anterior segment size and AL in 90% of eyes.[35]

These seven parameters when fed into the Holladay IOL consultant and surgical outcomes assessment program (HIC.SOAP) leads to calculation of IOL power. The program is available online at www.hicsoap.com. Like most formulae, the Holladay 2 also works better if the A-constants are personalized.

Artificial Intelligence-based Formulae

Although a form of regression, these formulae use huge databases and a sophisticated engineering based statistical model to identify relationships between variables.

Clarke neural network and Hill-RBF are two examples of such formulae.

Hill-RBF Calculator

Jointly developed by RBF calculator physician team, Haag-Streit Switzerland, and Mathworks, the Hill-RBF calculator is named after Dr Warren E Hill–one of the co-developers of this calculator. Unlike other methods of IOL power calculation, the Hill-RBF calculator is a sophisticated algorithm rather than a formula.

The Hill-RBF calculator relies on a sophisticated mathematical model consisting of an artificial neural network that uses radial basis functions as activation functions. The calculator recognizes patterns and learns to perform tasks based solely on data that it receives independent of previously known data–a property known as adaptive learning. The Hill-RBF calculator also has the ability to create its own organization, or representation of data. Unlike static formulae, the Hill-RBF calculator is constantly evolving and learning. It tends to get smarter at predicting IOL powers as it gets more data. It is also the only formula that gives a clue regarding the accuracy of the predicted IOL power. The calculator lets the operator know about how sure it is about the accuracy of predicted IOL power with in-bounds or out of bounds statement.

Version 2.0 of the Hill-RBF calculator was released in January 2018 and includes the facility to enter target refraction like regular vergence formulae.

It has been optimized for the Haag Streit Lenstar in combination with the Alcon SN60WF biconvex intraocular lens (IOL) and the Alcon MA60MA

Table 1: Holladay Schema- 9 types of eyes.

Anterior segment size				
	Large	Megalocornea + axial hyperopia	Megalocornea	Large eye, buphthalmos, megalocornea + axial myopia
	Normal	Axial hyperopia	Normal	Axial myopia
	Small	Small eye, nanophthalmos	Microcornea	Microcornea + axial myopia
	Axial length			

meniscus design intraocular lens for IOL powers from +30.00 D to +6.00 D for biconvex IOLs and from +5.00 D to −5.00 D for meniscus design IOLs. Though, it may be used with other optical biometers and other IOLs, the performance of the calculator may not be optimum.

Ray Tracing

Gaussian optics assumes that all components in an optical system are centered around a single optical axis and if the rays of interest have only very small angles relative to this axis. Phenomena like spherical aberrations cannot be explained with the help of Gaussian optics.

Third generation IOL formulae also make another assumption that the refractive components within the optical system of the eye are thin lenses. For example, the anterior and posterior corneal surfaces are not considered separately but as a single surface with a fictitious refractive index assuming that anterior and posterior corneal radii bear a fixed ratio to one another. Also the IOL is considered to be a thin lens.

Ray tracing is a calculation method for single rays passing through an optical system. It does not make the assumptions that are made by Gaussian optics based formula.

The Olsen formula, Okulix, and PhacoOptics are examples of ray tracing methods to calculate IOL power.[29,36]

Olsen Formula

This formula was developed by Dr Thomas Olsen. The Olsen formula uses paraxial and ray tracing techniques. The formula attempts to calculate true net corneal power and avoids the errors of a thin lens formula.

The postoperative anterior chamber depth is predicted using a regression formula. The effective lens position is determined from the ACD and lens thickness.

The Olsen formula uses a new constant called C-constant that describes the IOL position as a constant fraction of the capsular bag size. The C-constant determines where the IOL will rest within the eye. The variables that need to be entered in this formula are ACD, AL, lens thickness, and keratometry.[37]

Okulix

Okulix uses ray tracing optics rather than Gaussian optics to calculate IOL power. No assumptions are made regarding the ratio between anterior and posterior corneal radii. Hence, the anterior and posterior corneal surface must be topographically measured. Also the IOL is not considered to be a thin lens but is described by its anterior and posterior central curvature radius, asphericity (if any) of the surfaces, central thickness, and index of refraction. The true geometrical position of the IOL is estimated.

IOL power prediction does not differ too much between 3rd generation Gaussian optics formulae and ray tracing techniques. However, in eyes with abnormal anatomy and postrefractive surgery eyes ray tracing techniques hold an edge.[38]

PhacoOptics
PhacoOptics is also a software that uses ray tracing techniques to calculate IOL power. It also has all the advantages that ray tracing optics allow. It also incorporates a multiple-variable algorithm to predict the postoperative ACD, including the concept of the C-constant developed by Dr Thomas Olsen.

Newer Developments

Wang-Koch Modification
When IOL power is calculated for long eyes, often surgeons end with a postoperative hyperopic surprise. To avoid this Dr Li Wang and Dr Doug Koch suggested that the ALs more than 25.2 mm be modified in the following manner before they are entered into formulae such as SRK-T, Holladay 1, Holladay 2, Haigis, and Hoffer Q formulae (Table 2).

Full Monte IOL
This is a software based on an adaptive optimizing process called the Markov Chain Monte Carlo process. It gives a probability curve rather than a single emmetropic power that enables the surgeon to choose the appropriate IOL to implant. The software continuously optimizes itself as and when it receives new data. New variables such as sulcus-to-sulcus width and sulcus-to-sulcus perpendicular depth, obtained from ultrasound biomicroscopy have been added to the software.

UniversIOL Calculator
Developed by Dr Samir Sayegh, the UniversIOL calculator is an online calculator that provides the surgeon with a choice of IOL formulae or combinations of formulae for spherical and toric IOL power calculation, a choice of computational strategies and a choice of IOL ranking criteria that can be selected by the surgeon. It does not propose a new formula. The lens database of UniversIOL includes lenses from a variety of manufacturers of monofocal, aspheric, toric, and multifocal lenses.

Toric IOL Calculators
Several toric IOL calculators are available online as well as on board optical biometers. Some of the popular toric IOL calculators available are:

Assort Toric Calculator
It is a generic calculator that allows the surgeon to select the most appropriate IOL from various manufacturers based on the desired postoperative residual refraction. It makes available optimized IOL constants for commonly used

Table 2: Wang-Koch modification for IOL formulae.

Holladay 1 optimized axial length	0.829 x AL + 4.27
Haigis optimized axial length	0.929 x AL + 1.56
SRK-T optimized axial length	0.854 x AL + 3.72
Hoffer Q optimized axial length	0.853 x AL + 3.58

Where, AL is the IOLMaster determined axial length.[39]

formulae. It also takes into account the toricity induced by wound placement. Corneal topographic astigmatism (CorT Total) is a new parameter that is used in this calculator. It includes posterior corneal astigmatism.

In the event of a postoperative refractive surprise, the calculator can also estimate the correction that can be obtained from rotating the IOL, IOL exchange, or LASIK.[40]

Barrett Toric Calculator

It is available on http://www.ascrs.org/barrett-toric-calculator. The spherical equivalent is calculated from the Barrett universal 2 formula. A theoretical model is employed to derive posterior corneal curvature. Estimated lens position is obtained using vector calculations and cylindrical implant power needed for neutralizing the total corneal astigmatism is calculated. The Haag Streit Lenstar is recommended for obtaining the raw data required for this calculator.[40]

Holladay IOL Consultant Toric Preoperative Planner

The toric preoperative (PreOp) planner enables users to calculate the optimum cylindrical power and axis of placement for a toric implant using keratometry and the estimated surgically-induced astigmatism (SIA). Unlike some other calculators, it does not use a constant ratio of 1.46 to estimate the IOL toricity from the corneal astigmatism. This helps to prevent errors that can occur in the case of extremes of IOL power.[40]

Verion

The Verion from Alcon laboratories is a platform that incorporates tools for calculation of IOL power, toricity, and surgical planning. Its components are the Verion Reference Unit, the Verion Planner, and the Verion Digital Markers.

The Verion Reference Unit measures keratometry and pupil size. It captures a high resolution image of the eye. Anatomical landmarks such as limbus, scleral vessels, iris, and pupil features are detected. These are used for registration and intraoperative tracking.

The Verion Planner is a software for surgical planning. Data captured by the Verion Reference Unit is transferred to the Verion Planner. It has a number of commonly used IOL power calculation formulae.

The Verion Digital Marker is a tool that creates an overlay that is displayed through the oculars of the operating microscope. After all data is fed into the Verion Digital Marker, it generates a digital overlay that can be viewed by the surgeon in real time. Using iris registration the system provides automatic cyclotorsion control thus eliminating cumbersome preoperative marking and preventing errors during transcription of data.

Other Toric Calculators

Some of the other toric calculators available online are Alcon online toric calculator (https://www.myalcon-toriccalc.com), Acrysof toric calculator (www.acrysoftoriccalculator.com), AMO easy toric IOL calculator (https://www.amoeasy.com/calc), Care Group toric IOL calculator (http://toric1.

caregroupindia.com/toric/Default.aspx), and Appasamy Associates toric calculator (http://www.appasamy.com/toric.php).

astigmatismfix.com
This website features a tool called toric results analyzer, developed by John Berdahl and David Hardten, that helps the surgeon identify whether an implanted IOL is properly aligned or not. In case of a postoperative refractive surprise, this tool can predict whether IOL rotation will be beneficial in reducing residual astigmatism. It also suggests the optimum IOL alignment axis which can eliminate or reduce the remaining astigmatic error.

IOL Power Calculation in Eyes Post Corneal Refractive Surgery

In eyes that have undergone corneal refractive surgery, corneal curvature is altered. This induces error into measurement of corneal power and prediction of ELP. Hence, the standard methods of IOL power calculation are inadequate to measure IOL power in such eyes.

Standard keratometers only measure the corneal curvature of the anterior surface to calculate corneal power, assuming that the radii of curvature of the anterior and posterior corneal surfaces bear a fixed ratio to each other. Corneal refractive surgery changes only the anterior corneal curvature and leaves the posterior curvature unaltered. Thus, the ratio between the radii of curvature of the anterior and posterior surface is altered.

A number of methods have been devised to overcome this error in calculation. Many of them like these have been abandoned due to practical constraints and/or unreliability. Some of the current strategies used for IOL power calculation in eyes that have undergone corneal refractive surgery are discussed below.

Haigis- L Formula
The Haigis-L formula is obtained by modifying the standard Haigis formula.

The Haigis-L formula modifies the corneal radius of curvature (r corr) as measured by the IOLMaster in the following manner:

$$r\ corr = \frac{331.5}{-5.1625 \times r\ meas + 82.2603 - 0.35}$$

Where, r meas is the measured corneal radius of curvature.[41]

Masket Method
Developed by Samuel Masket, it is a postoperative regression formula. The Holladay 1 formula is used to calculate IOL power for eyes with AL greater than 23 mm and Hoffer Q formula is used to calculate IOL power for eyes with AL less than 23 mm. The simulated keratometry values are used.
The following formula is used

$$(LSE \times -0.326) + 0.101 = \text{Post-LASIK IOL power adjustment}$$

Where, LSE is the laser corrected spherical equivalent adjusted for vertex distance.[41]

Modified Masket Method
Dr Warren E Hill modified the Masket method as follows:

(LSE × −0.4385) + 0.0295 = Post-LASIK IOL power adjustment.[41]

Aphakic Refraction
Mackool et al., described this method to calculate IOL power in post refractive surgery eyes. After cataract extraction, no IOL is implanted immediately. After an hour refraction is performed. The following formula is used to calculate IOL power.[42]

IOL power (D) = Aphakic refraction × 1.75

This method was found to be more accurate when anterior chamber IOLs were implanted.[41]

Ianchulev and Leccisotti described another formula using a similar approach.

IOL power (D) = 0.07 × (2) + 1.27 × + 1.22, where x = aphakic refraction

This approach was found to be more accurate when the IOL was placed posteriorly.[42]

However, both of these approaches are cumbersome.

Intraoperative Aberrometry
Intraoperative aberrometers such as the ORA and Holos (discussed earlier) predict IOL power more precisely than conventional formulae in eyes that have undergone corneal refractive surgery.[41]

Ray Tracing
Okulix and PhacoOptics (discussed earlier) which use ray tracing rather than Gaussian optics are in general more accurate than conventional formulae when it comes to IOL power calculation in eyes that have undergone corneal refractive surgery.[41]

Because so many formulae are available for calculating IOL power in eyes that have undergone corneal refractive surgery, the whole process of IOL power calculation in such eyes can be cumbersome. This difficult task of is simplified by many web-based tools.

American Society of Cataract and Refractive Surgery Post Refractive Calculator
The American Society of Cataract and Refractive Surgery (ASCRS) post-refractive calculator (www.iolcalc.ascrs.org) makes use of several available formulae. Both historical and nonhistorical methods of IOL power calculation may be used. It provides the surgeon with an average of IOL powers calculated using several methods. The IOL power calculated using the ASCRS calculator is reasonably accurate.[41]

Hoffer-Savini LASIK IOL Power Tool
The Hoffer-Savini LASIK IOL power tool is a spreadsheet that can be downloaded from the web address www.iolpowerclub.org/post-surgical-iol-calc. Measured keratometry, AL, and other biometric data have to be entered in

the spreadsheet. The tool then provides modified biometric parameters that may be used in any of the commonly used formulae or the tool itself can give IOL power using various formulae that are available.[41]

Barrett True-K Formula

The Barrett True-K formula for IOL power calculation in post corneal refractive surgery eyes is provided by the Asia-Pacific Association of Cataract and Refractive Surgeons (www.apacrs.org). This formula provided results that were comparable to or better than those provided by the ASCRS online calculator in post corneal refractive surgery eyes.[43]

The McCarthy Post Refractive IOL Calculator

The McCarthy post refractive IOL calculator (www.mccarthyeye.com/post-refractive-iol-calculator) was designed based on a study conducted by McCarthy et al. on the refractive outcomes of biometry performed on 173 eyes that previously underwent LASIK or PRK.[41,44]

EyePro Application

The EyePro is an android app which makes use of two formulae—the BESt postrefractive IOL formula and the PAK postrefractive IOL formula. The keratometry values for the Borasio Edmondo Smith and Stevens (BESSt) formula have to be obtained from the Pentacam.[41, 45-47]

REFERENCES

1. Apple DJ, Sims J. Harold Ridley and the invention of the intraocular lens. Surv Ophthalmol. 1996;40(4):279-9
2. Mundt GH, Hughes WF. Ultrasonics in ocular diagnosis. Am J Ophthalmol. 1956;41(3):488-98.
3. Hoffmann PC, Hütz WW, Eckhardt HB, et al. Intraocular lens calculation and ultrasound biometry: immersion and contact procedures. Klin Monbl Augenheilkd. 1998;213(3):161-5.
4. Olsen T. Calculation of intraocular lens power: a review. Acta Ophthalmol Scand. 2007;85(5):472-85.
5. Drexler W, Findl O, Menapace R, et al. Partial coherence interferometry: a novel approach to biometry in cataract surgery. Am J Ophthalmol. 1998;126(4):524-34.
6. Eleftheriadis H. IOLMaster biometry: refractive results of 100 consecutive cases. Br J Ophthalmol [Internet]. 2003;87(8):960-3.
7. Kunavisarut P, Poopattanakul P, Intarated C, et al. Accuracy and reliability of IOL master and A-scan immersion biometry in silicone oil-filled eyes. Eye (Lond). 2012;26(10):1344-8.
8. Ghoraba HH, El-Dorghamy AA, Atia AF, et al. The problems of biometry in combined silicone oil removal and cataract extraction: a clinical trial. Retina (Philadelphia, Pa). 2002;22(5):589-96.
9. Nakhli FR. Comparison of optical biometry and applanation ultrasound measurements of the axial length of the eye. Saudi J Ophthalmol. 2014;28(4):287-91.
10. Shah M, Shah S, Shah K, et al. Biometry for IOL power calculation, which technology is better optical or acoustic? Sudan J Ophthalmol. 2014;6(1):6-9.
11. Holladay JT. Ultrasound and optical biometry. Cataract Refract Surg Today Europe; 2009. pp. 18-9.

12. Astbury N, Ramamurthy B. How to avoid mistakes in biometry. Community Eye Health. 2006;19(60):70-1.
13. Sheard R. Optimising biometry for best outcomes in cataract surgery. Eye. 2014;28(2):118-25.
14. McAlinden C, Wang Q, Gao R, et al. Axial length measurement failure rates with biometers using swept-source optical coherence tomography compared to partial-coherence interferometry and optical low-coherence interferometry. Am J Ophthalmol. 2017;173:64-9.
15. Findl O, Drexler W, Menapace R, et al. Optical biometry in cataract surgery. modern cataract surgery. 2002;34:131-40.
16. Schmid GF. Axial and peripheral eye length measured with optical low coherence reflectometry. J Biomed Opt. 2003;8(4):655-62.
17. Srivannaboon S, Chirapapaisan C, Chonpimai P, et al. Clinical comparison of a new swept-source optical coherence tomography–based optical biometer and a time-domain optical coherence tomography–based optical biometer. J Cataract Refract Surg. 2015;41(10):2224-32.
18. Leitgeb R, Hitzenberger CK, Fercher AF. Performance of fourier domain vs time domain optical coherence tomography. Opt Express. 2003;11(8):889-94.
19. Hill W, Angeles R, Otani T. Evaluation of a new IOLMaster algorithm to measure axial length. J Cataract Refract Surg. 2008;34(6):920-4.
20. Akman A, Asena L, Güngör SG. Evaluation and comparison of the new swept source OCT-based IOLMaster 700 with the IOLMaster 500. Br J Ophthalmol. 2016;100(9):1201-5.
21. Epitropoulos A. Axial length measurement acquisition rates of two optical biometers in cataractous eyes. Clin Ophthalmol. 2014;8:1369-76.
22. Melike O, Totuk G, Aykan U. Repeatability of the New Swept Source Optical Biometer IOLMaster®700 Measurements. EC Ophthalmol. 2017;7(3):78-85.
23. Kurian M, Negalur N, Das S, et al. Biometry with a new swept-source optical coherence tomography biometer: Repeatability and agreement with an optical low-coherence reflectometry device. J Cataract Refract Surg. 2016;42(4):577-81.
24. Mandal P, Berrow EJ, Naroo SA, et al. Validity and repeatability of the Aladdin ocular biometer. Br J Ophthalmol. 2014;98(2):256-8.
25. Aktas S, Aktas H, Tetikoglu M, et al. Refractive Results Using a New Optical Biometry Device. Medicine (Baltimore). 2015;94(48).
26. Tityal JS, Kaur M, Falera R, et al. Intraoperative aberrometry–assisted intraocular lens exchange in post-refractive surgery intraocular lens surprise. JCRS Online Case Reports. 2018;6(1):12-4.
27. Woodcock MG, William FW, Kerry A, et al. Uses for Intraoperative Wavefront Aberrometry. Cataract Refract Surg Today Europe. 2012:31-40.
28. Strobel J. Determination of Intraocular Lenses by Ultrasound. Ultrasono Ophthalmol. 1981;29:233-8.
29. Koch DD, Hill W, Abulafia A, et al. Pursuing perfection in intraocular lens calculations: I. Logical approach for classifying IOL calculation formulas. J Cataract Refract Surg. 2017;43(6):717-8.
30. Haigis W. The Haigis formula. In: Shammas H (Ed). Intraocular Lens Power Calculations. Thorofare (NJ): Slack Inc; 2003. pp. 41-57.
31. Ladas JG, Siddiqui AA, Devgan U, et al. A 3-D "Super Surface" combining modern intraocular lens formulas to generate a "Super Formula" and maximize accuracy. JAMA Ophthalmol. 2015;133(12):1431-6.
32. Barrett GD. An improved universal theoretical formula for intraocular lens power prediction. J Cataract Refr Surg. 1993;19(6):713-20.

33. Zhang Y, Liang XY, Liu S, et al. Accuracy of intraocular lens power calculation formulas for highly myopic eyes. J Ophthalmol. 2016;2016:1917268.
34. Roberts TV, Hodge C, Sutton G, et al. Comparison of Hill-radial basis function, Barrett Universal and current third generation formulas for the calculation of intraocular lens power during cataract surgery. Clin Experiment Ophthalmol. 2017.
35. Holladay JT. Standardizing constants for ultrasonic biometry, keratometry, and intraocular lens power calculations. J Cataract Refr Surg. 1997;23(9):1356-70.
36. Hoffer KJ. The Hoffer Q formula: a comparison of theoretic and regression formulas. J Cataract Refract Surg. 1993;19(6):700-12.
37. Olsen T, Hoffmann P. C constant: new concept for ray tracing-assisted intraocular lens power calculation. J Cataract Refract Surg. 2014;40(5):764-73.
38. Saiki M, Negishi K, Kato N, et al. Ray tracing software for intraocular lens power calculation after corneal excimer laser surgery. Jpn J Ophthalmol. 2014;58(3):276-81.
39. Wang L, Shirayama M, Ma XJ, et al. Optimizing intraocular lens power calculations in eyes with axial lengths above 25.0 mm. J Cataract Refract Surg. 2011;37(11):2018-27.
40. Alpins N, Barrett GD, Hansen MS, et al. Innovative Toric Iol calculators and how to use them. Cataract Refract Surg Today Europe. 2015.
41. Hodge C, McAlinden C, Lawless M, et al Intraocular lens power calculation following laser refractive surgery. Eye Vis. 2015;2:7.
42. Sheppard AL, Dunne MCM, Wolffsohn JS, et al. Theoretical evaluation of the cataract extraction-refraction-implantation techniques for intraocular lens power calculation. Ophthalmic Physiol Opt. 2008;28(6):568-76.
43. Abulafia A, Hill WE, Koch DD, et al. Accuracy of the Barrett True-K formula for intraocular lens power prediction after laser in situ keratomileusis or photorefractive keratectomy for myopia. J Cataract Refract Surg. 2016;42(3):363-9.
44. McCarthy M, Gavanski GM, Paton KE, et al. Intraocular lens power calculations after myopic laser refractive surgery: a comparison of methods in 173 eyes. Ophthalmol. 2011;118:940-4.
45. Savini G, Barboni P, Profazio V, et al. Corneal power measurements with the Pentacam Scheimpflug camera after myopic excimer laser surgery. J Cataract Refract Surg. 2008;34:809-13.
46. Saiki M, Negishi K, Kato N, et al. A new central-peripheral corneal curvature method for intraocular lens power calculation after excimer laser refractive surgery. Acta Ophthalmol. 2013;91:e133-9.
47. Ho JD, Liou SW, Tsai RJ, et al. Estimation of the effective lens position using a rotating Scheimpflug camera. J Cataract Refract Surg. 2008;34:2119-27.

CHAPTER 8

Custom Cataract Surgery

Rajiv Choudhary

■ INTRODUCTION

In the past five decades, there has been a dramatic evolution of cataract surgery resulting in high patient expectations. The development of phacoemulsification surgery, femtosecond laser, and good quality intraocular lenses (IOLs) are the three most significant strides that have been made in the cataract surgery. Ophthalmologists continually strive to give a near normal vision to patients. The custom cataract surgery generally provides better unaided visual acuity postoperatively than routine basic cataract surgery. The custom cataract surgery takes into consideration refractive targeting, biometry, IOL power calculation, customization of surgical modality, microincisional cataract surgery (MICS), choice of IOLs, and management of preexisting or postoperative astigmatism.[1] In the present article a comprehensive review is presented on these aspects of custom cataract surgery.

■ REFRACTIVE TARGETING

Cataract surgeons must assess the patient thoroughly and provide a logistic estimate of recovery of visual acuity. Sometimes, they become overenthusiastic and thus become victims of their own success causing great disappointment to the patient. Targeting emmetropia is usually common. However, in patients with high preexisting ametropia, high astigmatism and prior refractive surgery [radial keratotomy (RK) or laser-assisted in situ keratomileusis (LASIK)], cataract surgery may not yield required results in spite of advancement in surgical technique.

■ BIOMETRY

Accurate measurement of the power of IOLs to be implanted is another important step. Corneal power, anterior chamber depth (ACD), and axial length of the eye have to be measured. The error in the measurement of axial length results in a significant postoperative refractive error.[2] An axial eye length measurement error of 0.5 mm can induce a postoperative refractive error of up to 1.4 D.[3,4] The partial coherence interferometry (PCI), using a semiconductor diode laser, should be used to determine axial length and

ACD. Optical biometry has become the first choice for IOL power calculation. The technique is noncontact in nature and provides a high resolution of measurement of axial length.[5,6] It is accurate and reliable,[7,8] and improves the refractive results of cataract surgery[9,10] The calculation formulae of IOL power are dependent on the axial length and the dioptric power of the cornea. The effective lens position (ELP) can be calculated on these two variables (which yield the power of the IOL) to obtain emmetropia. The Haigis formula was found to be more accurate than Hoffer Q in a large series of cases of hyperopia.[11]

CUSTOMIZATION OF SURGICAL MODALITY

Phaco tip in conventional phaco moves linear and uses increased energy[12] resulting in corneal endothelial damage. The main aim of customization is to use less energy and surge control to get clearer cornea postoperatively. One can achieve it by:
- Power modulation
- Newer software
- Ultrasound other than longitudinal.

Power Modulation

It is breaking up the ultrasonic power into smaller packets of pulses and bursts which can be achieved in one of the following ways:

Continuous Mode

In continuous power setting, energy delivery is continuous with variation in power controlled by the amount of foot pedal depression (Fig. 1).

Pulse Mode

In pulse mode, the pulse power increases linearly by how far down the foot pedal is depressed. After each pulse of energy delivered, there is a period in which no energy is delivered (Fig. 2). It reduces heat and delivers half the energy into the eye.

Burst Mode

In burst mode, each burst has the same power but the interval between bursts decreases as the foot pedal is depressed (Fig. 3). As a result, at maximum foot pedal depression, the burst of energy will become continuous delivery of energy. The advantages of this upgraded range of programmability are the smoothness and precision of power delivery.

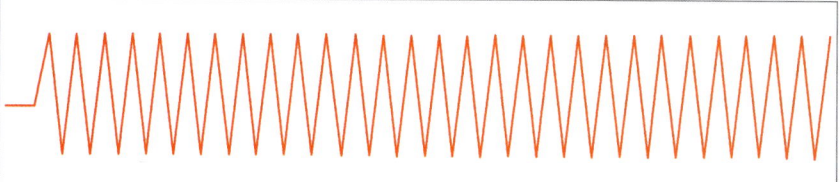

Fig. 1: Continuous mode power modulation.

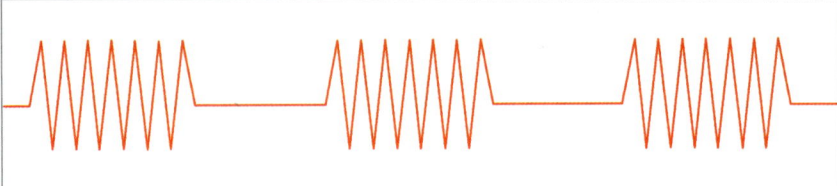

Fig. 2: Pulse mode power modulation.

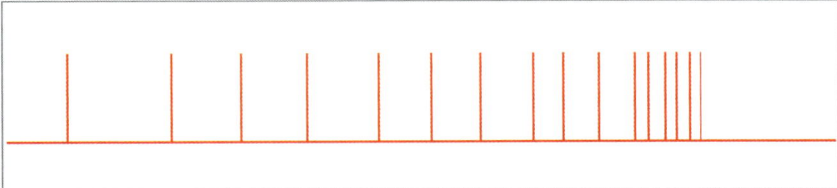

Fig. 3: Burst mode power modulation.

When to use which Power Modulation?
It depends on grade of nuclear sclerosis and stage of phacoemulsification. For nuclear sclerosis grade II-III, pulse mode usually works. For nuclear sclerosis grade IV continuous mode is required during sculpting and then pulse mode is required during chopping. In femtosecond laser-assisted nucleotomy, the phaco energy is minimized quite significantly even in nuclear cataracts.[13]

Newer Software
They tend to reduce temperature at wound site and provide better chamber stability even at high vacuum levels.

Ultrasound other than Longitudinal
Traditionally, the phacoemulsification probe delivers power only in a longitudinal manner with the phaco needle moving forward and backward. Recent innovation in phaco technology also allows for the delivery of power through a lateral motion which can increase cutting efficiency by reducing repulsion of lens material.

The lateral movements may be torsional or transversal:
- **Torsional (OZil):** Here, phaco tip oscillates in a rotational manner along its primary axis. It works best with angled-phaco needle. It provides oscillatory torsional amplitude which causes less repulsion of lens material and reduced thermal energy at incision. The advantages of this technology are better followability, less chattering and less of phaco energy consumption.[14]
- **Transversal:** Here, phaco tip moves in an elliptical path. It works equally well with a straight or angled needle. The advantages of this technology are no jack hammer effect, side to side movement and reduced chatter.

Ultrasound customization depends upon the density of nucleus. Grade II-III nuclear sclerosis is emulsified with torsional alone and low vacuum. Grade IV nuclear sclerosis would need both longitudinal and torsional ultrasound.

ROLE OF MICROINCISIONAL CATARACT SURGERY IN CUSTOMIZATION

Microincisional cataract surgery is not only achieving a smaller incision, but also about making a global transformation of the surgical procedure towards minimal aggressiveness.[15,16]

Why MICS to be the Preferred Choice in Customization?
The following advantages make it a preferred choice:
- Smaller incision
- Shorter tunnel
- More stable chamber during surgery
- Decreased surgical trauma
- Fast visual recovery and improved visual outcome
- Reduced anatomical healing time
- Reduced rate of complications
- Less postoperative inflammatory reaction and
- Less endothelial cell damage.

Advantages of MICS in Difficult Situations
It is very useful in small pupil as small incision induced decreased fluidics, steady-sized pupil, and deep anterior chamber will provide safe results. It is also helpful in nuclear cataract as modern phaco machines with new tips cause easy and efficient emulsification of hard nucleus. Posterior polar cataract can be managed efficiently with MICS as it does not allow sudden collapse of anterior chamber and hence there is better chamber stability. In intraoperative floppy iris syndrome (IFIS), MICS allows lower and smoother fluidics current which decreases volatility in AC thus, prevents iris from billowing and coming up to the phaco tip. In cataract with zonular laxity, MICS decreases flow and prevents movements of crystalline lens back and forth. In pseudoexfoliation syndrome because of better fluidics control and chamber maintenance in MICS, there is decreased risk of zonular dialysis, posterior capsule rent (PCR) and luxation of lens into vitreous. Cataract with shallow anterior chamber is managed well with stable fluidics and tight chamber achieved during MICS. In postradial keratotomy cataract, small incision of MICS is crucial to maintain the integrity of cornea as much as possible. In pediatric cataracts, leaking incisions and anterior chamber instability are taken care of by 1.8 mm incision and advanced fluidics.

Thus, MICS provides security, high efficiency, minimal invasiveness, improved wound strength and integrity, reduced endothelial cell loss, fast patient recovery time and less surgically induced astigmatism thereby achieving the purpose of customization.[17]

INTRAOCULAR LENS SELECTION
Currently, the goal of cataract surgery is to provide fast and complete visual rehabilitation without surgical complications and minimal postoperative refractive errors. Intraocular lens technology has evolved dramatically in

recent years with various premium IOLs improving the visual outcome.[18] The patients with preexisting ocular conditions, such as age-related macular degeneration (AMD), glaucoma, diabetic retinopathy, optic neuropathies, and Fuchs' dystrophy are poor candidates for premium IOLs.

The principal options in IOL selection are:
- Basic lens requiring glasses for distance and near
- Correction of astigmatism requiring glasses for near but not for distance
- Correction of astigmatism along with implantation of lifestyle IOL to yield good uncorrected distance, intermediate and near vision.

Multifocal Intraocular Lens

With respect to changing profile of cataract patients, multifocal IOL provides functional vision over a range of distances (near, intermediate and far distances) and is a good alternative (Fig. 4).[19,20]

Multifocal IOLs have specialized optical properties that can divide light to bring it into focus at more than one point at the same time. These IOLs are made up of concentric rings of varying optical power, each of which refracts or bends incoming light, bringing it into focus at different points simultaneously.

Multifocal IOL can be refractive, diffractive, and combination of refractive and diffractive. Refractive multifocal IOLs do not split the light precisely into two focal points; instead, there is a small spread of light around the near focal point area. The spread results in increased range of near visual acuity rather than the precise optical quality obtained with a single precise focal point. The diffractive technology seems somewhat more promising with a better performance.

A common complaint with multifocal IOL implantation is the lack of intermediate vision, and this is especially true with diffractive high-addition multifocal IOLs. A current trend in multifocal IOL design is to have a relatively lower reading addition. This results in a longer working distance for the patient but an improvement in intermediate vision.

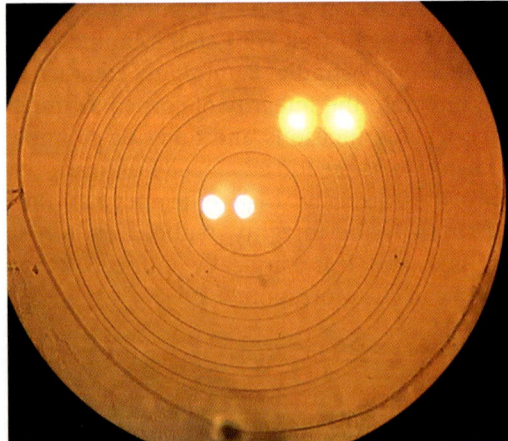

Fig. 4: Multifocal intraocular lens.

The latest IOLs in the multifocal armamentarium are:
- Tecnis multifocal [marketed by Abbott Medical Optics (AMO)]
- ReSTOR IOL (Alcon)
- Fine vision and AT-Lisa (trifocal MIOL)
- Symfony extended depth of focus IOL (Tecnis)
- AcrySof IQ PanOptix IOL

The compromises of multifocal (bifocal and trifocal) lenses include loss of contrast, halos, and glare.

The ongoing research on IOL results in new solution for presbyopia correction—*extended depth of focus (EDOF) IOLs* which delivers continuous, full range of high quality vision without the compromises of other multifocal IOLs. These EDOF IOLs offer optimal distance acuity and contrast sensitivity and some improved intermediate visual acuity.

Which Multifocal to Choose?

It depends on lifestyle and optical factors. Patients who work in dim light, Tecnis multifocal is better than ReSTOR because it is pupil independent. In patients with previous refractive surgery, severe dry eye and aberrations and high astigmatism one should avoid multifocal IOL. In patients with large pupil, Tecnis multifocal is better than ReSTOR. ReSTOR tends to perform better as the pupil comes down in patients with small pupil; ReSTOR + 3 is more helpful. In night drivers and pilots, one should avoid multifocal IOLs. Patients who did not like bifocal or progressive glasses are not good candidate for multifocal IOLs as the patients are accustomed to monovision.

Approximately 85% of people who receive multifocal IOLs find that they do not need glasses for distance or near activities. However, multifocal IOLs have some shortcomings in the form of being expensive and having chance of photic phenomena (about 5–10% of people receiving multifocal implants complain of some glare or halos around lights at night).

HOW TO MINIMIZE POSTOPERATIVE ASTIGMATISM AND CORRECT PREEXISTING ASTIGMATISM?

Various modalities for astigmatism management at the time of cataract surgery are:
- Proper incision placement and construction
- Limbal relaxing incisions (LRIs)
- Femtosecond laser-assisted arcuate keratotomy (FLAK)
- Toric IOL.

Incision Placement and Construction

Incision must be placed on a steeper axis and it should be in a proper plane (Fig. 5 and Table 1).[21,22]

Limbal Relaxing Incisions

These are peripheral corneal relaxing incisions which are made at 80–90% depth and at steeper axis meridian of cornea. The size, depth, and locations

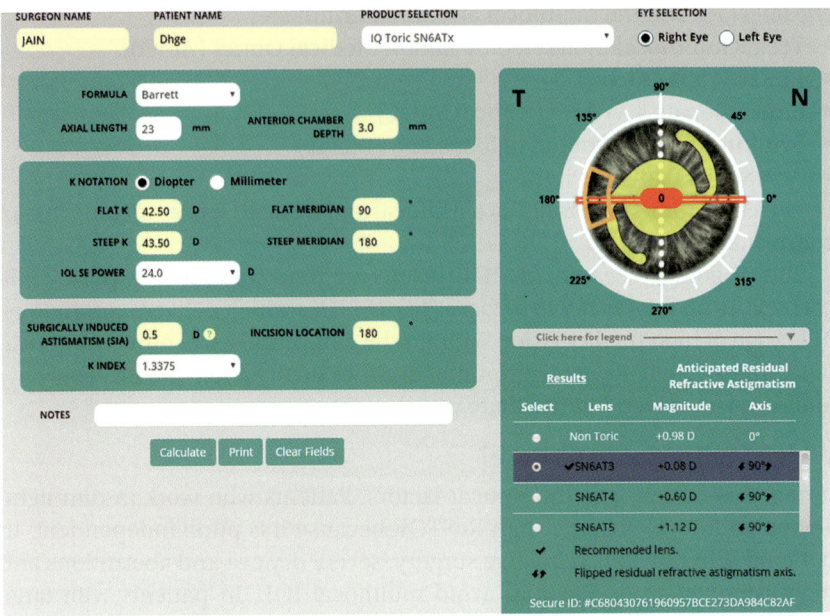

Fig. 5: Location of incision to reduce astigmatism; incision is planned at steeper axis, 180°.

Table 1: Location of incision to reduce astigmatism.

Preoperative corneal astigmatism	1.00 D 180°
Flat k	42.50 D 90°
Steep k	43.50 D 180°
Incision location	180°
SIA	0.50 D 90°
Anticipated residual astigmatism	0.50 D 180°

(SIA: surgically induced astigmatism)

are important to get accurate results. Nichamin and Koch nomogram can be used for making limbal relaxing incisions (LRIs). The relaxing incisions are easier to perform, less dependent on pachymetry, less likely to result in overcorrections and result in quicker postoperative stabilization of refraction. These incisions are very effective for low to moderate amount of astigmatism (<3 D). LRI combined with temporal corneal tunnel are more effective. The downside of LRIs is that they are less predictable. LRI are contraindicated in keratoconus, autoimmune disease, peripheral corneal disease, and cases with prior corneal surgery.

Femtosecond Laser-assisted Arcuate Keratotomy

Femtosecond laser-assisted cataract surgery is gaining popularity because it is more precise than traditional methods. It offers surgeons the opportunity to perform procedures that are not possible to be done manually. The femto laser machine has arcuate incision planning software. It auto-populates incision parameters based on surgeon reference and surgically-induced astigmatism and recommends the placement of lens incision based on preoperative data (Figs. 6A and B). The steep axis corneal marking adds to surgeon's ability to manage astigmatism. The incisions are made to depth of 85% of corneal thickness. Astigmatism less than 1 D can be typically treated with placement LRIs. Astigmatism between 1 D and 3 D can be treated with LRIs or FLAK or Toric IOL.

Indications of FLAK are
- Cataract patients with astigmatism who decline toric IOL.
- If manual LRIs are not predictable, FLAK is advantageous in the sense that it has a good precision with regular depth of incision, the arc length and the diameter at which incision is made.

Toric Intraocular Lens
The most commonly available toric IOLs are Tecnis toric IOL, Staar Toric IOL, AcrySof IQ, and Rayner I-flex.

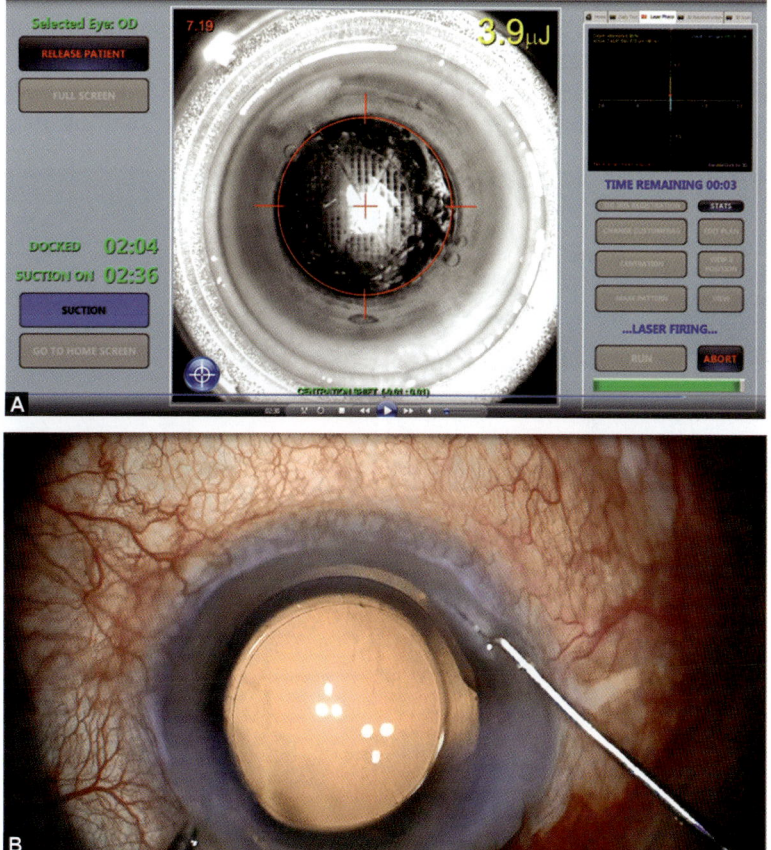

Figs. 6A and B: (A) Femto laser-assisted arcuate keratotomy; (B) Arcuate incision being opened after completion of surgery.

When the LRIs are not sufficient to correct astigmatism, or predictable enough and if astigmatism is greater than 1 D, use of toric IOL is indicated. Toric IOLs are regarded to give more reliable results. Astigmatism greater than 3 D may be corrected with combination of toric IOL, LRIs or FLAK.

Toric IOL power calculation includes precise keratometry and consideration of surgically-induced astigmatism. Keratometry can be done with automated keratometer or corneal topography. For accurate toric IOL power calculation, online calculator is available.

For toric IOL implantation, preoperatively reference marking is done with patient in upright position. Two reference marks are placed at limbus 180° apart. Reference marking can also be done on slit lamp (Figs. 7A to C). Femtosecond laser may also be utilized for reference marking on corneal or anterior capsule. Reference markings are used to align placement on axis marks.

Surgery for toric IOL implantation is a standard phacoemulsification surgery. The IOL alignment is a three step procedure: First is gross alignment, then removal of viscoelastic substance and finally alignment.

Axis alignment can be judged by latest Verion and Callisto technology. As compared to LRI and arcuate incisions, toric IOL implantation is more effective and predictable.[23,24]

The rotational stability is critical to effectiveness of toric IOL. One degree rotation of toric IOL results in 3.3% IOL power loss, 30° rotation negates

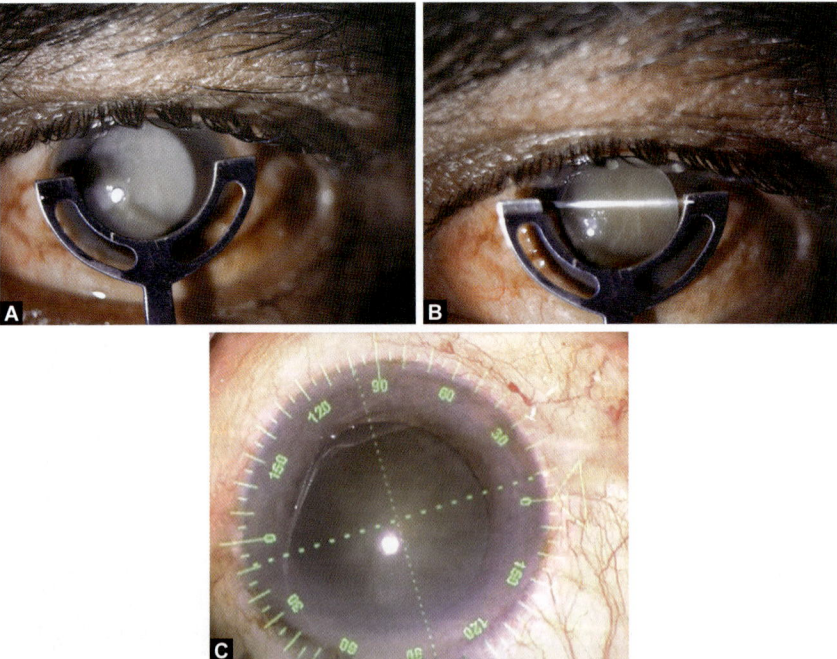

Figs. 7A to C: Placement of reference marks by different techniques. (A) Reference marking in sitting position; (B) Reference marking on slit lamp (C) Reference marking by version.

the cylindrical correction of toric IOL and further rotation induces more astigmatism.[25] Recently, introduced loop and plate toric lenses seldom rotate more than 15°.[26]

CONCLUSION

Custom cataract surgery is the order of the day. The appropriate power modulation, newer software, and newer ultrasound techniques provide use of less energy, shorten phaco time and give clear cornea postoperatively with successful visual outcome. Addressing astigmatism appropriately, customization of surgical procedure and IOL selection result in better visual outcome with the least possible spectacle aid.

REFERENCES

1. Ashwin PT, Shah S, Wolffsohn JS. Advances in cataract surgery. Clin Exp Optom. 2009;92:333-42.
2. Olsen T. Sources of error in intraocular lens power calculation. J Cataract Refract Surg. 1992;18:125-9.
3. Olsen T. Calculation of intraocular lens power: a review. Acta Ophthalmol Scand. 2007;85:472-85.
4. Hitzenberger CK. Optical measurement of the axial eye length by laser Doppler interferometry. Invest Ophthalmol Vis Sci. 1991;32:616-24.
5. Hill W, Angeles R, Otani T. Evaluation of a new IOL Master algorithm to measure axial length. J Cataract Refract Surg. 2008;34:920-4.
6. Parravano M, Oddone F, Sampalmieri M, et al. Reliability of the IOL Master in axial length evaluation in silicone oil-filled eyes. Eye (Lond). 2007;21:909-11.
7. Packer M, Fine IH, Hoffman RS, et al. Immersion A-scan compared with partial coherence interferometry: outcomes analysis. J Cataract Refract Surg. 2002;28:239-42.
8. Németh J, Fekete O, Pesztenlehrer N. Optical and ultrasound measurement of axial length and anterior chamber depth for intraocular lens power calculation. J Cataract Refract Surg. 2003;29:85-8.
9. Eleftheriadis H. IOL Master biometry: refractive results of 100 consecutive cases. Br J Ophthalmol. 2003;87:960-3.
10. Rose LT, Moshegov CN. Comparison of the Zeiss IOL Master and applanation A-scan ultrasound: biometry for intraocular lens calculation. Clin Experiment Ophthalmol. 2003;31:121-4.
11. MacLaren RE, Natkunarajah M, Riaz Y, et al. Biometry and formula accuracy with intraocular lenses used for cataract surgery in extreme hyperopia. Am J Ophthalmol. 2007;143:920-31.
12. McNeill JI. Flared phacoemulsification tips to decrease ultrasound time and energy in cataract surgery. J Cataract Refract Surg. 2001;27:1433-6.
13. Sachdev MS, Sachdev G. Femtosecond Laser-assisted Cataract Surgery. In: Nema HV, Nema N (Eds). Cataract Surgery. New Delhi: Health Sciences Publishers; 2018. pp. 397-406.
14. Walkow T, Anders N, Klebe S. Endothelial cell loss after phacoemulsification: relation to preoperative and intraoperative parameters. J Cataract Refract Surg. 2000; 26:727-32.
15. Agarwal A, Agarwal A, Agarwal S, et al. Phakonit: phacoemulsification through a 0.9 mm corneal incision. J Cataract Refract Surg. 2001;27:1548-52.

16. Weikert MP. Update on bimanual microincisional cataract surgery. Curr Opin Ophthalmol. 2006;17:62-7.
17. Alió JL, Rodriguez-Prats JL, Vianello A, et al. Visual outcome of microincision cataract surgery with implantation of an Acri. Smart lens. J Cataract Refract Surg. 2005;31:1549-56.
18. Bauer NJ, de Vries NE, Webers CA, et al. Astigmatism management in cataract surgery with the AcrySoftoric intraocular lens. J Cataract Refract Surg. 2008;34:1483-8.
19. de Vries NE, Nuijts RM. Multifocal intraocular lenses in cataract surgery: literature review of benefits and side effects. J Cataract Refract Surg. 2013;39(2):268-78.
20. Shah S, Cristina Peris-Martinez C, Reinhard T, et al. Visual outcomes after cataract surgery: multifocal versus monofocal intraocular lenses. J Refract Surg. 2015;31(10):658-66.
21. Kaufmann C, Peter J, Ooi K, et al. Limbal relaxing incisions versus on-axis incisions to reduce corneal astigmatism at the time of cataract surgery. J Cataract Refract Surg. 2005;31:2261-5.
22. Khokhar S, Lohiya P, Murugiesan V, et al. Corneal astigmatism correction with opposite clear corneal incisions or single clear corneal incision: comparative analysis. J Cataract Refract Surg. 2006;32:1432-7.
23. Bauer NJ, de Vries NE, Webers CA, et al. Astigmatism management in cataract surgery with the AcrySoftoric intraocular lens. J Cataract Refract Surg. 2008;34:1483-8.
24. Mendicute J, Irigoyen C, Aramberri J, et al. Foldable toric intraocular lens for astigmatism correction in cataract patients. J Cataract Refract Surg. 2008;34:601-7.
25. Novis C. Astigmatism and toric intraocular lenses. Curr Opin Ophthalmol. 2000;11:47-50.
26. Chang DF. Comparative rotational stability of single-piece open-loop acrylic and plate-haptic silicone toric intraocular lenses. J Cataract Refract Surg. 2008;34:1842-7.

CHAPTER 9

Astigmatism Management in Cataract Surgery

Gitansha Shreyas Sachdev, D Ramamurthy

■ INTRODUCTION

Cataract surgery today is fast evolving into a refractive procedure. With the advent of technological advancements including the femtosecond laser for cataract surgery and premium intraocular lenses (IOLs), improved surgical outcomes and postoperative emmetropia can now be achieved. Accurate biometry and IOL power calculation is imperative for correction of spherical refractive errors. Postoperative astigmatism however, may result in suboptimal visual outcomes. While cataract extraction eliminates the lenticular component of astigmatism, corneal astigmatism remains unaffected. The incidence of preexisting corneal astigmatism in patients undergoing cataract extraction is greater than 1 diopter (D) in approximately 30% of the eyes, wherein one-third have an astigmatism exceeding 2 D.[1-4]

Various techniques for the management of coexisting corneal astigmatism have been described including placement of corneal incisions on the steep keratometry axis, paired opposite clear corneal incisions (OCCI), limbal relaxing incision (LRI) or arcuate keratotomies (AK), toric IOL implants, and bioptics. This chapter will provide a comprehensive overview of the available techniques, methods for accurately measuring preoperative corneal astigmatism and intraoperative principles for obtaining optimal refractive outcomes.

■ PREOPERATIVE ASSESSMENT

Preoperative assessment entails determination of the magnitude and axis of corneal astigmatism. Important prerequisites for obtaining accurate measurements include a healthy ocular surface with a stable tear film, absence of corneal epitheliopathy and discontinuation of contact lenses for a minimum period of 5-14 days.

Various devices have been described for the measurement of corneal curvature including manual keratometry, partial coherence interferometry (IOL Master), optical low coherence reflectometry (Lenstar), slit scanning corneal topography (Oculus-Pentacam, Optikgerate GmBH), Dual

Scheimpflug analyzer (Galilei, Ziemer, Switzerland), Fourier domain optical coherence topography and aberrometry ray tracing technology (I trace, Tracey technologies). Keratometry (manual and automated) and placido-based devices provide measurement of the anterior corneal curvature only. An assumed fixed anterior versus posterior corneal curvature ratio is used to calculate the total corneal power.

Corneal tomography measures global corneal astigmatism, identifies the steep and flat meridians, detects subclinical corneal ectasia, such as keratoconus and pellucid marginal degeneration and demonstrates the nature of astigmatism (symmetric versus irregular).

Studies evaluating the repeatability and comparability of corneal astigmatism measurement using different devices demonstrated similar results in certain cohorts,[5,6] while other studies demonstrated significant variability.[7,8]

Ideally, preoperative data should be obtained from a minimum of two devices with different principles of data acquisition.[9]

POSTERIOR CORNEAL ASTIGMATISM

Total corneal astigmatism is a resultant of the contribution from both anterior and posterior corneal surfaces. Anterior corneal astigmatism (ACA) is with-the-rule (WTR) with a drift toward against-the-rule (ATR) with advancing age. Posterior corneal astigmatism (PCA) is generally ATR and demonstrates stability over time. The mean magnitude of PCA is –0.30 D with 9% of the eyes demonstrating an astigmatism in excess of –0.50 D. A maximal value of PCA greater than –0.8 D was demonstrated in corneas with WTR ACA. Correlation between anterior and posterior corneal astigmatism was moderate when steep anterior meridian was aligned vertically, weak when it was oriented obliquely and absent for horizontal alignment.[10]

Traditional devices including keratometry and placido-disc measure only the ACA. Not accounting for the PCA, results in overcorrection of WTR astigmatism by a factor of 1.38 and undercorrection of ATR astigmatism by a factor of 0.65.[11]

The difference is more pronounced in corneal ectatic disorders like keratoconus which elicit a greater effect on the PCA with an average magnitude of 0.95 D in eyes with WTR astigmatism and 0.55 D for ATR astigmatism. Utilizing the ACA only will overestimate the total corneal astigmatism by 0.16 D in WTR and 0.22 D for ATR astigmatism.[12]

PREOPERATIVE CORNEAL MARKING

A precise preoperative corneal marking is an important step to achieve ideal postoperative outcomes. Cyclotorsion of two to three degrees is common from sitting to supine position, with some eyes demonstrating a cyclotorsion of up to 15°.[13] Preoperative corneal marking is therefore imperative to avoid intraoperative errors of misalignment.

Both manual and automated methods are available. *Manual methods* include slit lamp marking with the coaxial thin slit rotated along the horizontal meridian (Fig. 1), pendular marker, bubble marker (Fig. 2) and

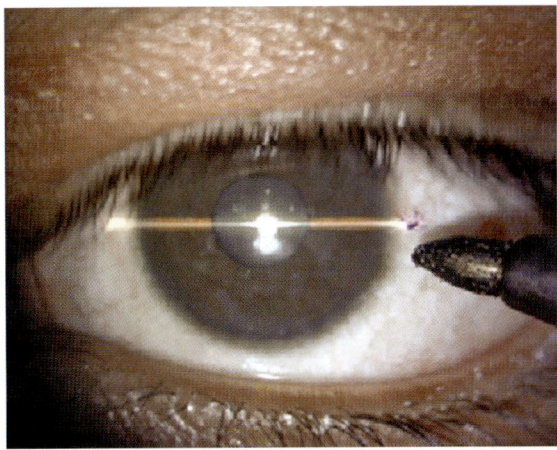

Fig. 1: Slit lamp marking with coaxial thin slit rotated along the horizontal meridian.

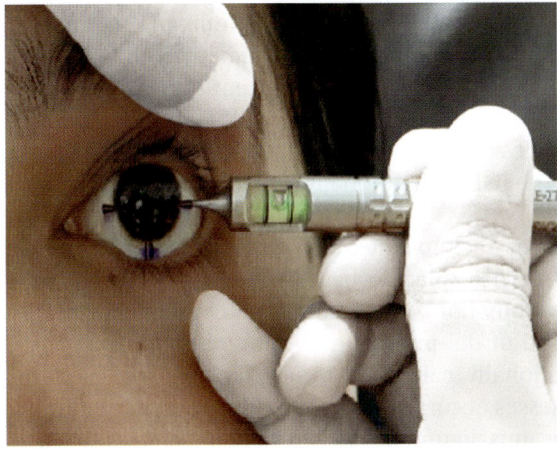

Fig. 2: Nuijts-Solomon bubble marker.

tonometer marker. The marking should be performed while the patient is seated and fixating on a distant target. An adequate topical anesthesia would afford patient comfort. The corneal surface should be dry to prevent the ink marks from spreading. Although the slit lamp marking has least vertical misalignment, the rotational accuracy is greatest with the pendular marker.[14] The three step procedure is described most commonly and entails preoperative ocular marking at the horizontal meridian, intraoperative alignment of the marks to a device with angular gradations [such as Mendez gauge or limbal relaxing incision (LRI) marker] and corneal marking at desired angle of alignment.

Automated methods include image guided systems (Callisto, Carl Zeiss, Germany; True Vision, Goleta, CA and Verion, Alcon, Houston, Texas) and aberrometry-guided devices (ORA, Alcon, Irvine, CA and Holos, Clarity Medical Systems, Pleasanton, CA).

Ocular response analyzer (ORA) is based on the principle of Talbot-Moire interferometry. It allows precise measurement of IOL including spherical and cylindrical power, as well as refinement of the axis by providing the direction and magnitude of rotation required. This is particularly useful in eyes wherein the IOL power calculation is challenging, such as pediatric eyes and post keratorefractive procedures. Precise measurements are obtained in the aphakic mode once the anterior chamber is well formed with viscoelastic. Ocular surface instability, corneal opacities, excessive pressure from the eyelid speculum, unsteady patient fixation and insufficient intraocular pressure (lower than 25 mm Hg) are factors that may compromise accuracy in measurement.[15]

Digital image-guided systems including Callisto and Verion, capture high resolution images of the eye including iris landmarks, limbus, and scleral blood vessels. These serve as reference markers and any change in the position intraoperatively determines the extent of cyclotorsion. Intraoperative overlay additionally provides guidance for placement of corneal incisions, capsulorhexis construction and IOL positioning (Figs. 3A to C). The Verion system includes a comprehensive astigmatism planning software which allows the surgeon to determine the extent of astigmatism to be corrected at the corneal (LRIs) and lenticular plane (toric IOLs). Based on this, the software provides the length and the placement of the LRIs and toricity and alignment of the IOL. It additionally provides an estimated residual manifest error.

I trace (Tracey Technologies, Houston, Texas) combines ray tracing aberrometry and corneal placido-based topography. Preoperative assessment includes determination of the corneal curvature, angle alpha estimation and calculation of the internal and total ocular aberrations. The toric IOL planner additionally calculates toricity and axis of implantation of toric implants, assesses accuracy of preoperative corneal marking and calculates postoperative misalignment and required rotation to achieve optimal outcomes.

SURGICAL METHODS FOR TREATING CORNEAL ASTIGMATISM

Various surgical methods for correction of astigmatism during cataract surgery have been described. Important caveats to remember include aggressive correction of ATR astigmatism, undercorrection of WTR astigmatism and caution to prevent flipping of axis.

Astigmatic Effect of Surgical Incision

Surgically-induced astigmatism (SIA) is the astigmatic effect secondary to the corneal incision. A clear corneal incision results in a flattening effect at the meridian of placement, and a coupling effect steepens the perpendicular axis. Various factors determine the SIA including the site, dimensions, and type of incision.

The induced astigmatism is lowest for temporal incisions and greater following superior incisions. This is because the optical center does not

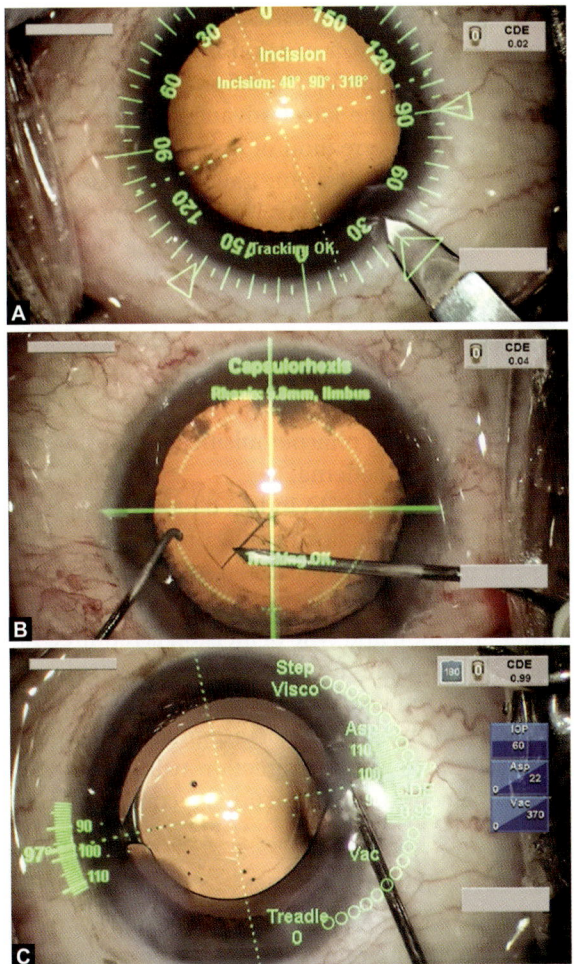

Figs. 3A to C: (A) Verion intraoperative overlay for placement of corneal incisions; (B) Capsulorhexis construction; (C) Intraocular lens positioning.

coincide with the geometric center but is present more nasally and inferiorly. Thus, temporal incisions being the farthest induce the least impact on the corneal curvature in the optical zone. The eyelid induced pressure on the superior incision may further increase its astigmatic effect. Limbal incisions produce lower flattening effect vis-à-vis clear corneal incisions due to greater distance from the optical center. Additionally, faster healing response secondary to limbal vascularity results in earlier stabilization and lower astigmatic effect.

Numerous studies have demonstrated similar astigmatic effect for incision lengths of 2 mm or lower with an average SIA of 0.2–0.3 D. An additional change of 0.25 D in corneal curvature is noted with every subsequent increase of 0.5 mm, and an average SIA of 0.5 D is seen for a 3.2 mm incision. Wound architecture distortion secondary to intraocular lens implantation, should also be considered with an increase in incision size as high as 11%.[16,17] A smaller, temporal, and chevron incision induces least astigmatism effect following sclera-corneal incision in manual small incision cataract surgery.[18]

The femtosecond laser is the latest advancement in the field of cataract surgery. The laser allows the creation of precisely-shaped incisions of pre-determined shape and size. This would theoretically translate into a lower SIA in comparison to manual incisions.[19] However, the data published thus far demonstrated no significant difference between the two groups, while one study demonstrates a greater astigmatism following femtosecond incisions.[20-22] Limitations in imaging and subsequent eye movements during laser delivery can result in a more anterior placement with greater astigmatic effect. Additionally, the inability of the laser to cut through opaque media limits the creation of limbal incisions. Moreover, precise wound geometry would lead to a snug fit of the phacoemulsification probe with subsequent wound distortion and corneal edema.

Surgeons should calculate the SIA induced for different types of incisions. The online SIA calculator (www.doctor-hill.com) determines the astigmatic effect of the incision by evaluating the differences between preoperative and postoperative keratometry values and meridians. A minimum cohort of 30 eyes with consistent location and type of incision is required for analysis.

However, recent improvements in astigmatism calculation include the replacement of SIA by centroid surgical-induced astigmatism. Traditional mean SIA relies on the magnitude of astigmatism alone. Centroid SIA considers the magnitude as well as direction using vector analysis to find the geometric mean. A centroid value of 0.1 is recommended for 2.2-2.4 mm incisions.

Opposite Clear Corneal Incisions

In eyes with astigmatism greater than 0.5 D, opposite clear corneal incisions (OCCI) can be fashioned. The mechanism is based on the assumption that healing tissue forms between the two incisions, and the tissue additive effect results in corneal flattening.

First introduced by Lever and Dahan in 2000, the study demonstrated a mean astigmatic reduction of 2.06 D.[23] However, other studies have demonstrated a mean flattening of 1-1.6 D at 3-months' postoperative visit.[24,25]

Peripheral Corneal or Limbal Relaxing Incisions

Limbal relaxing incisions as a modality for astigmatic correction was first described in 1898. LRIs maintain a coupling ratio of 1:1, wherein the magnitude of flattening observed in the incised meridian is equal to the corresponding steeping in the perpendicular axis. Therefore, no variation is induced in the spherical equivalent obviating the need to compensate the spherical power.

The incisions are created at the outset of the surgical procedure as the epithelial disruptions are minimal and the intraocular pressure consistent.

Moreover, the corneal surface should be relatively dry to assess egress of aqueous fluid in the event of an inadvertent full thickness incision. Precise preoperative corneal marking is imperative as an axis deviation of 5, 10, or 15° results in a 17, 33, and 50% reduction in effect, respectively (Euler's Theorem).[1]

Paired incisions are constructed in the clear cornea, 0.5 mm within the limbus, using a diamond blade at a preset depth of 600 microns or pachymetry adjusted variable depth (90% of the thinnest reading obtained over the entire arc length of the intended axis). The length of the incision depends on the SIA, magnitude, and location of corneal astigmatism and the age of the patient. A number of nomograms have evolved, the Donnenfield and NAPA (Nichamin age and pachymetry-adjusted nomogram) being the most popular (available at www.LRIcalculator.com).

The femtosecond laser allows the creation of precise AK at a predetermined corneal depth (Fig. 4). The placement can either be anterior penetrating (anterior 80% depth cut, posterior 20% uncut) or intrastromal (anterior and posterior 10% uncut, central 80% cut). As these incisions are placed more centrally (8 mm zone), as a general rule of thumb the length of the arc is reduced by 20% vis-à-vis LRIs. Potential advantage of AK includes selective opening allowing postoperative titration of the astigmatic effect.

Although LRIs are a cost-effective and easy method for astigmatism management, the precision of refractive outcomes is limited with risk of irregular astigmatism, over- or undercorrection. Toric IOLs provide greater precision in comparison to corneal-based approach for astigmatism management. Long-term stability is an additional advantage, whereas corneal incisions are prone to regression over time.[26,27]

Toric Intraocular Lenses

Toric IOLs were first introduced in 1992 by Shimizu, as a nonfoldable polymethylmethacrylate (PMMA) material inserted through a 5.7 mm incision.[28]

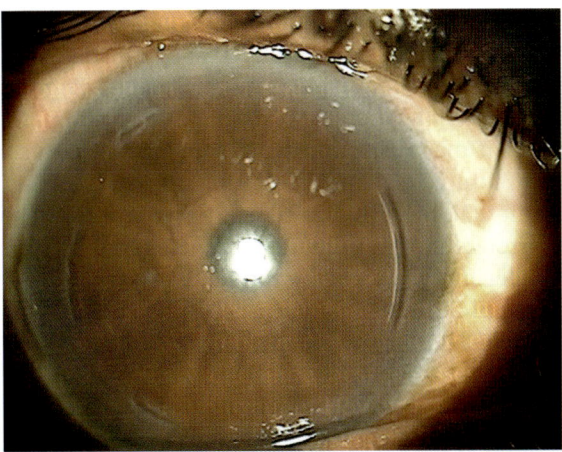

Fig. 4: Femtosecond laser-assisted arcuate keratotomy.

Since then various advancements have resulted in increased predictability and enhanced safety with toric IOL implantation. Toric IOLs are indicated in patients with preoperative corneal astigmatism greater than 1.50 D. A postoperative residual cylindrical error of greater than 0.75 D with multifocal IOLs leads to suboptimal visual outcomes secondary to loss of contrast.[29] Therefore, multifocal toric implants are preferred in cases of preoperative astigmatism greater than 1.0 D. At present, standard toric IOLs are available in cylindrical powers of 1.5 D to 6.0 D (1.03–4.11 D at the corneal plane) and are intended to correct corneal astigmatism from 0.75 D to 4.75 D.[30]

Patient Selection
Preoperative workup entails a comprehensive ocular examination to rule out comorbidities. Eyes with irregular astigmatism secondary to corneal scarring or ectatic disorders should be counseled regarding the possibility of residual error. Toric IOLs should be considered in patients with mild-to-moderate amount of irregular astigmatism who can be satisfactorily corrected with spectacles. Zonular instability and posterior capsular dehiscence are considered contraindications for toric implants.

Intraocular Lens Power Calculation
Earlier nomograms for toric IOL power include Alcon and Holladay toric calculator. Newer nomograms have evolved with greater understanding of corneal astigmatism. Baylor nomogram incorporates the PCA while calculating the IOL power.[10] Barrett formula additionally incorporates the effective lens position, by considering the anterior chamber depth and axial length. The new Alcon toric calculator incorporates the Barrett formula. The total corneal astigmatism is estimated as a vector based on keratometry values from optical low coherence reflectometry using Abulafia-Koch linear regression formula.[31]

Surgical Procedure
The various methods for corneal marking and intraoperative IOL positioning have been discussed. A well-centered capsulorhexis providing an adequate 360° IOL overlap is essential to ensure IOL stability. The correct placement of the IOL involves gross and fine positioning. Following in the capsular bag implantation, the IOL should be placed 10–20° short of the intended axis, as the implant may rotate during subsequent viscoelastic removal. It is imperative to completely remove the ophthalmic viscosurgical device (OVD) behind the IOL to minimize risk of postoperative rotation. The IOL is subsequently rotated to the intended axis using the irrigation-aspiration probe or IOL dialer. The marks of the toric IOL indicate the flat meridian or plus cylinder axis of the toric IOL and should be aligned with the marked alignment axis. An adequate wound hydration should be achieved to maintain a stable anterior chamber.

Stability of Toric Intraocular Lens
Long-term stability of toric implants is necessary as postoperative rotation results in suboptimal visual outcomes. Every degree of misalignment induces

a 3.3% loss of astigmatic correction with a complete nullification following a 30° rotation.[32]

Toric IOL rotation can be seen as early as 1 hour postoperative and is more common within the first 10 days.[33] Early rotation can occur secondary to incomplete OVD removal. Late rotation is associated with IOL design and material, inadequate capsulorhexis overlap, larger axial length and vertical axis of implantation.[34,35] Toric IOLs are available in various materials including hydrophilic acrylic, hydrophobic acrylic, silicone and PMMA. Additionally, both aspheric and spherical implants are commercially available. Maximum rotational stability is observed with hydrophobic acrylic material. This is secondary to the development of strong adhesions between the IOL material and the lens capsule in the early postoperative period. Extracellular matrix proteins especially fibronectin play a major role in IOL capsular bag adhesion. Acrylic IOLs explanted from human autopsy eyes contained significantly more fibronectin in comparison to PMMA and silicone.[36] Silicone IOLs demonstrated the least stability with plate-haptics performing slightly better than conventional three piece lenses.[37]

Significant rotation requiring IOL repositioning should ideally be performed 1 week after IOL implantation. A negative correlation has been established between the interval from cataract surgery to repositioning procedure and the degree of residual misalignment.[38]

On the other hand, excessive delay beyond a couple of weeks may pose difficulties during the second intervention, as adhesions may form between the IOL and capsular bag.[39]

Online toric IOL calculators (Berdahl and Hardten) are available at www.astigmatismfix.com to determine the ideal position in case of malrotation. The calculation is derived from the postoperative manifest refraction and the power and axis of the toric implant. An alternate method includes wavefront aberrometry to calculate the internal aberrations to determine the correct orientation of the toric implant.[40,41]

Cases with large residual error not amenable to correction by repositioning would require IOL exchange, piggyback IOLs or keratoablative refractive correction (bioptics).

Bioptics

The eye offers the surgeon two distinct planes, the lenticular and the corneal on which to engineer refractive improvements. Sometimes a correction on just one plane is insufficient to achieve clear vision. The concept of bioptics was introduced by Zaldivar in 2002, when he performed laser in situ-keratomileusis (LASIK) to correct residual refractive error in eyes with phakic implants.[42]

A detailed anterior segment evaluation is mandatory, with special attention to the ocular surface health. Preoperative dry eye, persistent epithelial erosions, meibomian gland dysfunction or blepharitis if present should be treated. Systemic disorders like diabetes should be well-controlled as they may interfere with wound healing. Preoperative corneal tomography to determine the ideal refractive procedure should be done. Available options include surface ablation, microkeratome-assisted LASIK and femtosecond-laser assisted LASIK. While using a microkeratome the intraocular pressure is elevated in an eye that has recently undergone a penetrating corneal incision. One should ideally wait for a period of 3 months to achieve wound healing and refractive stability.

Surface ablation is the preferred modality for eyes with lower pachymetry, such as those with prior refractive surgery. The advantages include earlier intervention in comparison to flap based procedures. Disadvantages include postoperative patient discomfort and increased risk of infection and haze.

CONCLUSION

In conclusion, a meticulous preoperative evaluation and intraoperative execution are imperative to achieve optimal visual outcomes. The importance of PCA should be recognized, and investigative modalities calculating both anterior and posterior corneal curvature should be standard of care. Various advancements have been seen in the methods for preoperative marking including image-guided and aberrometry-guided devices, resulting in increased intraoperative precision. Improvements in the design and material of toric implants afford greater rotational stability and superior refractive outcomes.

REFERENCES

1. Nichamin LD. Astigmatism control. Ophthalmol Clin North Am. 2006;19:485-93.
2. Chen W, Zuo C, Chen C, et al. Prevalence of corneal astigmatism before cataract surgery in Chinese patients. J Cataract Refract Surg. 2013;39:188-92.
3. Ferrer-Blasco T, Montes-Mico R, Peixoto-de-Matos SC, et al. Prevalence of corneal astigmatism before cataract surgery. J Cataract Refract Surg. 2009;35:70-5.
4. Hoffman PC, Hutz WW. Analysis of biometry and prevalence data for corneal astigmatism in 23,239 eyes. J Cataract Refract Surg. 2010;36:1479-85.
5. Lee H, chung JL, Kim EK, et al. Univariate and bivariate polar value analysis of corneal astigmatism measurements obtained with 6 instruments. J Cataract Refract Surg. 2012;38:1608-15.
6. Shirmaya M, Wang L, Weikert MP, et al. Comparison of corneal powers obtained from 4 different devices. Am J Ophthalmol. 2009;148:528-35.
7. Visser N, Berendschot TT, Verbakel F, et al. Comparibility and repeatibilty of corneal astigmatism measurements using different measurement technologies. J Cataract Refract Surg. 2012;38:1764-70.
8. Crawford AZ, Patel DV, McGhee CN. Comparison and repeatability of keratometric and corneal power measurements obtained by Orbscan II, Pentacam, and Galilei corneal tomography systems. Am J Ophthalmol. 2013;156:53-60.
9. Browne AW, Osher RH. Optimizing precision in toric lens selection by combining keratometric techniques. J Refract Surg. 2014;30:67-72.
10. Koch D, Ali SF, Weikert MP, et al. Contribution of posterior corneal astigmatism to total corneal astigmatism. J Cataract Refract Surg. 2012;38:2080-87.
11. Goggin M, Zamora-Alejo k, Esterman A, et al. Adjustment OF anterior corneal astigmatism values to incorporate the likely effect of posterior corneal curvature for toric intraocular lens calculation. J Refract Surg. 2015;31:98-102.

12. Savini G, Naeser K, Schiano-Lomoriello D, et al. Influence of posterior corneal astigmatism on total corneal astigmatism in eyes with keratoconus. Cornea. 2016;35:1427-33.
13. Chang J. Cyclotorsion during laser in situ keratomileusis. J Cataract Refract Surg. 2008;34(10):1718-23.
14. Popp N, Hirnschall N, Maedel S, et al. Evaluation of 4 corneal astigmatic marking methods. J Cataract Refract Surg. 2012;38:2094-9.
15. Stringham J, Pettey J, Olson RJ. Evaluation of variables affecting intraoperative aberrometry. J Cataract Refract Surg. 2012;38:470-4.
16. Febbraro JL, Wang L, Borasio E, et al. Astigmatic equivalence of 2.2 mm and 1.8 mm superior clear corneal cataract incision. Graefes Arch Clin Exp Ophthalmol. 2015;253:261-5.
17. Gross RH, Miller KM. Corneal astigmatism after phacoemulsification and lens implantation through unsutured scleral and corneal tunnel incisions. Am J Ophthalmol. 1996;121:57-64.
18. Jauhari N, Chopra D, Chaurasia RK, et al. Comparison of surgically induced astigmatism in various incisions in manual small incision cataract surgery. Int J Ophthalmol. 2014;7(6):1001-4.
19. Steinert RF. Application of the Femtosecond Laser in Cataract Surgery for the Creation of Multi-Planar, Self-Sealing Incisions, ASCRS 2010, Boston.
20. Diakonis VF, Yesilirmak N, Cabot F, et al. Comparison of surgically induced astigmatism between femtosecond laser and manual clear corneal incisions for cataract surgery. J Cataract Refract Surg. 2015;41:2075-80.
21. Nagy Z, Dunai A, Kranitz K, et al. Evaluation of femtosecond laser assisted and manual clear corneal incisions on surgically induced astigmatism and higher order aberrations. J Refract Surg. 2014;30:522-25.
22. Zhu S, Qu N, Wang W, et al. Morphologic features and surgically induced astigmatism of femtosecond laser versus manual clear corneal incisions. J Cataract Refract Surg. 2017;43(11):1430-5.
23. Lever J, Dahan E. Opposite clear corneal incision to correct preexisting astigmatism in cataract surgery. J Cataract Refract Surg. 2000;26:803-5.
24. Khokhar S, Lohiya P, Murugiesan V, et al. Corneal astigmatism correction with opposite clear corneal incision or single clear corneal incision. J Cataract Refract Surg. 2006;32:1432-7.
25. Nemeth G, Kolozsvari B, Berta A, et al. Paired opposite clear corneal incision: time related changes of its effects and factors on which these changes depend. Eur J Ophthalmol. 2014;0:2-14.
26. Poll JT, Wang L, Koch DD, et al. Correction of astigmatism during cataract surgery: toric intraocular lens compare to peripheral corneal relaxing incisions. J Refract Surg. 2011;27:165-71.
27. Mingo-Botin D, Munoz-Negrete FJ, Won Kim HR, et al. Comparison of toric intraocular lens and peripheral corneal relaxing incisions to treat astigmatism during cataract surgery. J Cataract Refract Surg. 2010;36:1432-7.
28. Shimizu K, Misawa A, Suzuki Y. Toric intraocular lenses: correcting astigmatism while controlling axis shift. J Cataract Refract Surg. 1994;20:523-6.
29. Pepose JS. Maximizing satisfaction with presbyopia correcting intraocular lenses: the missing links. Am J Ophthalmol 2008;146:641-8.
30. Khan MI, Chang SW, Muhtaseb M. The use of toric intraocular lens to correct astigmatism at the time of cataract surgery. Oman J Ophthalmol. 2015;8:38-43.
31. Abulafia A, Koch DD, Wang L, et al. New regression formula for toric intraocular lens calculations. J Cataract Refract Surg. 2016;42:663-71.

32. Ma JJ, Tseng SS. Simple method for accurate alignment in toric phakic and aphakic intraocular lens implant. J Cataract Refract Surg. 2008;34:1631-6.
33. Miyake T, Kimaye K, Amano R, et al. Long term clinical outcomes of toric intraocular lens impl antation in cataract cases with preexisting astigmatism. J Cataract Refract Surg. 2014;40:1654-60.
34. Ruhswurm I, Scholz U, Zehetmayer M, et al. Astigmatism correction with foldable toric intraocular lens in cataract patients. J Cataract Refract Surg. 2000;26:1022-7.
35. Shah GD, Praveen MR, Vasavada AR, et al. Rotational stability of a toric intraocular lens: influence of axial length and alignment in the capsular bag. J Cataract Refract Surg. 2012;38:54-9.
36. Linnola RJ, Werner L, Pandey SK, et al. Adhesion of fibronectin, vitronectin, laminin, and collagen type IV to intraocular lens material in pseudophakic human autopsy eyes. Part 1: histological sections. J Cataract Refract Surg. 2000;26:1792-806.
37. Paul CK, Ormonde S, Rosen PH, et al. Postoperative intraocular lens rotation: A randomised comparison of plate and loop haptic implants. Ophthalmol. 1999;106:2190-5.
38. Oshika T, Inamura M, Inoue Y, et al. Incidence and outcomes of repositioning surgery to correct misalignment of toric intraocular lens. Ophthalmol. 2018;125:31-5.
39. Chang DF. Repositioning technique and rate for toric intraocular lenses. J Cataract Refract Surg. 2009;35(7):1315-6.
40. Berdahl JP, Hardten DR. Residual astigmatism after toric intraocular lens implanataion. J Cataract Refract Surg. 2012;38:730-1.
41. Lockwood JC, Randelman JB. Toric intraocular lens rotation to optimize refractive outcome despite appropriate intraoperative positioning. J Cataract Refract Surg. 2015;41:878-83.
42. Zaldiver R, Oscherow S, Piezzi V. Bioptics in phakic and pseudophakic intraocular lens with the Nidek EC- 500 excimer laser. J Refract Surg. 2002;18:S336-9.

CHAPTER 10

Pseudoexfoliation Cataract: Management

Prakrati Gupta, Sirisha Senthil

■ INTRODUCTION

Pseudoexfoliation syndrome (PXF) was first described by John Lindberg, a Finnish ophthalmologist.[1] It is an age-related fibrillopathy, with manifestations primarily in the eye.[2]

Dandruff like white deposits accumulates progressively in the anterior chamber (AC), its angle, anterior surface of the lens, zonules, ciliary processes, trabecular meshwork and the pupillary margin. One of the earliest sites for clinically evident exfoliation to be observed is on the anterior capsule of the lens and on the margin of the pupil. The prevalence of PXF is variable across the populations with highest prevalence in Scandinavian population.[3]

In southern India in individuals aged 40 years or more, the prevalence of PXF ranges from 3.01% to 6.0%.[4] Weak zonular support and poor pupillary dilatation can lead to complications during cataract surgery in eyes with PXF. A thorough preoperative assessment and intraoperative care is needed to avoid cataract surgical complications and have a good surgical outcome in eyes with PXF.

■ PREOPERATIVE EVALUATION

Preoperative evaluation of patients with PXF syndrome is essential in preventing devastating complications during cataract surgery. Often, the PXF deposits may be subtle and the condition can be missed. Strong index of suspicion, meticulous pre- and post-pupillary dilatation examination with the help of slit lamp and using higher magnification and oblique illumination would help to identify PXF on various ocular structures.

Foreseeing potential difficulties is important to prepare the surgeon for a safe surgery. Preoperatively all the risks and benefits of the surgery should be explained to the patient.

Corneal Evaluation

Endothelial deposits of pseudoexfoliation material may be seen,[5] which may range from tiny deposits to large flakes. These eyes may be associated with endothelial cell loss which may lead to early endothelial decompensation.[6] This can occur spontaneously or with minimal increase in intraocular pressure (IOP) even in phakic eyes or following an uncomplicated cataract surgery.

Anterior Chamber Depth

Anterior chamber depth is a strong indirect indicator of lens subluxation. Careful assessment of the depth of the AC in all the quadrants is important and should always be compared between the two eyes. The AC can become shallow or deep depending upon the lens subluxation. Anterior subluxation will lead to shallowing, whereas posterior subluxation of the lens will cause deepening of the AC (with asymmetry in the two eyes).

Asymmetry may be evident on gonioscopy, with unilateral closed angles or wide-open angle with excess trabecular meshwork pigmentation.

In PXF eyes, zonular instability may cause unilateral shallowing of the AC. This may increase the risk of complications. In a study by Kuchle et al.,[7] 13.4% intraoperative complications occurred in eyes with PXF and AC depth of less than 2.5 mm as compared to 6.9% over all incidences and 2.8% incidence of complications when AC depth was 2.5 mm or more.

Preoperative counseling about the possible complications and additional interventions that may be needed in the presence of PXF with lens subluxation is very important.

Pupillary Ruff

Pseudoexfoliation is classically associated with peripupillary iris transillumination and pupillary ruff defects.[8] In PXF eyes, the assumption is that the anterior surface of the lens and pigment layer of the iris are in close proximity with resultant pigment dispersion.

Gradual release of pigment occurs due to rubbing of iris against the rough lens capsule during physiologic pupillary movements or in presence of cataract or subluxated lens with anterior displacement of the lens[9] (Figs. 1A to F).

Pupil Size

Pupils of patients with pseudoexfoliation show poor pupillary dilatation with mydriatic agents though this is not a pathognomonic sign for PXF. This happens due to excessive accumulation of the exfoliated material into the extracellular matrix of the iris stroma, which prevents mydriasis of the pupil by mechanical obstruction. Also, the iris pigment epithelium is adherent to the anterior lens surface due to the exfoliation material, causing restriction of pupillary movements. In addition, in PXF, the iris muscle fibers undergo degenerative and atrophic changes, which occur due to tissue hypoxia, which also contribute to inadequate pupillary dilatation.[10]

Cataract Density

Lens opacification and predominantly nuclear sclerosis is more common in PXF patients.[11,12] One of the important distinctive signs of PXF is deposition

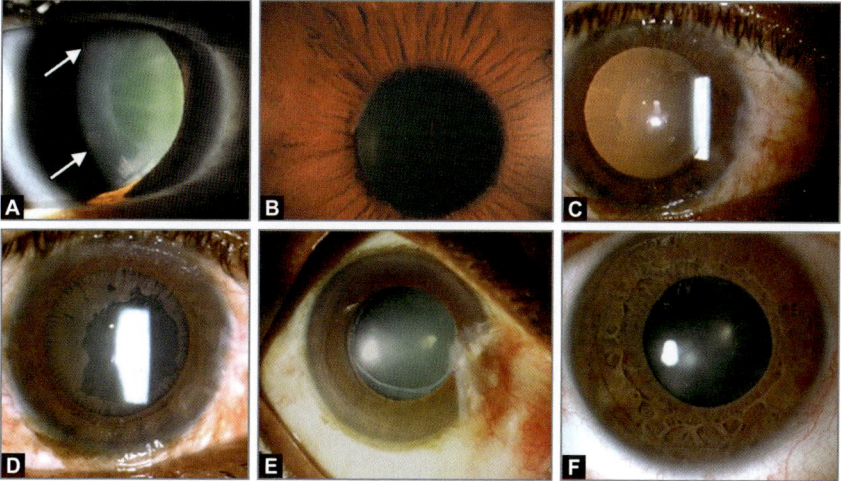

Figs. 1A to F: (A) Slit lamp examination showing brown radial pigments in the periphery suggestive of pigmentary form of pseudoexfoliation (arrows); (B) Diffuse slit lamp examination showing white dandruff like pseudoexfoliation deposits on the pupil; (C) Diffuse slit lamp examination showing white dandruff like pseudoexfoliation deposits on the anterior lens capsule in retroillumination; (D to F) Slit lamp examination showing white dandruff like pseudoexfoliation peripheral ring with anterior curling edges of the deposits on the lens capsule and pterygium with hyalinization of the iris vessels.

of dandruff like material on the anterior lens surface that may be present in the classic trizonal distribution. The changes of exfoliation can be very subtle and can be easily missed in undilated pupil. Hence, meticulous examination is very important to diagnose the condition early. Dilated examination under high magnification and retroillumination would help pick up early signs of PXF of the anterior lens capsule.

The typical presentation of PXF has three different areas after dilatation:
1. **Central zone** is a homogenous white sheet usually corresponding approximately to the diameter of the pupil. It can be absent in almost 20% of the cases.
2. **Peripheral zone** is often layered, granular and always present.
3. **The intermediate clear zone:** The movement of the iris above the anterior lens surface causes a clear intermediate zone.

Phacodonesis

In PXF, phacodonesis is not uncommon. This happens due to zonular instability. During cataract surgery, the weak zonules may lead to increased complication rates. In these eyes cataractous lenses may subluxate with anterior or posterior displacement or may dislocate either completely or partially. Maximum pupillary dilatation best assesses zonular instability, phacodonesis, and signs of subluxation. However, since these eyes do not often dilate well, there is a likelihood of missing phacodonesis preoperatively.

Zonular Instability

Exfoliative material depositing on the zonular fibers and ciliary processes lead to proteolytic disintegration of the zonules leading to zonular instability. This proteolytic disintegration is caused by lysosomal enzymes, which has been demonstrated in pseudoexfoliative aggregates immunohistochemically.[13] In cases of zonular dehiscence, preoperatively identification of the severity and the number of clock hours of dehiscence are critical in determining the safe surgical approach.

There are certain direct and indirect signs of zonular instability:
- **Direct signs:** Phacodonesis, lens subluxation, iridodonesis and zonular dialysis.
- **Indirect signs:** Small pupil with either a shallow or hyper-deep AC (compared to the other eye).

Phacodonesis, iris flutter, or subtle iridodonesis are the earliest signs of zonulopathy. Iridodonesis can be detected by relaxing the zonules with the help of 2% pilocarpine. For phacodonesis, a grading scale from +1 to +4 exists which helps the surgeon to plan the technique to cataract extraction.

Intraocular Pressure

The pigments released from the iris and fibrillar deposits cause clogging of the trabecular meshwork, thus leading to increased IOP in eyes with PXF. These patients need close monitoring as the IOP can rise dramatically within months. The diurnal control of IOP is worse in pseudoexfoliation eyes as compared to other primary glaucomas.[14] In unilateral PXF eyes, the IOP is higher as compared to the contralateral eye without PXF.[15] In a study by Shingleton et al.,[16] IOP reduction after phacoemulsification is proportional to the preoperative IOP. Higher the preoperative IOP, greater is the postoperative IOP reduction. They also noted that in PXF eyes, the postoperative day one spikes were 30 mm Hg or higher. Hence, due precaution should be taken while operating on PXF eyes with advanced disc and field damage. Postoperative aqueous suppressants, oral or topical are recommended postoperatively in eyes with elevated IOP and/or advanced disc damage.

■ PSEUDOEXFOLIATION AND CATARACT SURGERY

During cataract surgery, there is an increased risk of intraoperative complications in PXF eyes. Most common ones are posterior capsular rent, vitreous loss, and zonular dehiscence.

In a publication by Lumme et al.,[17] eyes with PXF had more intraoperative complications. The vitreous loss was fourfold and there was tenfold AC intraocular lens (ACIOL) placement compared to non-PXF eyes.

However, with the recent modified surgical techniques, better instrumentation and understanding the complication rates are far less.[18] In pseudoexfoliation eyes, phacoemulsification is a good choice of surgery for cataract extraction with the use of specialized adjunctive devices.[19] In India, small incision surgery is a safe and effective alternative for patients with pseudoexfoliation which offers the advantage of being economical and being applicable in low resource settings. However care has to be taken to perform certain steps that would make the cataract surgery safe.

Intraoperative Challenges

Small Pupil

Crucial prerequisite for a good surgical outcome is the adequately dilated pupil throughout cataract surgery. In eyes with PXF, small pupil poses the greatest risk for increased intraoperative complications. The small pupil can be dilated with the help of various techniques.

- **Viscodilatation:** This is done with a high molecular weight cohesive viscoelastics or pseudodispersive viscoelastics, such as Healon GV or Healon 5.
- Mini-sphincterotomies with microscissors (Figs. 2A to C)
- Pupil expansion devices:
  - **Two-instrument iris stretch:**[20] This is done with the help of Kuglen or Y-hooks. Viscoelastic is used for AC deepening. Two hooks are used to stretch the pupillary margin. This is achieved by hooking the iris margin with the hooks from opposite paracentesis ports, and is moved 180° apart towards the limbus and held in a stretched position for a moment (at least 30 seconds). If necessary this can be repeated

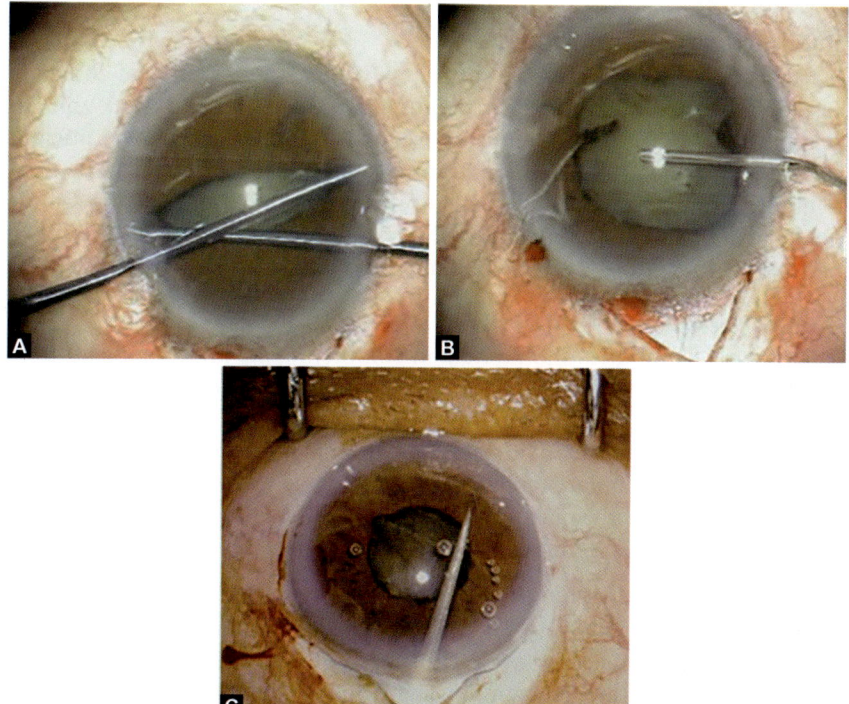

Figs. 2A to C: Pupillary stretch with Kuglen hooks (A and B) and multiple sphincterotomies (C) during cataract surgery.

90° apart for additional stretch avoiding damage to the lens and corneal endothelium (Fig. 2). This causes tears in the pupillary margin and helps with dilatation.
- **Retractors:** Iris retractors can be used to enlarge the pupil, often in a diamond configuration. The retractors are placed through 3 or 4 paracentesis ports and the pupillary margin is hooked and beaded after adequate stretching. Always avoid the main incision for placing the retractors.[20]
- **Ring:** Pupil expander ring or Malyugin ring,[21] can also be used to dilate the pupil. This can be inserted through the main incision and can avoid additional paracentesis.

Capsulorhexis
In eyes with PXF, adequately sized and well-centered continuous curvilinear capsulorhexis (CCC) should be planned. CCC is more challenging in cases with weak zonules as zonular counter traction is compromised.[19]

Hydrodissection
Good hydrodissection is extremely important. This helps to relieve the capsulo-cortical and capsule-nuclear adhesions there by decreasing the resistance to nuclear rotation. This also helps to facilitate free movement of the nuclear fragments during phacoemulsification, thus minimizing undue stress on the zonules.[22]

Small Incision Cataract Surgery
Manual small incision cataract surgery (SICS) is a better surgical choice in cases of the hard nucleus with poor pupillary dilatation and weak zonules (Figs. 3A to D). Appropriate incision size based on the size of the nucleus should be planned. Mini sphincterotomies with micro-scissors can be used to enlarge the pupil size. Large capsulorhexis, good hydrodissection, gentle nuclear rotation, careful nucleus delivery, and cortical aspiration should be performed. In-the-bag intraocular lens (IOL) is a good option even with SICS.

Phacoemulsification Technique
Nucleotomy techniques should help in completing the phacoemulsification safely. Some of the tips are, gentle nuclear rotation, direct chop technique or stop and chop may help to minimize zonular stress, and two instruments can be used for nuclear rotation. However, this is based on the density of the cataract and zonular stability. Vertical chop is useful particularly when working in an eye with small pupil and zonular instability, when the cataract is not very hard (Figs. 4A and B).

Removal of Cortical Material
Cortical aspiration is a very critical step and can worsen the pre-existing zonular weakness in these eyes. During cortical aspiration, identification of subtle signs that indicate zonular instability is very important to prevent serious complications. During the cortical aspiration, capsule equator collapse, peripheral posterior capsular folds or visibility of the peripheral

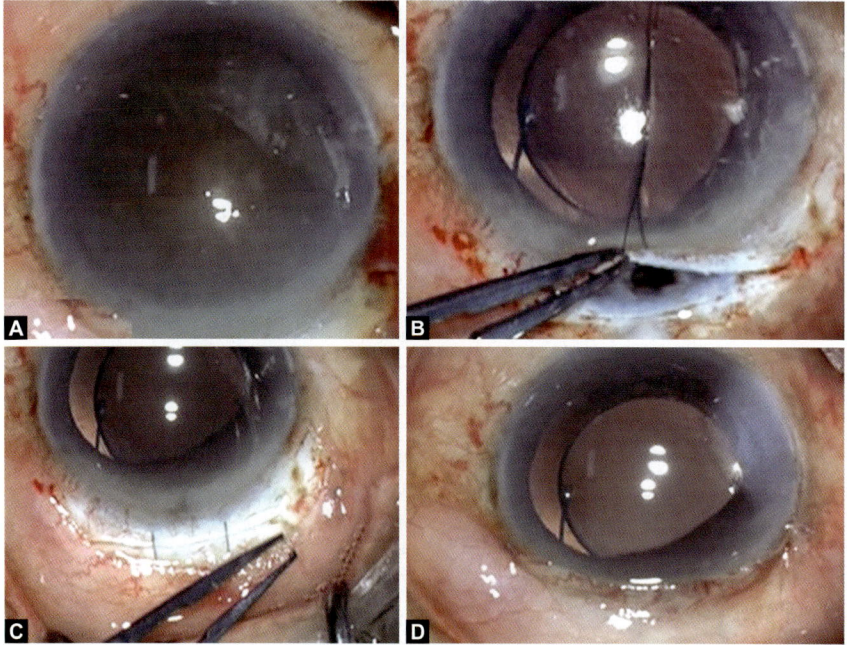

Figs. 3A to D: Intraoperative photographs showing steps of small incision cataract surgery with trabeculectomy in an eye with brown cataract.

capsular fornix indicates zonular instability. Tangential stripping of the cortex under low flow conditions reduces undue tension on zonules during and can prevent further worsening of zonular dialysis.

Adjunctive Devices for Zonular Weakness

Several capsular support devices are available to provide support to the weak capsular bag and zonular apparatus. The device selection depends upon progressive and static zonulopathy, the integrity of the capsule and number of clock hours of zonular dialysis.

Capsular Tension Ring

A capsular tension ring (CTR) is an open-ring device, C-shaped and made up of polymethyl methacrylate (PMMA) material. It comes in various sizes, with suturing eyelets at either end of the rings. It stretches the posterior capsule as it is slightly larger than the capsular bag and provides uniform radial forces to the bag. These forces act to recenter a decentered capsular bag. Thus, CTR ensures safe and effective surgery.

CTR's also reduces decentration of the IOL and thus helps to improve visual acuity.[23] In addition, it decreases postoperative capsular contraction (phimosis) and posterior capsular opacification.[24] A CTR can be inserted at any time after the capsulorhexis, before or after nucleus removal or after cortical wash. However, epinucleus or cortical wash may be difficult after CTR insertion.[25] A CTR is contraindicated, if there is a tear in the anterior or posterior capsule, as the tear will almost certainly extend given the force

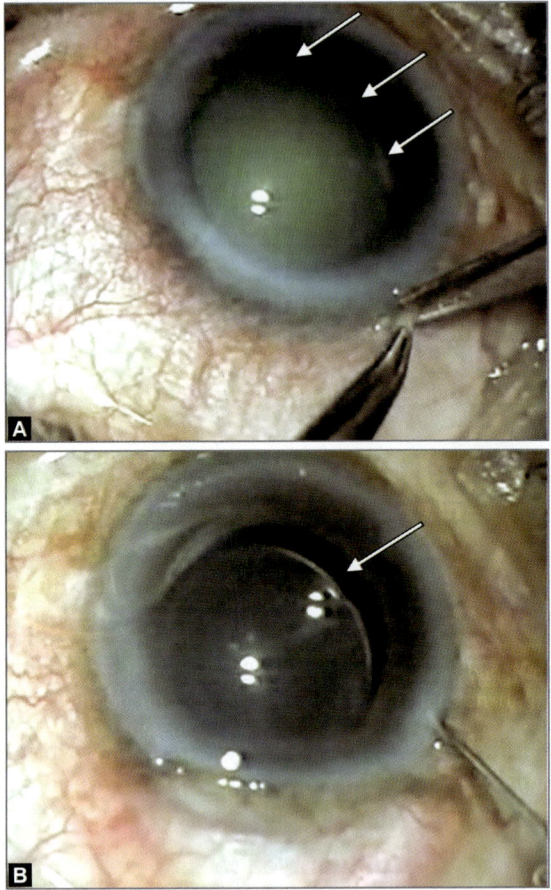

Figs. 4A and B: Intraoperative photographs showing subluxated lens (A) (arrows) at the start of phacotrabeculectomy and (B) in-the-bag intraocular lens with subluxation (arrow).

placed on the capsular bag during insertion. In cases of progressive zonular weakness, severe subluxation of more than 180°, a modified CTR or Cionni ring is the best option.

It has scleral fixation hook which can be fixed using transscleral fixation suture.[26]

Capsule Tension Segment

Capsule tension segment (CTS) is indicated in cases with severe zonular instability, typically greater than four clock hours or profound generalized zonular weakness and phacodonesis. It is made of PMMA and is a partial ring design spanning 90° with a raised single eyelet centrally, which remains above the anterior capsule. It can be inserted into the capsular bag any time after capsulorhexis.

One or two CTS devices may be used depending on the degree of zonular instability. In contrast to CTR, it can be placed in the area of greatest zonular weakness even in the presence of small posterior or anterior capsular tear.[27]

Capsule Retractors

In cases of severe zonulopathy, capsule retractors center the capsular bag and provide additional anteroposterior support. While using the capsule retractors one should avoid anterior capsule edge tear or equatorial capsule puncturing.[28,29]

Intraocular Lens Selection

The IOL selection in PXF eyes depends upon stability of the capsule.

Silicon IOL which are flexible should be avoided because they cause anterior capsule opacification and increase risk of capsular contraction syndrome.[30]

Single piece foldable IOLs may be a better choice in these eyes as they need less manipulation during implantation and hence less chance of damage to the capsule and zonules.

Sulcus placed IOL in the absence of zonular support should be avoided. Using toric or multifocal IOLs may be avoided as zonular instability and capsule contraction may result in decentration of the IOL and visual disturbance.[22]

Intraocular Lens Fixation

When endocapsular placement is not possible, the most widely used approaches are:
- Scleral fixated lens (with or without sutures)
- Iris claw lens
- AC angle supported IOLs (ACIOL)

Glued-scleral IOL is a good surgical choice in cases of severe zonular instability in PXF eyes.[31] Due to higher endothelial cell loss in PXF eyes, ACIOL can lead to corneal decompensation and hence should be avoided.[19]

POSTOPERATIVE COMPLICATIONS

Postoperatively, PXF eyes may show early and late complications.

Early Postoperative Complications

- As the blood-aqueous barrier is altered in PXF eyes, inflammation in the AC is severe and prolonged.[29]
- Inflammation also causes capsule contraction and cystoid macular edema (CME).[32] Topical nonsteroidal anti-inflammatory drugs (NSAIDs) may be beneficial in these cases. Compared to non-PXF eyes IOP spikes postoperatively are higher and more common in PXF eyes.[33]

Late Postoperative Complications (Figs. 5A and B)

- Anterior capsular phimosis—the anterior capsule contracts leading to tilt or decentration of the IOL.[34]
- This can be treated either by Nd:YAG (Neodymium: yttrium aluminum garnet) laser relaxing incisions or can be cut surgically with the help of microscissors. At the earliest sign of fibrosis,[22] Nd:YAG laser should be used to release capsular traction and prevent IOL displacement.

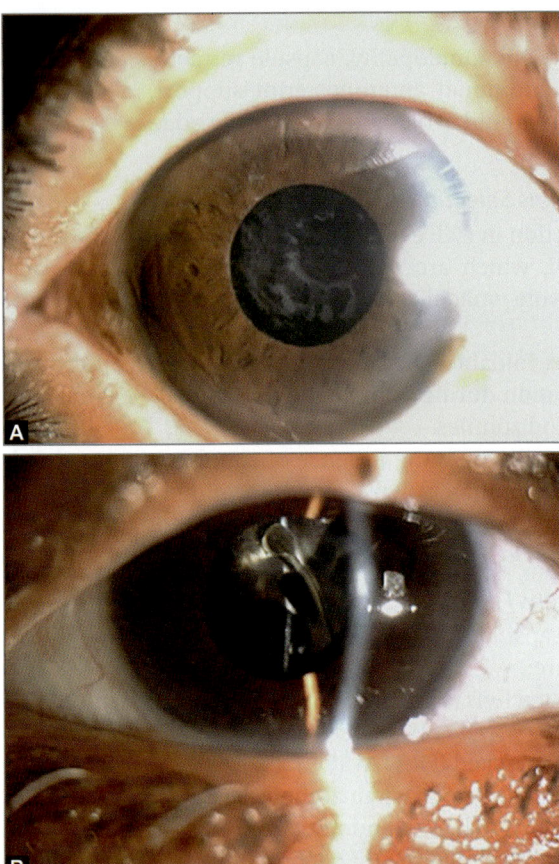

Figs. 5A and B: (A) Slit lamp photograph showing pseudoexfoliation deposits on the intraocular lens; (B) Capsular phimosis with displacement of haptic of intraocular lens in an eye with pseudoexfoliation.

- *IOL instability:* In eyes with PXF, the incidence of subluxation or dislocation of IOL postoperatively is higher (mean 8.5 years after initial surgery) as compared to non-PXF eyes.[35] Progressive disintegration of the zonules and contraction of the capsule can lead to IOL instability and may occur many years postoperatively even with uneventful surgery.[19]
- When the entire capsular bag IOL complex is dislocated, it can be sutured to the sclera, however is technically challenging and is associated with serious complications.[36] Some cases may need explanation of the IOL-bag complex by an anterior or posterior approach.

CONCLUSION

Cataract surgery in eyes with pseudoexfoliation is challenging. The high incidence of intraoperative complications during surgery warrant proper preoperative evaluation and planning. Meticulous surgery can prevent serious complications and ensures good outcome. Long-term follow-up even after uneventful cataract surgery is recommended in view of associated late complications like elevated IOP and IOL displacement.

REFERENCES

1. Tarkkanen A, Kivela T, John G. Lindberg and the discovery of exfoliation syndrome. Acta Ophthalmol Scand. 2002;80(2):151-4.
2. Ritch R, Schlotzer-Schrehardt U. Exfoliation syndrome. Surv Ophthalmol. 2001;45(4):265-315.
3. Desai MA, Lee RK. The medical and surgical management of pseudoexfoliation glaucoma. Int Ophthalmol Clin. 2008;48(4):95-113.
4. Thomas R, Nirmalan PK, Krishnaiah S. Pseudoexfoliation in southern India: the Andhra Pradesh eye disease study. Invest Ophthalmol Vis Sci. 2005;46(4):1170-6.
5. Ariga M, Nivean M, Utkarsha P. Pseudoexfoliation syndrome. J Curr Glaucoma Pract. 2013;7(3):118-20.
6. Naumann GO, Schlotzer-Schrehardt U. Keratopathy in pseudoexfoliation syndrome as a cause of corneal endothelial decompensation: A clinicopathologic study. Ophthalmol. 2000;107(6):1111-24.
7. Kuchle M, Viestenz A, Martus P, et al. Anterior chamber depth and complications during cataract surgery in eyes with pseudoexfoliation syndrome. Am J Ophthalmol. 2000;129(3):281-5.
8. Prince AM, Ritch R. Clinical signs of the pseudoexfoliation syndrome. Ophthalmol. 1986;93(6):803-7.
9. Aasved H. Incidence of defects in the pigmented pupillary ruff in eyes with and without fibrillopathia epitheliocapsularis (so-called senile exfoliation or pseudoexfoliation of the anterior lens capsule). Acta Ophthalmol (Copenh). 1973;51(5):710-5.
10. Asano N, Schlotzer-Schrehardt U, Naumann GO. A histopathologic study of iris changes in pseudoexfoliation syndrome. Ophthalmol. 1995;102(9):1279-90.
11. Hietanen J, Kivela T, Vesti E, et al. Exfoliation syndrome in patients scheduled for cataract surgery. Acta Ophthalmol (Copenh). 1992;70(4):440-6.
12. Puska P, Tarkkanen A. Exfoliation syndrome as a risk factor for cataract development: five-year follow-up of lens opacities in exfoliation syndrome. J Cataract Refract Surg. 2001;27(12):1992-8.
13. Schlotzer-Schrehardt U, Naumann GO. A histopathologic study of zonular instability in pseudoexfoliation syndrome. Am J Ophthalmol. 1994;118(6):730-43.
14. Bayraktar S, Alton T, Kucuksumer Y, Yilmaz OF. Capsular tension ring implantation after capsulorhexis in phacoemusification of cataracts associated with pseudoexfoliation syndrome. Intraoperative complications and early postoperative findings. J Cataract Refract Surg. 2001;27:1620-8.
15. Hiller R, Sperduto RD, Krueger DE. Pseudoexfoliation, intraocular pressure, and senile lens changes in a population-based survey. Arch Ophthalmol. 1982;100(7):1080-2.
16. Shingleton BJ, Laul A, Nagao K, et al. Effect of phacoemulsification on intraocular pressure in eyes with pseudoexfoliation: single-surgeon series. J Cataract Refract Surg. 2008;34(11):1834-41.
17. Lumme P, Laatikainen L. Exfoliation syndrome and cataract extraction. Am J Ophthalmol. 1993;116(1):51-5.
18. Shingleton BJ, Heltzer J, O'Donoghue MW. Outcomes of phacoemulsification in patients with and without pseudoexfoliation syndrome. J Cataract Refract Surg. 2003;29(6):1080-6.

19. Drolsum L, Ringvold A, Nicolaissen B. Cataract and glaucoma surgery in pseudo-exfoliation syndrome: A review. Acta Ophthalmol Scand. 2007;85(8):810-21.
20. Malyugin B. Cataract surgery in small pupils. Indian J Ophthalmol. 2017;65(12):1323-8.
21. Hashemi H, Seyedian MA, Mohammadpour M. Small pupil and cataract surgery. Curr Opin Ophthalmol. 2015;26(1):3-9.
22. Shingleton BJ, Crandall AS, Ahmed, II. Pseudoexfoliation and the cataract surgeon: preoperative, intraoperative, and postoperative issues related to intraocular pressure, cataract, and intraocular lenses. J Cataract Refract Surg. 2009;35(6):1101-20.
23. Lee DH, Shin SC, Joo CK. Effect of a capsular tension ring on intraocular lens decentration and tilting after cataract surgery. J Cataract Refract Surg. 2002;28(5):843-6.
24. D'Eliseo D, Pastena B, Longanesi L, et al. Prevention of posterior capsule opacification using capsular tension ring for zonular defects in cataract surgery. Eur J Ophthalmol. 2003;13(2):151-4.
25. Ahmed, II, Cionni RJ, Kranemann C, et al. Optimal timing of capsular tension ring implantation: Miyake-Apple video analysis. J Cataract Refract Surg. 2005;31(9):1809-13.
26. Cionni RJ, Osher RH. Management of profound zonular dialysis or weakness with a new endocapsular ring designed for scleral fixation. J Cataract Refract Surg. 1998;24(10):1299-306.
27. Hasanee K, Butler M, Ahmed, II. Capsular tension rings and related devices: current concepts. Curr Opin Ophthalmol. 2006;17(1):31-41.
28. Lee V, Bloom P. Microhook capsule stabilization for phacoemulsification in eyes with pseudoexfoliation-syndrome-induced lens instability. J Cataract Refract Surg. 1999;25(12):1567-70.
29. Schumacher S, Nguyen NX, Kuchle M, et al. Quantification of aqueous flare after phacoemulsification with intraocular lens implantation in eyes with pseudoexfoliation syndrome. Arch Ophthalmol. 1999;117(6):733-5.
30. Werner L, Pandey SK, Escobar-Gomez M, et al. Anterior capsule opacification: a histopathological study comparing different IOL styles. Ophthalmol. 2000;107(3):463-71.
31. Ragam A, Ritterband DC, Waisbren EC, et al. Clinical outcomes and intraocular pressure control after Scleral-glued Intraocular lens insertion in eyes with pseudoexfoliation. J Glaucoma. 2018;27(2):164-9.
32. Ursell PG, Spalton DJ, Whitcup SM, et al. Cystoid macular edema after phacoemulsification: relationship to blood-aqueous barrier damage and visual acuity. J Cataract Refract Surg. 1999;25(11):1492-7.
33. Pohjalainen T, Vesti E, Uusitalo RJ, et al. Intraocular pressure after phacoemulsification and intraocular lens implantation in nonglaucomatous eyes with and without exfoliation. J Cataract Refract Surg. 2001;27(3):426-31.
34. Davison JA. Capsule contraction syndrome. J Cataract Refract Surg. 1993;19(5):582-9.
35. Jehan FS, Mamalis N, Crandall AS. Spontaneous late dislocation of intraocular lens within the capsular bag in pseudoexfoliation patients. Ophthalmol. 2001;108(10):1727-31.
36. Ostern AE, Sandvik GF, Drolsum L. Late in-the-bag intraocular lens dislocation in eyes with pseudoexfoliation syndrome. Acta Ophthalmol. 2014;92(2):184-91.

CHAPTER 11

Femtosecond Laser-assisted Cataract Surgery in Posterior Polar Cataracts

Mahipal S Sachdev, Gitansha Shreyas Sachdev, Rashmi Deshmukh, Hemlata Gupta

INTRODUCTION

Posterior polar cataract (PPC) remains a challenge due to its propensity for posterior capsular dehiscence and subsequent vitreous loss during cataract extraction. This is secondary to a preexisting capsular defect or an abnormal adhesion of the posterior polar opacity to the capsular bag. Principles described to minimize intraoperative complications include maintenance of a closed chamber technique, hydrodelineation to create an epinuclear plate for mechanical protection, and steps to prevent excessive hydraulic pressure within the capsular bag. The use of various surgical adjuncts such as dispersive ophthalmic viscoelastic devices and triamcinolone acetate has been described, allowing optimal intraoperative management in the event of a complication. The advent of the femtosecond laser is the latest advancement in the field of cataract surgery, further enhancing the safety and efficacy of conventional phacoemulsification in PPCs.

POSTERIOR POLAR CATARACT

Posterior polar cataract is believed to develop from the remnants of the tunica vasculosa lentis (TVL), a structure that provides nutrition to the developing lens.[1] The name is derived from the typical location at the posterior pole of the lens. Incidence ranges from 3 to 5 per 1000.[2,3] Though the cataract becomes clinically symptomatic around 35–50 years of age, the development begins during embryonic life or early childhood. Bilateral presentation is common with dominant inheritance, whereas sporadic cases present unilaterally.[4]

Classification of Posterior Polar Cataract
- **Duke-Elder's classification:**[5]
  - **Stationary:** Circular posterior capsular opacity, well circumscribed in nature.

- **Progressive:** Whitish opacification of the posterior cortex in the form of radiating opacities that progress to involve the posterior capsule.
- **Singh's classification:**[6]
  - **Type 1:** Posterior subcapsular opacity in addition to the posterior polar plaque.
  - **Type 2:** Well-demarcated posterior polar opacity with "onion-ring" appearance, with or without greyish spots at the edge.
  - **Type 3:** Clearly demarcated posterior opacity with associated dense white spots at the edge, indicative of a capsular thinning, fragility or absence in some cases.
  - **Type 4:** Type 1, 2, or 3 in combination with nuclear sclerosis.
- **Schroeder classification:**[7]
  Classification for pediatric polar cataracts:
  - **Grade 1:** Polar opacity with no impact on the optical quality of the surrounding clear lens.
  - **Grade 2:** Obstruction of the red reflex in two-thirds of the pupillary aperture. No associated optical distortion.
  - **Grade 3:** Absence of red reflex in undilated pupil. Optical distortion associated with polar opacity, extending beyond the area of cataract.
  - **Grade 4:** The opacity is totally occlusive. Loss of red reflex in dilated pupil.

Timing of Surgery

Early surgical intervention is advisable especially in visually significant pediatric cataracts, with an associated amblyogenic effect. A lower complication rate and easier surgical removal are associated with a softer nucleus. The risk of a posterior capsular defect development increases over time in cases having an intact capsule initially.

Phacoemulsification in Posterior Polar Cataract

Phacoemulsification in posterior polar cataract (PPC) poses a challenge for the surgeon. The incidence of posterior capsular dehiscence during cataract extraction ranges from 7.1% to 36%.[8-10] An excessive adherence between the plaque and a normal posterior capsule, a weakened capsule secondary to thinning or a preexisting congenital capsular defect are predisposing risk factors. Additionally, an association of the size of the polar opacity with the occurrence of intraoperative posterior capsular rent (PCR) has been demonstrated. Polar opacities that measured >4 mm in diameter had a higher chance of PCR compared to those <4 mm.[11] Further, age younger than 40 years has also been reported to be an independent risk factor for PCR.[12]

Maintenance of a closed chamber technique, avoiding rapid build-up of hydraulic pressure within the capsular bag and providing an epinuclear cushion for the posterior capsule are the principles for performing a safe phacoemulsification. In order to achieve this, cortical-cleaving hydrodissection is avoided and instead hydrodelineation is performed to separate the nuclear fibers from the polar opacity.[9] A successful hydrodelineation is characterized by the presence of a golden ring (Fig. 1).

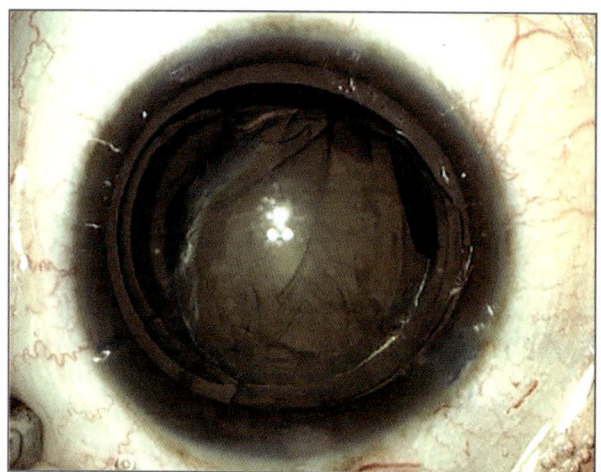

Fig. 1: "Golden ring" following hydrodelineation.

Nuclear rotation is avoided and utmost care is taken to maintain the anterior chamber dynamics. Phacoemulsification is performed using low parameters. Cortical removal is done with low bottle height and the posterior cortex is removed at the end. Capsular polishing is best avoided.

FEMTOSECOND LASER-ASSISTED CATARACT SURGERY

A solid state laser, the femtosecond operates in the near infrared range (wavelength 1053 nm) using pulses with a duration of 10^{-15} seconds. The laser energy results in photo disruption of stromal tissue through plasma formation and subsequent expansion into cavitation bubbles. Since the first indication for flap creation in LASIK, improvements in technology have led to an increase in pulse frequency with subsequent decrease in energy and collateral damage.[13,14] The femtosecond laser in cataract surgery is indicated for creation of corneal incisions (penetrating and partial thickness), capsulotomy construction, and lens fragmentation.

Optimizing Outcomes in Femtosecond Laser-assisted Cataract Surgery

Although the femtosecond laser has greatly increased the precision and accuracy of cataract surgery, it comes with its own host of unique challenges. Following are certain caveats to optimize outcomes with the femtosecond laser.

An optimal dock is of paramount importance for successful laser delivery. Counseling the patient to keep both eyes open, relaxes the facial muscles allowing easy insertion of the patient interface. The non-applanating interface can be slid under the upper lid followed by the lower lid while asking the patient to look in the opposite direction. Avoiding tilt is crucial to reduce the risk of suction loss and incomplete capsulotomies. The patient's nose should be moved sideways by tilting the head to the opposite side.

It is not uncommon to notice pupillary constriction following completion of the dock. A reduction of as much as 30% in the mean pupil area has been reported.[15] The release of prostaglandins and inflammatory cytokines subsequent to laser delivery has been hypothesized as the cause. The extent of miosis following femtosecond delivery showed positive correlation to the duration of lens fragmentation, and primary incision creation, the patients' age and the capsulotomy margin-pupil distance. Preoperative nonsteroidal anti-inflammatory administration counters the action of inflammatory mediators and prevents pupillary constriction.[16]

The femtosecond laser delivery leads to a build-up of gas bubbles within the capsular bag. Prior to performing a hydrodelineation, it is imperative to release the trapped bubbles by nudging the nucleus from side to side or using the "rock and roll technique." This prevents excessive build-up of pressure within the bag which may lead to capsular block syndrome or on a rare occasion a capsular blowout.[17-19]

Femtosecond Laser-assisted Cataract Surgery in Posterior Polar Cataracts

The level of planning and customization available with the femtosecond laser platforms has brought about an unparalleled accuracy, predictability and repeatability in surgical outcomes. Moreover, the femtosecond laser offers distinct advantages over conventional phacoemulsification in challenging cases such as PPCs.

Creation of a Precise Capsulotomy

Anterior capsulotomy is the first step in all femtosecond platforms apart from the Femto-LDV. It is completed prior to lens fragmentation, as the subsequent cavitation bubble release results in capsular displacement from the initial position. The femtosecond laser enables a precise cut within the anterior lens capsule, creating capsulotomies of exact shape, size, and location.[20] Achieving a well-centered capsulotomy enables a subsequently perfect intraocular lens overlap, resulting in a more precise effective lens position and improved refractive outcomes (Fig. 2). This is of paramount importance in the event of a posterior capsular dehiscence, where an adequate sulcus support is required for intraocular lens implantation. A greater vertical spot spacing may improve the quality of the capsulotomy cut, resulting in fewer capsular tags. Increased vertical spot spacing reduces the laser delivery time, with a subsequent decrease in the number of aberrant and misplaced laser spots secondary to eye movements.[21]

Anterior Segment Optical Coherence Tomography Imaging

The laser platforms include an inbuilt anterior segment imaging system and a live video display, to allow precise docking and overlay of the surgical planning. It provides a high definition image of the ocular anterior segment, up till the area of the posterior lens capsule. While the remaining platforms utilize the high definition anterior segment optical coherence tomography (AS-OCT), the Victus incorporates an integrated swept source OCT system.

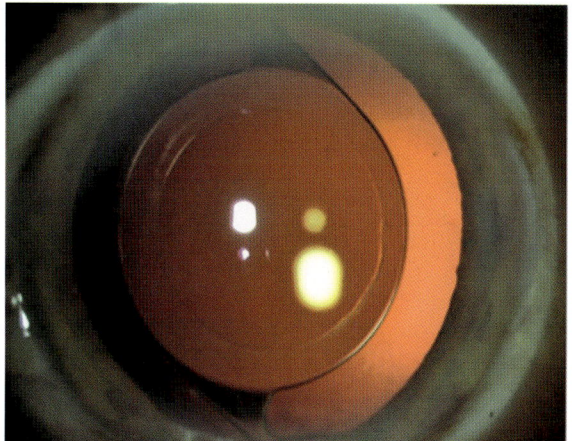

Fig. 2: Well-centered capsulotomy resulting in a precise effective lens position.

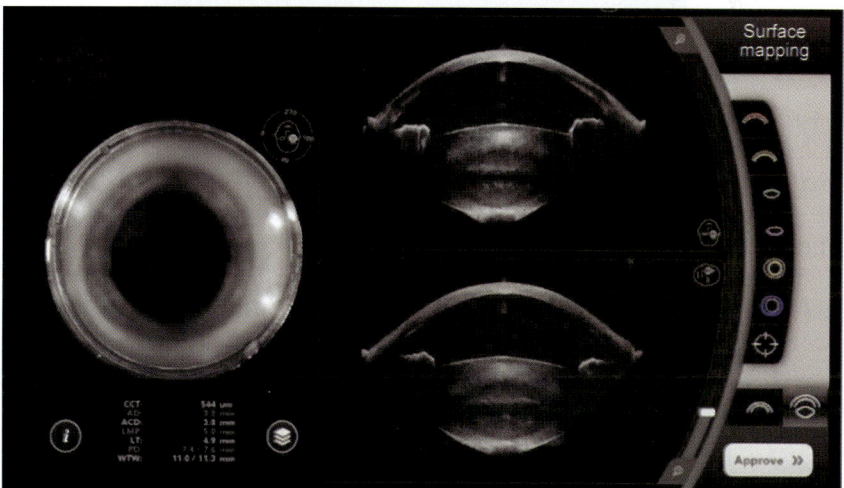

Fig. 3: Posterior capsular defect on anterior segment optical coherence tomography (OCT).

In PPCs, the anterior segment imaging helps demonstrate preexisting capsular defects not detectable by slit lamp evaluation (Fig. 3). This anatomical finding is of critical importance in determining the surgical planning and likelihood of intraoperative complications. Various classifications have been described to determine the status of the posterior capsule on AS-OCT and subsequent incidence of posterior capsular dehiscence. The presence of a clear space between the posterior capsule and the nucleus along with the continuity of the posterior capsule, has been described for segregation of true PPC from a posterior subcapsular plaque.[22] Another grading system was based on the morphology of the posterior capsule and its relation to the PPC.[23] Grade 1 represents an area of clearance of 50% or more between the lenticular opacity and the posterior capsule, whereas a clearance of less than half is classified as grade 2. Grade 3 represents the absence of an intact

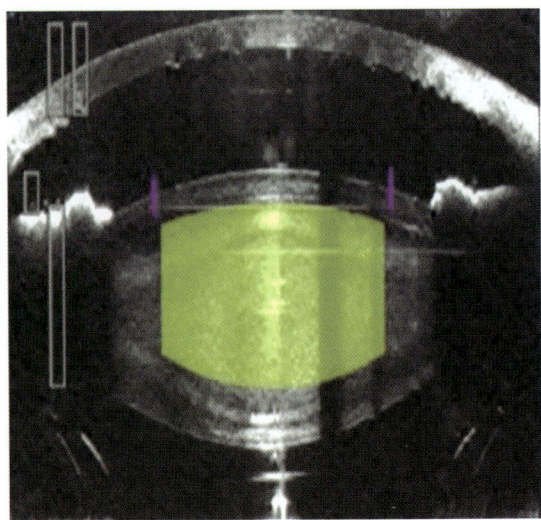

Fig. 4: Increase in posterior offset in the case of a posterior polar cataract (PPC). The offset is increased to 750–800 μ from 500 μ.

posterior capsule or inability to identify the posterior capsule posterior to the polar plaque. The incidence of posterior capsular dehiscence was significantly greater with grade 2 and 3 polar cataract. Patients with these defects should be counseled regarding the increased risk of intraoperative complications and possible delayed visual recovery.

The width of the posterior safety zone, i.e., the distance of the laser cut from the posterior capsule can be adjusted to increase the epinuclear cushion over the posterior capsule. The important caveat to remember is to align the posterior most plane of femtosecond dissection 800 to 1000 μ above the plane of the posterior capsule (Fig. 4). This helps reduce the energy delivered close to the posterior polar plaque and prevents subsequent splitting of the capsule. The cavitation bubbles form a cleavage plane separating the nucleus from the polar opacity.

Lens Fragmentation

Another advantage the femtosecond laser offers is lens fragmentation. Several studies indicate a reduction of as much as 30% in the effective phaco-emulsification time. This translates into lower endothelial cell damage due to shorter phacoemulsification time and less fluid entering the eye during surgery.[24]

Additionally, the laser fragmentation aids subsequent nuclear removal without excessive manipulation or rotation, which is of utmost important in PPCs. Various patterns of nucleus fragmentation have been described, especially in cases of hard nucleus with a coexisting posterior polar opacity.

The *femtodelineation* technique entails creation of a cylindrical pattern of nuclear division to segregate the nucleus into concentric cylinders of varying diameters, depth, and number based on the surgeon's preference.[25] This cylindrical pattern divides the nucleus into distinct concentric layers from the center of the nucleus to the periphery with the outermost layer of epinucleus providing a cushioning effect to the weak posterior capsule (Figs. 5A to C). An increase in the posterior offset from 500 µ to 750 µ enables the creation of a thick epinuclear layer. Emulsification is carried out using low parameters and nuclear removal is done layer by layer from inward without. This ensures a systematic removal of the nuclear core with an epinuclear cushion that remains till the end.

Subsequently, the epinucleus is removed from the fornixes and the central portion is removed at the end. This technique prevents transmission of the fluid turbulences and the mechanical forces to the posterior capsule. Each layer acts as a shock absorber and protects the outermost polar opacity. The elimination of hydro procedure additionally reduces the risk of hydraulic pressure build-up within the bag.

Another technique described known as the hybrid technique[26] utilizes the cylindrical as well as the chop patterns for nuclear division. Three chops 6 mm each, and three concentric cylinders of 2, 4, and 6 mm respectively are created using the femtosecond laser. Hydrodissection procedures are avoided and nucleus is removed along the preexisting cleavage planes. The nuclear fragments are emulsified in the first, second, and third tier. The outer

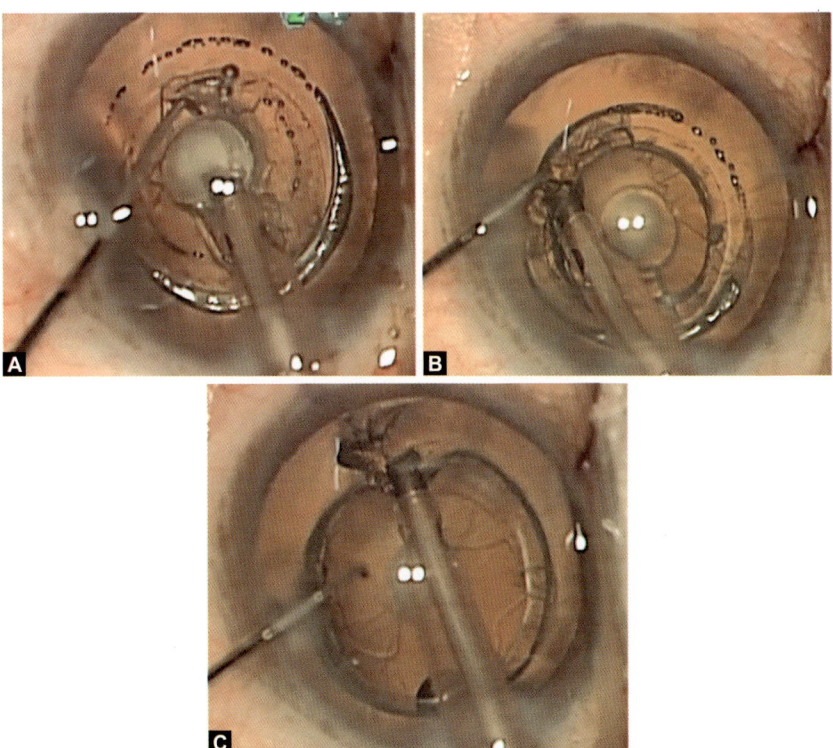

Figs. 5A to C: Femtodelineation technique: (A) An initial image demonstrating the femtosecond nucleotomy; (B) Subsequent removal of the inner core demonstrating the outer layers; (C) Removal of epinuclear cushion.

tiers form a cushion for the inner ones with the epinuclear plate being the outermost cushion. The epinuclear plate is the last to be aspirated gently. This technique is particularly helpful in cases of PPC with dense nuclear sclerosis.

CONCLUSION

In conclusion, femtosecond laser-assisted cataract surgery in PPC has its own advantages and limitations. The ability to perform a real-time OCT to create a cleavage plane above the polar opacity, and the techniques of femtodelineation and hybrid nucleotomy have made it possible to enhance the safety of the surgical procedure and protect the posterior capsule. At the same time, the possibility of capsular block syndrome should be kept in mind and necessary steps taken to avoid the same. By approaching crucial steps with utmost care, the incidence of complications in PPC can be significantly reduced.

REFERENCES

1. Gifford SR. Congenital anomalies of the lens as seen with the slit lamp. Am J Ophthalmol. 1924;7(9):678-85.
2. Lee MW, Lee YC. Phacoemulsification of posterior polar cataracts—a surgical challenge. Br J Ophthalmol. 2003;87(11):1426-7.
3. Vogt G, Horváth-Puhó E, Czeizel E. A population-based case-control study of isolated congenital cataract. Orv Hetil. 2006;147(23):1077-84.
4. Kalantan H. Posterior polar cataract: A review. Saudi J Ophthalmol. 2012;26(1): 41-9.
5. Duke-Elder S. Congenital deformities. System of Ophthalmology [Internet]. St. Louis, Mosby; 1964. pp. 723-6.
6. Masket S. Cataract surgical problem. J Cataract Refract Surg. 19971;23(6):819-24.
7. Schroeder HW. The management of posterior polar cataract: The role of patching and grading. Strabismus. 2005;13(4):153- 6.
8. Osher RH, Yu BC, Koch DD. Posterior polar cataracts: A predisposition to intra-operative posterior capsular rupture. J Cataract Refract Surg. 1990;16(2):157-62.
9. Vasavada A, Singh R. Phacoemulsification in eyes with posterior polar cataract. J Cataract Refract Surg. 1999;25(2):238-45.
10. Hayashi K, Hayashi H, Nakao F, et al. Outcomes of surgery for posterior polar cataract. J Cataract Refract Surg. 2003;29(1):45-9.
11. Kumar S, Ram J, Sukhija J, et al. Phacoemulsification in posterior polar cataract: Does size of lens opacity affect surgical outcome? Clin Exp Ophthalmol. 2010;38(9):857-61.
12. Das S, Khanna R, Mohiuddin SM, et al. Surgical and visual outcomes for posterior polar cataract. Br J Ophthalmol. 2008;92(11):1476-8.
13. Binder PS. Femtosecond applications for anterior segment surgery. Eye Contact Lens. 2010;36(5):282-5.
14. Hjortdal J, Nielsen E, Vestergaard A, et al. Inverse cutting of posterior lamellar corneal grafts by a femtosecond laser. Open Ophthalmol J. 2012;6:19-22.
15. Jun JH, Hwang KY, Chang SD. Pupil-size alterations induced by photodisruption during femtosecond laser assisted cataract surgery. J Cataract Refract Surg. 2015;41:278-85.

16. Schultz T, Joachim SC, Szuler M, et al. NSAID pretreatment inhibits prostaglandin release in femtosecond laser assisted cataract surgery. J Refract Surg. 2015;31(12):791-2.
17. Roberts TV, Sutton G, Lawless MA, et al. Capsular block syndrome associated with femtosecond laser-assisted cataract surgery. J Cataract Refract Surg. 2011;37(11):2068-70.
18. Yeoh R. Hydrorupture of the posterior capsule in femtosecond-laser cataract surgery. J Cataract Refract Surg. 2012;38(4):730.
19. Yeoh R, Theng J. Capsular block syndrome and pseudoexpulsive hemorrhage. J Cataract Refract Surg. 2000;26(7):1082-4.
20. Friedman NJ, Palanker DV, Schuele G, et al. Femtosecond laser capsulotomy. J Cataract Refract Surg. 2011;37:1189-98.
21. Schultz T, Joanchim SC, Noristani R, et al. Greater vertical spot spacing to improve femtosecond laser capsulotomy quality. J Cataract Refract Surg. 2017;43:353-7.
22. Das S, Kummelil MK, Kharbanda V, et al. Microscope integrated intraoperative spectral domain optical coherence tomography for cataract surgery: Uses and applications. Curr Eye Res. 2016;41(5):643-52.
23. Chan TC, Li EY, Yau JC. Application of anterior segment optical coherence tomography to identify eyes with posterior polar cataract at high risk for posterior capsular rupture. J Cataract Refract Surg. 2014;40(12):2076-81.
24. Conrad-Hengerer I, Hengerer FH, Shultz T, et al. Effect of femtosecond laser fragmentation of the nucleus with different softening grid sizes on effective phaco time in cataract surgery. J Cataract Refract Surg. 2012;38:1888-94.
25. Vasavada AR, Vasavada V, Vasavada S, et al. Femtodelineation to enhance safety in posterior polar cataracts. J Cataract Refract Surg. 2015;41(4):702-7.
26. Titiyal JS, Kaur M, Sharma N. Femtosecond laser-assisted cataract surgery technique to enhance safety in posterior polar cataract. J Refract Surg. 2015;31(12):826-8.

CHAPTER 12

Posterior Capsular Rupture Recognition and Management

Mohan Rajan, M Ravishankar, Sriram

■ INTRODUCTION

Cataract surgery is the most commonly performed surgical procedure in ophthalmology and despite tremendous technical and technological advancements, posterior capsular rent still occurs.

Early recognition combined with advances in instrumentation has enabled effective management of posterior capsule rupture during phacoemulsification. However, improper management may lead to serious complications with a higher incidence of permanent visual disability.

Stages at which posterior capsular rupture can occur: Posterior capsular rupture (PCR) can occur in any stage of phacoemulsification cataract surgery. The following are the stages in which you should anticipate and prevent PCR.
- During hydrodissection
- During nucleus removal
- During cortex removal
- During posterior capsule vacuuming
- During intraocular lens (IOL) implantation.

■ IMPROPERLY MANAGED POSTERIOR CAPSULAR RUPTURE

If PCR is not managed properly it can lead to severe complications and cause impairment of vision and even visual loss. The complications which may occur are:
- Cystoid macular edema (Fig. 1)
- Retinal detachment (Fig. 2)
- Endophthalmitis (Fig. 3)
- Secondary glaucoma.

■ EARLY SIGNS OF POSTERIOR CAPSULAR RUPTURE

During phacoemulsification procedure the surgeon may experience a few signs and some changes in the intraocular environment which may be very early signs of PCR. They are:

Posterior Capsular Rupture Recognition and Management

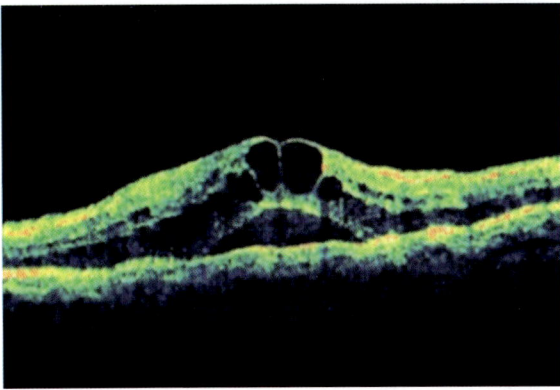

Fig. 1: Cystoid macular edema.

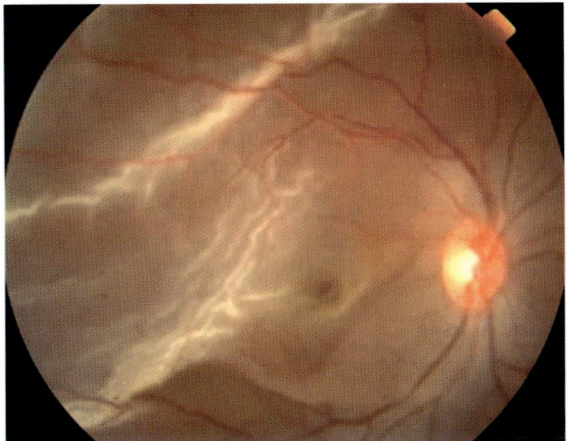

Fig. 2: Retinal detachment.

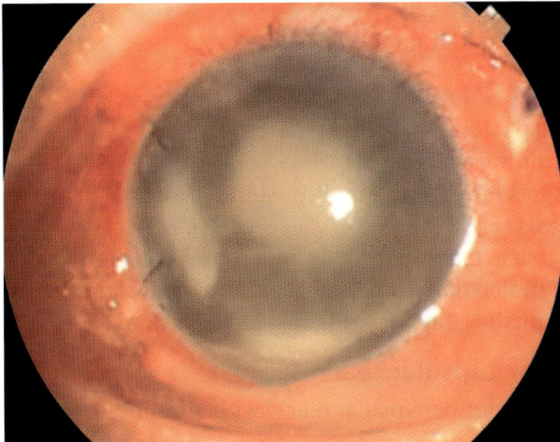

Fig. 3: Endophthalmitis.

- Sudden deepening of anterior chamber
- Loss of nucleus followability
- Lens tilt or deepening of the posterior chamber.

PREVENTION OF POSTERIOR CAPSULAR RUPTURE

Following measures should be taken for preventing and managing posterior capsule rupture.

Anticipation of Posterior Capsular Rupture

Posterior capsular rupture should be anticipated in the following conditions[1] where it is commonly seen in:
- Traumatic cataract (Fig. 4)
- Post vitrectomized eyes (Fig. 5)
- Posterior polar cataracts (Fig. 6)
- Hard brown cataract (Fig. 7).

Recognition of Posterior Capsular Rupture

The posterior capsular rupture has to be recognized very early to prevent the further complications which may arise intraoperative or postoperatively. The following signs are to be recognized during the procedure.
- Sudden deepening of anterior chamber and posterior chamber (Fig. 8)
- Loss of nucleus followability
- During hydrodissection beware of "Pupil Snap Sign": First tell-tale sign, and sudden constriction of the pupil
- Tilting of the nucleus may also be noticed.

Important Clinical Pearls

It is always better to avoid hydrodissection in certain complicated cataracts where the posterior capsule may have a preexisting dehiscence[2] or tear like:
- Posterior polar cataract[3,4]
- Traumatic cataract
- Previous vitreoretinal surgery.

Small Posterior Capsular Tear

In case of small posterior capsular tear,[5,6] the following steps are to be taken to prevent it becoming a large tear:
- It is wiser to convert the small posterior capsular tear into a posterior capsulorhexis (Fig. 9).
- It is better to use the microrhexis forceps or Utrata forceps.
- Inject high molecular viscoelastic, sodium hyaluronate to tamponade the tear; it also pushes the posterior capsule backward.

Large Posterior Capsular Tear

In case of large posterior capsular tear[4-6] with vitreous loss the following steps are to be done.
- It is important to always perform bimanual vitrectomy (Fig. 10) and also bimanual irrigation and aspiration

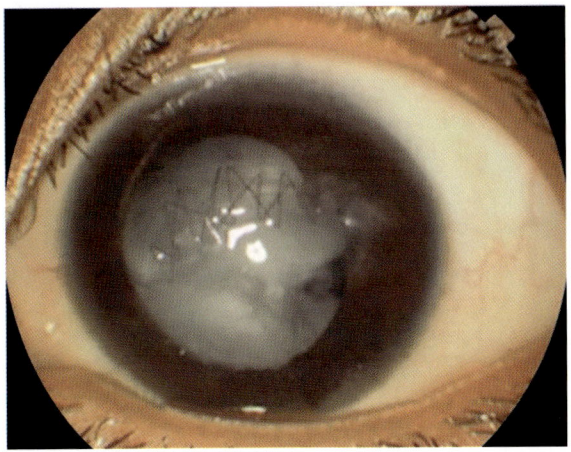

Fig. 4: Traumatic cataract.

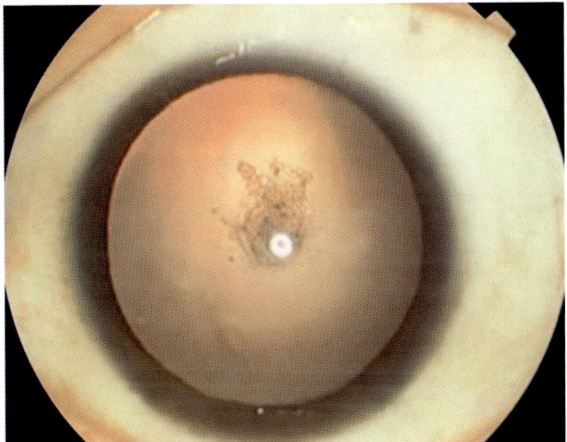

Fig. 5: Cataract postvitrectomy.

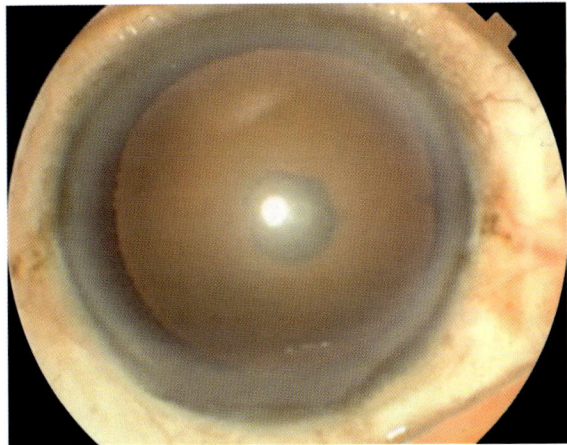

Fig. 6: Posterior polar cataract.

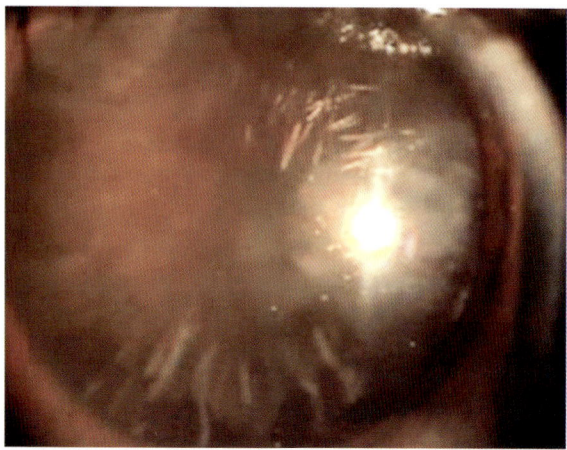

Fig. 7: Hard brown cataract.

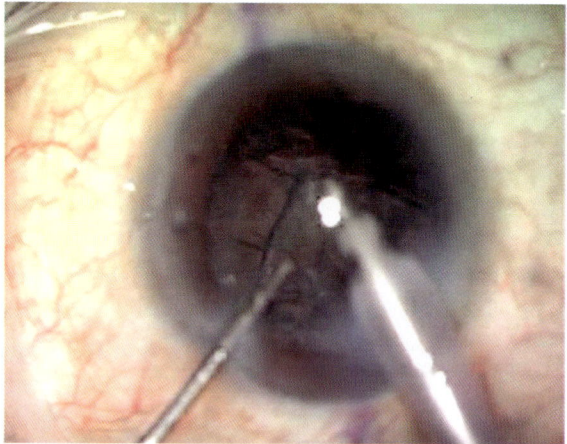

Fig. 8: Sudden deepening of anterior chamber.

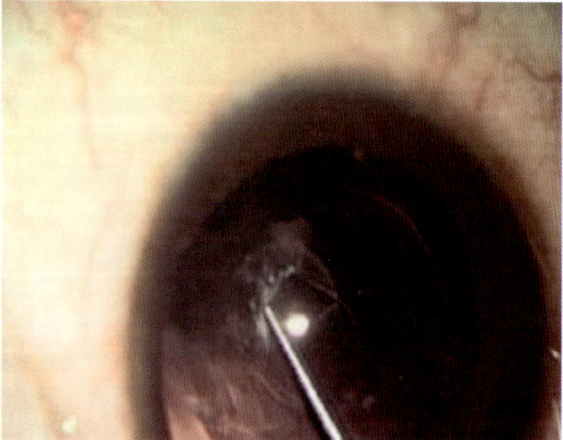

Fig. 9: Posterior capsulorhexis.

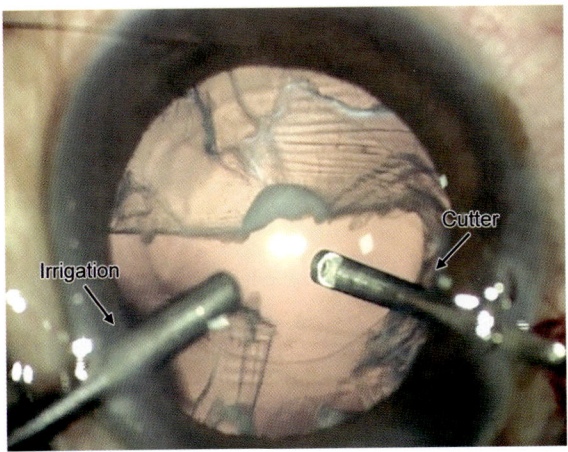

Fig. 10: Bimanual vitrectomy.

- In such situations the vitreous acts like a slinky
- Use separate infusion and aspiration as well as cutting the vitreous with the vitrector
- AC maintainer should always be used in such situation
- Do a complete central core vitrectomy. Remove the vitreous from the anterior chamber and also from behind the posterior capsular tear.
- The AC maintainer tamponades[7] break and prevent the tear from extending further and decreases hydration of vitreous.
- The IOL is implanted in the sulcus area if posterior capsular support is inadequate.

Vitrectomy Technique

- Anterior vitrectomy is to be performed adequately when there is vitreous loss
- Use always automated vitrector which is much safer and makes life easy for the surgeon
- During vitrectomy, bimanual technique is to be employed to prevent hydration of vitreous and enlargement of the break
- Use high cutting rate around 2,000–3,000/min
- The suction level should be low about 100–150 mm Hg
- Do not pull the vitreous, but it should be cut in place and allowed to fall back
- Always avoid excessive movement of vitrectomy probe.

Do Not Pull Out Phaco Probe

Do not panic when you see any signs of a posterior capsular tear, it is very important not to withdraw the phaco probe (Figs. 11A to C) immediately, which will lead to extension of the tear and even loss of nuclear fragments into the vitreous cavity.

A high molecular weight viscoelastic (preferably Viscoat) is injected through the side port (Fig. 12), which allows the anterior chamber to be well formed and prevents the extension of the posterior capsular tear.

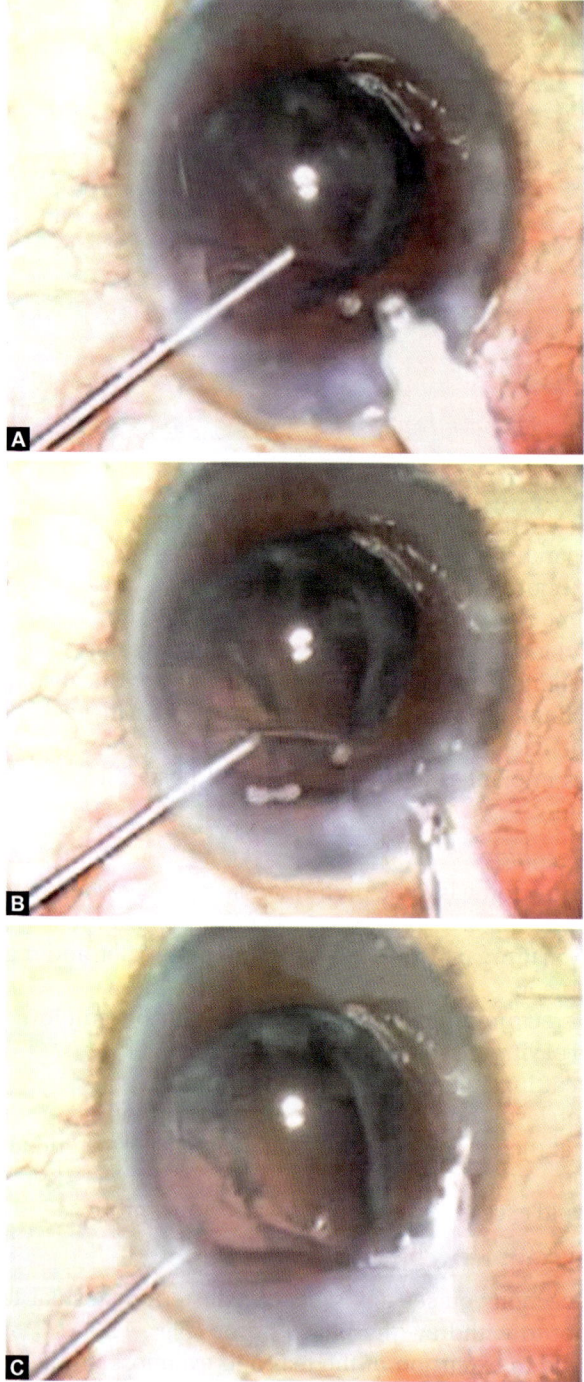

Figs. 11A to C: Posterior capsular tear is enlarging due to sudden withdrawal of the phaco probe.

Gentle Withdrawal of the Phaco Probe

After the chamber is well formed with viscoelastic, the phaco probe is to be removed gently (Figs. 13A to C) and then the operating surgeon should assess the situation and plan further course of action.

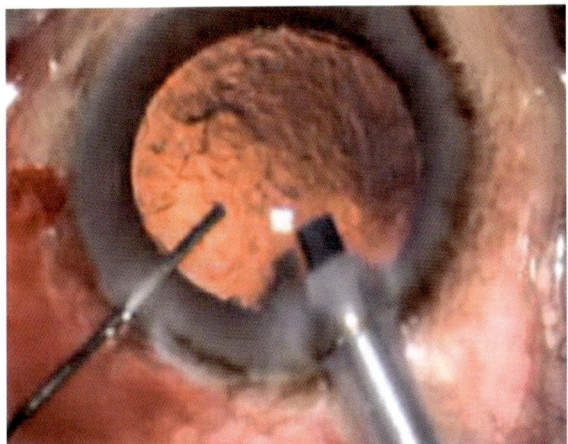

Fig. 12: Injecting viscoelastic.

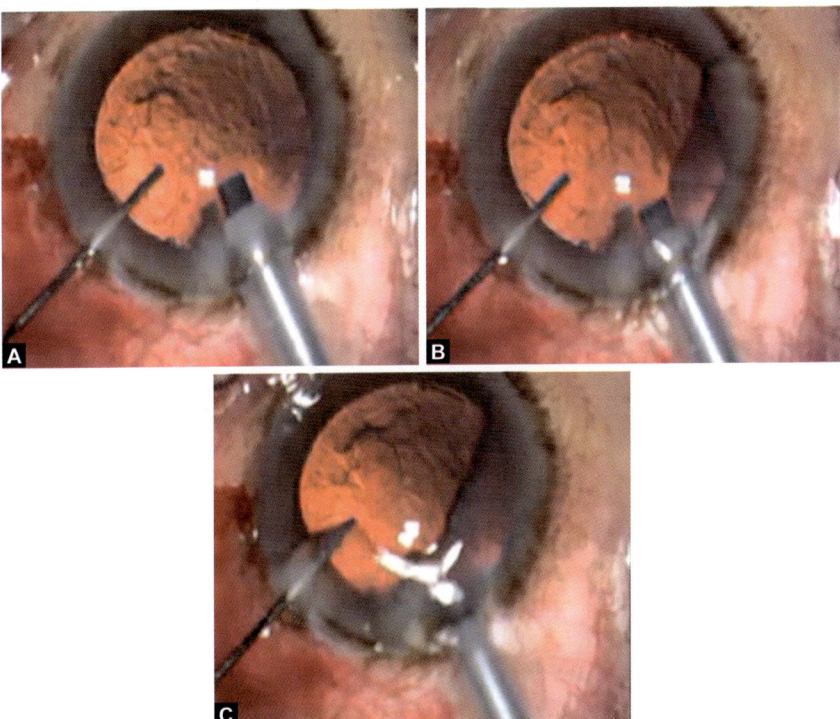

Figs. 13A to C: Gentle removal of the phaco probe.

Bimanual Irrigation and Aspiration

Bimanual irrigation and aspiration is done to remove the residual cortex as it has an advantage over coaxial irrigation and aspiration. Because the coaxial technique leads to increase in vitreous hydration, probable enlargement of the tear and even cause further loss of vitreous (Figs. 14A and B).

Central Anterior Vitrectomy

Preservative-free triamcinolone (Figs. 15A and B) to be used to stain the vitreous in order to ensure there is no vitreous strands extending into the anterior chamber and the incision wound area.

It is mandatory to use the vitreous cutter in the right sided port and the irrigation in the left sided port. Now check for capsule integrity.

Anterior vitrectomy can also be done through the pars plana using a 20 gauge system or by placing a trocar and cannula using a 23 gauge/25 gauge vitreous cutter (Figs. 16A and B).

Careful Assessment of the Capsule

It is very important to assess the 360° structural integrity and the strength of the anterior capsule (Fig. 17) and as well as the posterior capsule. This assessment would make the surgeon understand the exact support of the IOL to be implanted.

Decision Regarding Intraocular Lens Implantation

A foldable single piece IOL (Fig. 18) can be implanted into the bag if the posterior capsular rupture is small in size, after converting it into a posterior capsulorhexis, provided there is adequate capsular support the IOL.

If the posterior capsular tear is large, a multipiece IOL can be placed in the sulcus and supporting it by capturing the rhexis margin[8] (Fig. 19) with the optic of the IOL.

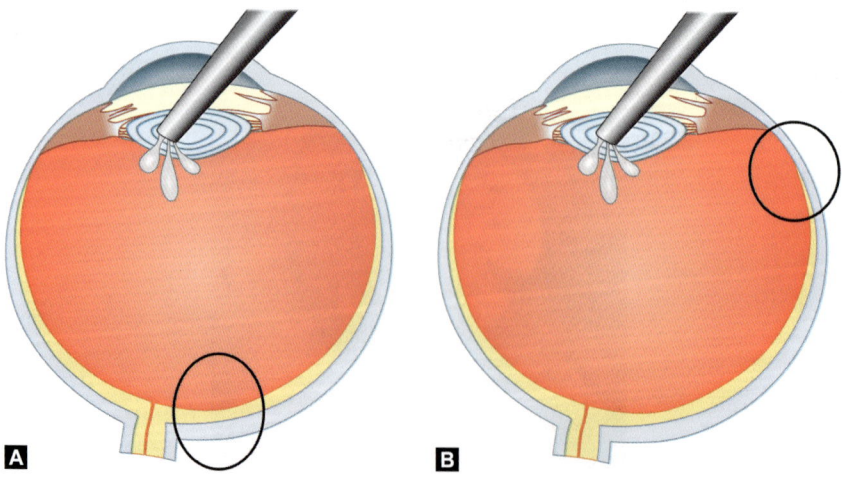

Figs. 14A and B: Coaxial irrigation aspiration.

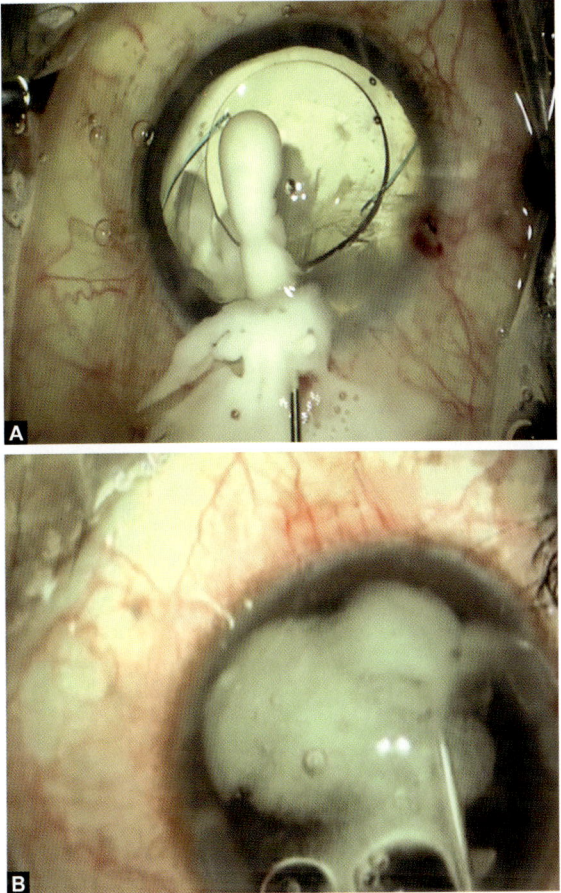

Figs. 15A and B: Triamcinolone is used to stain vitreous.

If there is deficiency or total absence of capsular support then the following IOL implantation can be considered appropriately on individual case basis:
- Anterior chamber IOL (Fig. 20)
- Iris claw (retro fixated) (Fig. 21)
- Sutured scleral-fixated IOL (Fig. 22)
- Glued IOL (Fig. 23).

Nucleus Drop

If whole nucleus drop occurs (Fig. 24), do not chase the nucleus with the phaco probe.

Perform a three port pars plana vitrectomy and make the nucleus mobile. Then use the fragmatome to emulsify the nucleus in the mid vitreous cavity.

If the nucleus is still seen in the anterior vitreous or pupillary area then one may attempt the following techniques for safe removal:
- Anterior assisted levitation (AAL) (Fig. 25) through the limbus
- Posterior assisted levitation (PAL) (Fig. 26) through the pars plana

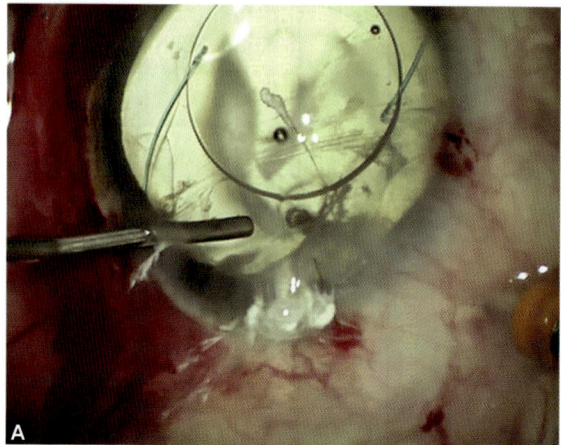
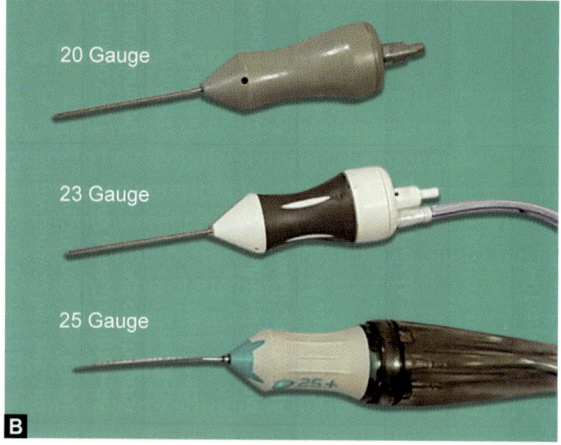

Figs. 16A and B: (A) Pars plana vitrectomy; (B) Vitrectomy cutter.

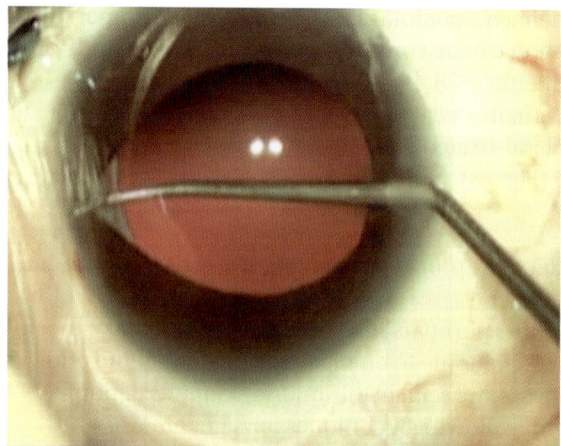

Fig. 17: Assessment of the capsule.

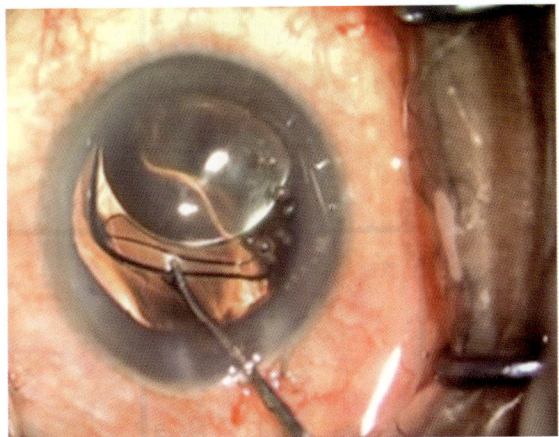

Fig. 18: Single piece intraocular lens.

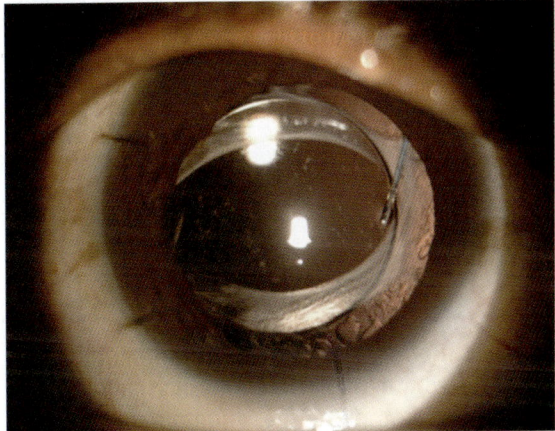

Fig. 19: Three piece intraocular lens.

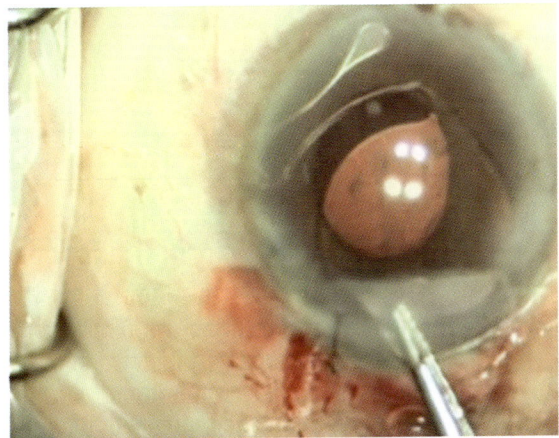

Fig. 20: Anterior chamber intraocular lens.

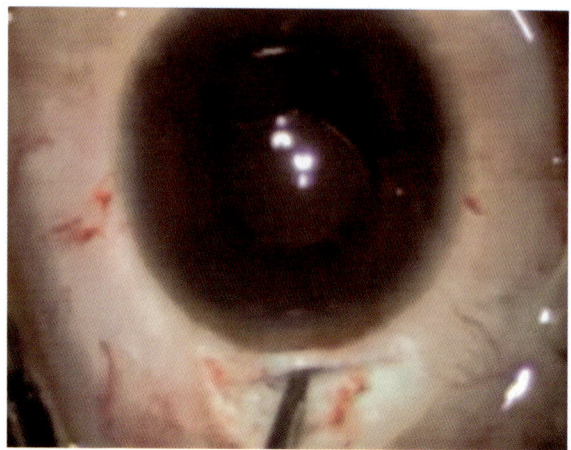

Fig. 21: Iris claw lens.

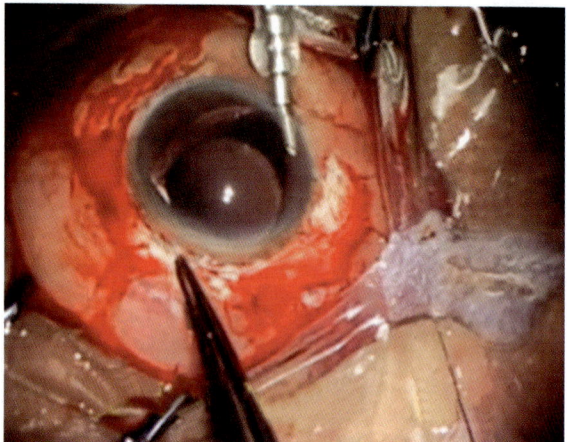

Fig. 22: Sutured scleral-fixated intraocular lens implantation.

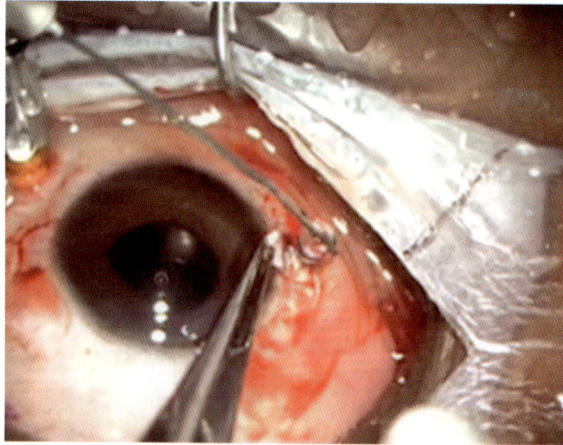

Fig. 23: Glued intraocular lens.

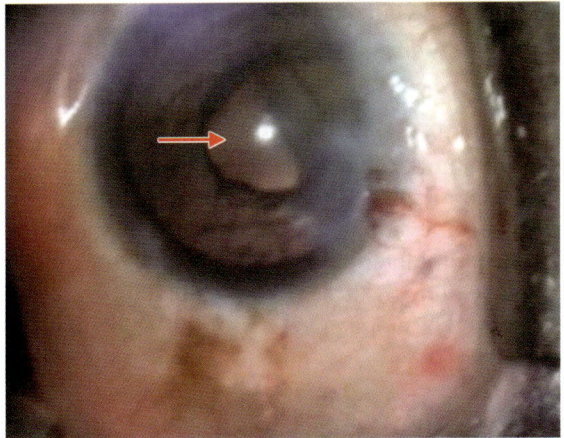

Fig. 24: Whole nucleus drop.

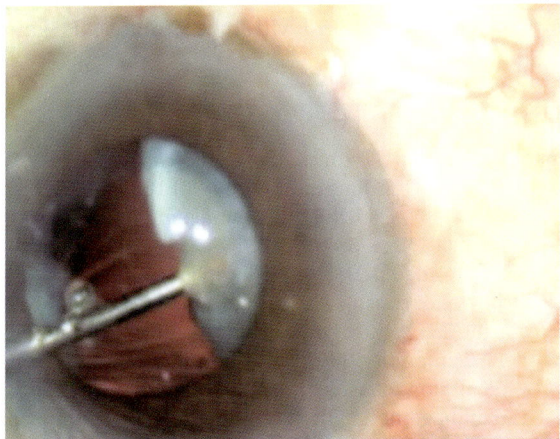

Fig. 25: Anterior assisted levitation.

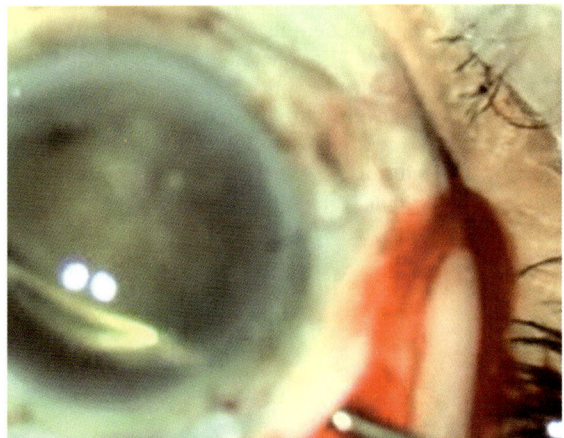

Fig. 26: Posterior assisted levitation.

- Do not attempt PAL in young patients and high myopics as the incidence of retinal tear and retinal detachment is high in the group.

Appropriate Nucleus Management

Anterior chamber should be reformed with viscoelastic, if the nuclear pieces are in the anterior chamber they should be removed with the phaco probe after lowering all parameters. If the nuclear fragments are in the anterior vitreous they can be removed by PAL[9] through pars plana route.

If the nucleus has completely descended into the posterior vitreous further management is to be done by three port, pars plana vitrectomy and nucleus fragments are removed by a phaco fragmatome.

SUMMARY

The incidence of PCR can be decreased significantly by identifying the presence of predisposing factors and appropriate modification of the surgical plan. Early recognition of posterior capsular tear along with prompt management of capsular tear and vitreous prolapse is key to the good postoperative outcome.

REFERENCES

1. Chakrabarti A, Nazneen Nazm N. Posterior capsular rent: Prevention and management. Indian J Ophthalmol. 2017;65(12):1359-69.
2. Bajpayee RB, Sharma N, Dada T, et al. Management of posterior capsule tears. Surv Ophthalmol. 2001;45:473-88.
3. Osher RH, Yu BC, Koch DD. Posterior polar cataracts: A predisposition to intraoperative posterior capsular rupture. J Cataract Refract Surg. 1990;16:157-62.
4. Rongé LJ, Contributing Writer. Posterior capsular rupture during cataract surgery. EyeNet Magazine. September, 2005.
5. Gimbel HV. Posterior capsule tears using phaco-emulsification causes, prevention and management. Euro J Implant Refract Surg. 1990;2:63-9.
6. Traianidis P, Sakkias G, Avramides S. Prevention and management of posterior capsule rupture. Euro J Ophthalmol. 1996;6(4):379-82.
7. Androudi S, Brazitikos PD, Papadopoulos NT, et al. Posterior capsule rupture and vitreous loss during phacoemulsification with or without the use of an anterior chamber maintainer. J Cataract Refract Surg. 2004;30:449-52.
8. Lee JE, Ahn JH, Kim WS, et al. Optic capture in the anterior capsulorhexis during combined cataract and vitreoretinal surgery. J Cataract Refract Surg. 2010;36:1449-52.
9. Lifshitz T, Levy J. Posterior assisted levitation: Long-term follow-up data. J Cataract Refract Surg. 2005;31:499-502.

CHAPTER
13

Phacoemulsification in Subluxated Lenses

Suhas Haldipurkar, Zain Khatib

■ INTRODUCTION

Performing phacoemulsification in subluxated lenses is extremely challenging even for an experienced surgeon, with a risk of potential complications at almost every step of surgery.[1-5] Even if phacoemulsification is successfully completed, long-term stability and fixation of the capsular bag remains a problem especially in cases with progressive zonulopathy.[6] The predisposing risk factors for subluxation of the crystalline lens include:
- Weak zonules (zonulopathy)—pseudoexfoliation, blunt trauma, advancing age, high myopia and systemic diseases like Marfan syndrome, homocystinuria
- Torn zonules (zonulodialysis)—blunt and penetrating trauma, iatrogenic (during surgery).

■ CAPSULAR SUPPORT DEVICES FOR SUBLUXATED LENSES

There are a number of devices that can be used during surgery for temporary and long-term stabilization of the capsular bag in zonular weakness.

Temporary Support Devices

These are only meant to be used intraoperatively to support the bag during capsulorhexis, hydrodissection and phacoemulsification. They include: iris hooks and capsular hooks.

Iris Hooks

Reusable 4-0 polypropylene iris hooks/retractors (available from various Indian manufacturers along with Katena Products, Denville, NJ, and FCI Ophthalmics) which are mostly used as pupillary expansion devices during phacoemulsification. They also work as effective devices to support the capsular bag when the zonules are weak (Figs. 1A and B). One or more retractors can be inserted depending on the degree of zonular defect, each through a separate paracentesis. In extreme subluxation, one may be required to use as many as 6 or 7 hooks to support the bag to remove the

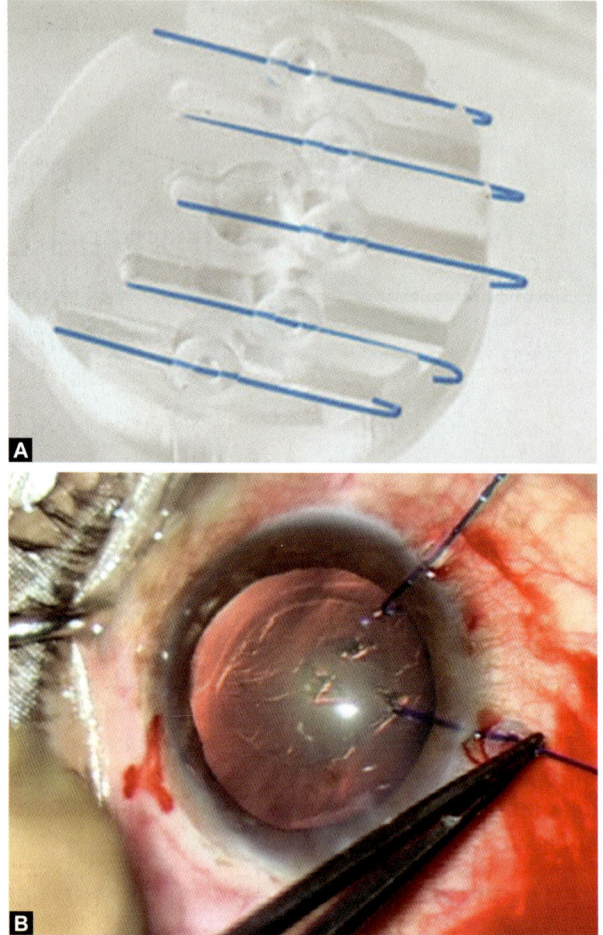

Figs. 1A and B: Iris hooks to support capsular bag in zonular weakness.

nucleus. However, since the hooked ends are very short and flexible, they may tend to slip off the anterior capsular edge during phacoemulsification and do not support the equator of the capsular bag. Also, excessive tightening of these hooks may tent up capsulorhexis edge which becomes vulnerable to tear once phacoemulsification is started.

Capsular Hooks

Disposable nylon capsular retractors/hooks [MicroSurgical Technology (MST), Redmond, WA] are specially designed to support the capsular bag in weak zonules. They feature a double-stranded design that creates a long blunt loop at the tip, which is meant to reach all the way up to equator once hooked around the capsular edge (Figs. 2A and B). Since they are slightly bulky with a long loop, they may be more difficult to insert as compared to the iris retractors, but once inserted correctly, they provide excellent stability and also have a much lower risk of tearing the capsulorhexis edge.

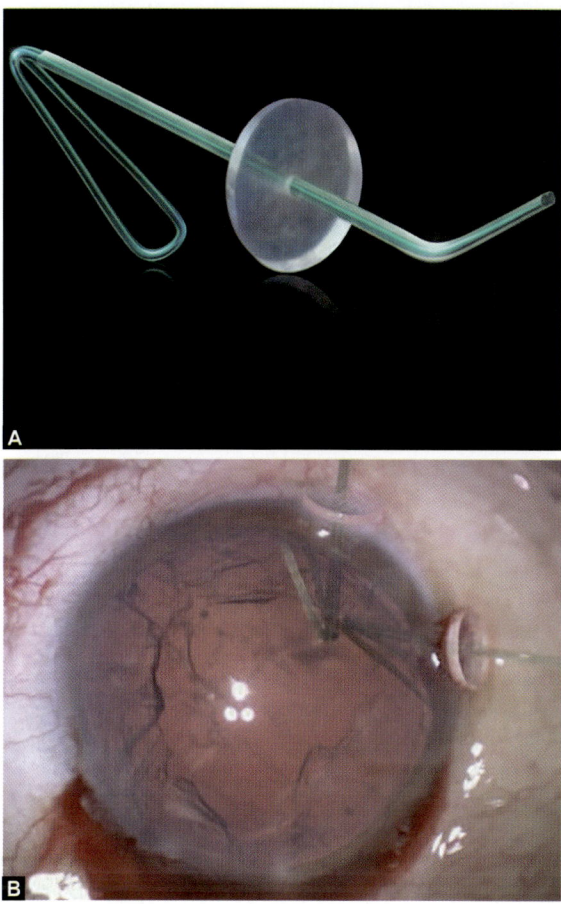

Figs. 2A and B: Capsular hooks with long blunt loop like tip, designed to reach up to the capsular fornix.

Long-term Stabilization

These include the capsule tension rings (CTRs) and the scleral fixation devices; Cionni ring and Ahmed capsule tension segment (Figs. 3A to D).

Capsule Tension Rings

These polymethylmethacrylate (PMMA) rings are the most commonly used devices for cases of mild to moderate zonular weakness (Morcher, FCI Ophthalmics, Marshfield Hills, MA; Ophtec along with several Indian manufacturers). They can be inserted using a forceps through the side port, or through the main port by a preloaded injector system (Geuder, Ophtec, Boca Raton, FL) at any stage following the completion of capsulorhexis.[7] At times one may be prompted to use it half way through the procedure to stabilize the bag for safer nucleus management. Fish-tail technique is often used for insertion of the ring.[8] The CTR works in several ways to counter zonular weakness:[9-15]

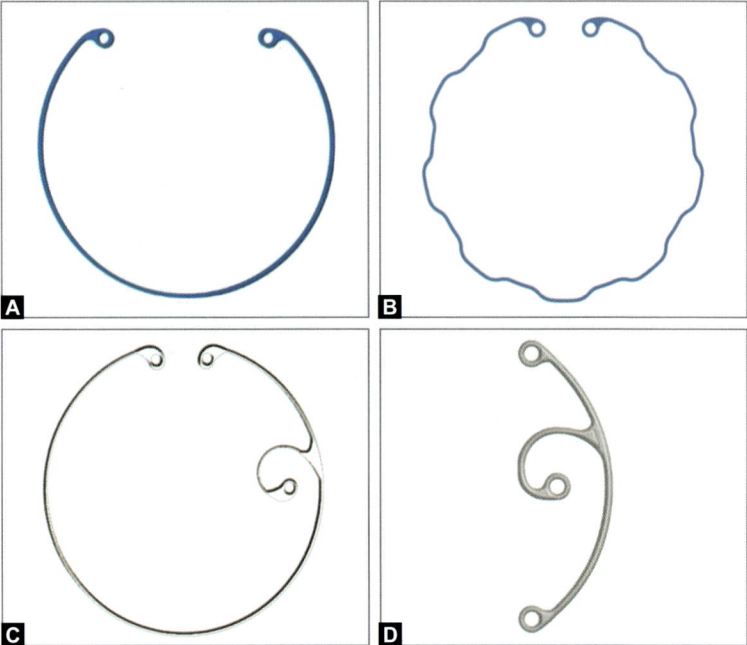

Figs. 3A to D: Devices for long-term stabilization of capsular bag (from left to right). (A) Morcher capsule tension ring; (B) Henderson capsule tension ring; (C) Cionni ring; (D) Ahmed capsule tension segment.

- Redistribution of mechanical forces such as that of nuclear sculpting or intraocular lens (IOL) insertion from areas of focal zonular weakness to the areas of stronger zonular support. However, this effect is lost if more than 180° of zonular weakness exists in the first place.
- The outward centrifugal force applied by the ring makes the flaccid bag taut (Fig. 4), thus preventing the capsular fornices from collapsing toward the aspirating instrument tip and also preventing the posterior capsule from trampolining forward.
- Resistance to postoperative capsular shrinkage and contraction.

Morcher CTRs are available in three sizes, larger diameter rings to be used for eyes with greater axial lengths and vice versa (Table 1).

Capsule tension rings have two distinct disadvantages.

1. Significant compression is required to implant the ring into the capsular bag because of its larger size. This may stretch the capsulorhexis and potentially shear zonules by distorting or decentering the bag. Because of this compressive force, CTRs should never be inserted in the presence of an anterior or posterior capsule tear.
2. A second drawback to CTRs is that they may impede cortical aspiration by pinning and trapping cortex in the capsular fornix. For this reason, surgeons should consider using iris/capsule retractors instead of a CTR to stabilize the bag during phacoemulsification. Ideally, CTR insertion can then be delayed until after the cortex has been removed.

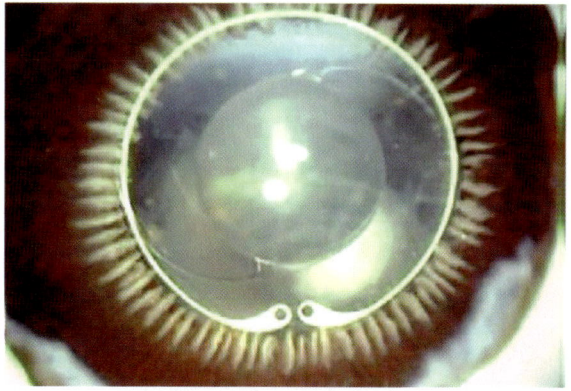

Fig. 4: Miyake-Apple view of a CTR showing effect of stretching of capsular equator and making a flaccid bag taut.

Table 1: Different sizes of capsule tension rings (CTRs).

CTR type	Actual diameter	Diameter when compressed	Indication based on axial length
Size 14	12.3 mm	10.0 mm	<24 mm
Size 14A	14.5 mm	12.0 mm	>28 mm
Size 14C	13.0 mm	11.0 mm	24–28 mm

The Henderson-modified CTR (FCI Ophthalmics) has a scalloped contour that facilitates cortical removal following placement.[16] If one area of cortex is difficult to remove because the Henderson CTR impinges on it, the ring can be rotated slightly until one of the gaps overlies the cortex.

For more severe forms of zonular weakness and frank subluxations, just a CTR alone will not suffice, and the capsular bag needs to be anchored to the sclera. It is for these cases that the Cionni-modified CTR and Ahmed capsule tension segment were designed.[17-19]

Cionni Ring
The Cionni rings are modified CTRs that have an additional fixation hook with an islet to allow a suture to be passed through thereby attaching the capsular bag to the sclera. The additional islet is positioned just above the plane of the ring so that it can come out of the rhexis margin when being fixed to the sclera. During surgery, the islet is to be placed near the area of maximum zonular weakness. There is also a double islet Cionni ring that allows scleral fixation at two points in cases of a more severe generalized zonular weakness.

Ahmed Capsule Tension Segment
The Ahmed CTS is a modified design of the Cionni ring, comprising of an arc of PMMA, with an islet for scleral fixation. It usually covers about one quadrant. It is intended to be used along with a conventional CTR in cases of severe subluxations. Since it is a smaller device than Cionni ring, it may be placed with lesser trauma and earlier on during the course of surgery. In fact, it can

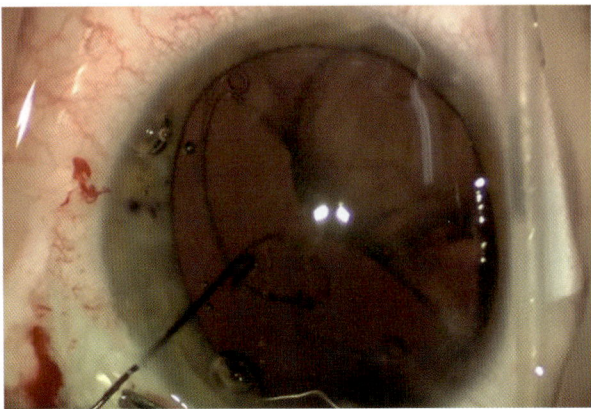

Fig. 5: Single iris retractor with an Ahmed CT segment used as temporary support for the capsular bag.

also be used as a temporary capsular support during phacoemulsification, by hooking an iris retractor in the islet of the CTS. This allows only a single iris retractor to be used and still provides a broad support to the capsular bag (Fig. 5).

■ PREOPERATIVE WORKUP

Clinical Examination

A thorough preoperative evaluation helps the surgeon to anticipate the challenges to be dealt with in the operating room. Sometimes there is an obvious subluxation of the lens that can easily be picked on slit-lamp examination. In such cases the surgeon should characterize and grade the zonular deficiency, describing it in terms of location, number of clock hours involved, presence or absence of phacodonesis and presence or absence of any vitreous disturbance. Phacodonesis is better appreciated in an undilated pupil as dilatation stabilizes the ciliary body and iris and dampens the lens movement.

In the absence of any obvious phacodonesis or visible zonular dialysis, the extent of zonular weakness is usually not known until the initiation of surgery. However, there are a few subtle signs of zonular weakness that can be picked up with careful examination. These include a wider iridolenticular gap (space between the iris and the anterior lens surface), a decentered nucleus, focal iridodonesis, and visibility of the peripheral lens equator upon lateral gaze.[20] In pseudoexfoliation, the zonulopathy is progressive and the whitish deposits are found not only on the zonules but also on the anterior lens surface and pupillary margin. The most ominous sign with pseudoexfoliation, however, is a shallow anterior chamber (AC) despite a normal axial length; this invariably indicates extremely weak zonules.[21] In some cases, there may be no signs of zonular weakness at all, but still warrant a high index of suspicion. These include a history of trauma to the eye in any patient with lenticular opacity

Flowchart 1: Showing choice of capsular bag support.

```
                        Choice of capsular bag support
                                    │
        ┌───────────────────────────┼───────────────────────────┐
        ▼                           ▼                           ▼
   Based on              Any zonulopathy                   Based on
   degree of     ──────► with phacodonesis                 etiology
   zonular
   weakness
```

- **Based on degree of zonular weakness:**
  - Mild to moderate (3-4 clock hrs or less) → **CTR**
  - Severe focal or diffuse zonulopathy → **Scleral fixation +/- (best decide on table)**
  - Tilted or decentered capsular bag → **Scleral fixation**

- **Any zonulopathy with phacodonesis:** Scleral fixation

- **Based on etiology:**
  - Traumatic and iatrogenic zonulodialysis: even if up to 6 hours, only CTR may work well, since rest of zonules are healthy
  - Generalized zonulopathy:
    - Pseudoexfoliation
    - Marfan syndrome
    - Severe blunt trauma
  - → Scleral fixation if moderate to severe subluxation

(CTR: capsular tension ring)

especially in the presenile age group, and brunescent hard cataracts in old-aged patients.

Patient Counseling

It is important preoperatively to counsel the patient about the complicated nature of the surgery. Even though all attempts should be made to preserve the capsular bag and place a preferred IOL in the bag, this may not be possible in all cases. Patients need to be made aware of the possibility of having to implant a nonroutine IOL (iris clip, scleral fixated, glued IOL). Informed consent should be modified from the routine cataract consent and should specifically include consent for placement of a CTR, or a nonroutine IOL. Many patients with Marfan syndrome have significant systemic problems that increase the risk of death or morbidity. These patients must be evaluated by the physician and cardiologist prior to surgery.

Planning for Surgery

The choice of whether to use a CTR only, or scleral fixation with Cionni ring/Ahmed CTS for capsular support is best decided on table during surgery, but a tentative decision can be made preoperatively based on the etiology and degree of zonular weakness (Flowchart 1), presence or absence of vitreous in the AC and the presence of phacodonesis.

■ SURGICAL PROCEDURE

Anesthesia

Peribulbar block is preferred over topical anesthesia due to the complicated nature of these cases. Massage of the globe after block is to be avoided as this may further compromise zonular integrity.

Incision

The main incision should be placed away from the zone of subluxation, preferably 90° away. This prevents further enlargement of the subluxation and minimizes traction on the zonules. The surgeon should work with the smallest possible incision without compromising the ability to perform necessary maneuvers, to maintain good fluidics during phacoemulsification and should be ready to enlarge the size of the incision for insertion of Cionni ring or segment.

Intraoperative Assessment

Before starting with capsulorhexis, it is important to assess the subluxated zone and grade it in terms of severity. If pre-existing vitreous disturbance is noted, a bimanual anterior vitrectomy can be performed at this stage itself, after staining with triamcinolone, and clearing the AC of all vitreous completely. A dispersive ophthalmic viscosurgical device (OVD) should be injected over the subluxated zone to tamponade the vitreous and prevent it from getting disturbed during the course of surgery. This step may be required to be repeated once or twice during the procedure as well.

Capsulorhexis

It is the capsulorhexis step that provides the first opportunity to directly assess the zonular integrity. The following two signs are strong indicators of the presence of a definite zonular weakness:
1. On trying to puncture the capsule, the cystitome just depresses rather than nicking the capsule, resulting in radiating capsular folds originating from the point of attempted puncture (Fig. 6).
2. *Pseudoplasticity phenomenon*: As the rhexis edge passes the area of zonular defect, the peripheral capsule which is generally immobile, also moves along the direction of the tearing capsular flap, thus providing no counter traction and making the capsulorhexis extremely difficult.

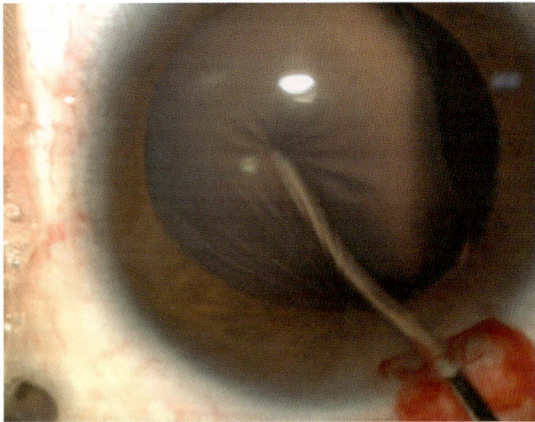

Fig. 6: Attempting rhexis in weak zonules: Cystitome depresses rather than nicking the capsule, resulting in radiating capsular folds originating from the point of attempted puncture.

Strategies for Capsulorhexis
- The capsulorhexis should be initiated in an area away from the weak zonules, where the capsule offers sufficient resistance.
- To puncture the capsule, use a straight tip 26-G needle and direct it tangentially with bevel up into the lens matter.
- Advancement of the flap is best done with forceps rather than a cystitome for better control. In cases of severe subluxation, a bimanual technique with a second forceps or spatula can be used to provide sufficient counter traction. Alternatively, counter traction can also be provided by using iris/capsule retractors to engage the rhexis margin.
- The sizing of the rhexis is important here. Although a large diameter rhexis would be preferable in these cases to counter the tendency for capsular contraction, making a smaller opening reduces the risk of a peripheral extension if one is struggling to control the tear. Cionni ring/Ahmed segment if required will need a peripherally placed rhexis edge to remain conspicuous in the undilated pupil.

Hydrodissection
A gentle but thorough cortical cleaving hydrodissection should be performed carefully so as to free the nucleus maximally and lessen the stress on zonules during phacoemulsification. Always ensure the nucleus is rotating freely prior to starting phacoemulsification. Using two instruments to bimanually rotate the nucleus is more effective in this case as opposed to a single instrument rotation.

Timing and Choice of Insertion of Capsular Support Device
The timing of when to insert the device depends on the condition of the zonules noted on table, choice of device, and expertise of the surgeon. Iris/capsule retractors can be inserted even before completion of rhexis whereas CTRs can only be used after completion of rhexis.

To provide temporary support during phacoemulsification, iris/capsule retractors are significantly more effective than CTRs because CTRs can only redistribute instrument and mechanical forces to the remaining intact zonules. The greater the zonular defect is, the less effective is a CTR to stabilize the bag. For severe subluxations, iris/capsule retractors are preferred (Fig. 7), but a CTR can be used along with the retractors if the capsular equator is tending to collapse toward the instrument.

Phacoemulsification
Phacoemulsification should be carried out with low bottle height, low aspiration flow rate and low vacuum. Care should be taken to minimize the movement of the nucleus while sculpting, with the emphasis on cutting through the nucleus even if that involves a somewhat higher power setting. If direct chop is used, it is preferable to lift the nucleus clear of the posterior capsule and then chop. At no point should downward force be used, as this gets transmitted to the posterior capsule and from there to the zonules. For soft nuclei, phacoaspiration or "chip and flip" technique should be used.

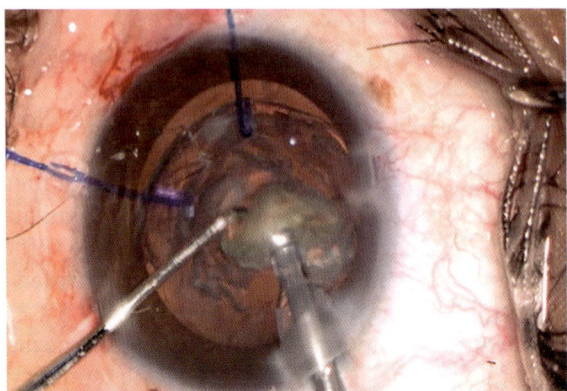

Fig. 7: Iris retractors used to support the bag during phacoemulsification.

Cortical Aspiration

Bimanual irrigation-aspiration is better than coaxial in these cases, as it provides finer control. Tangential aspiration should be performed rather than radial aspiration, to minimize pull on the weak zonules.

Technique of Capsule Tension Ring Insertion (Figs. 8A to E)

Before insertion of the CTR, the capsular bag should be well inflated with cohesive OVD. For manual insertion, a McPherson's forceps is used to gently insert the CTR through the side port, while a Y hook can be used through the second side port to guide the placement of the CTR into the bag. Once the proximal islet is inside the bag, a Sinskey hook or blunt tip chopper can be used to direct the distal end across the rhexis margin and into the capsular bag. The distal end should only be released when it is well below the rhexis margin because if it is lost in the ciliary sulcus or AC angle, it becomes difficult to retrieve it. The CTR can also be injected from a preloaded injector system. Once inserted, it should be dialed to a position such that the convex part of the ring abuts the area of zonular weakness. In situations where integrity of the bag is in doubt, a suture can be passed through the distal end of the islet as a safety measure to retrieve the ring if it takes a dip in the vitreous.

Technique of Scleral Fixation with Cionni Ring and Ahmed Segment (Figs. 9 A to F)

The insertion of Ahmed segment into the eye is fairly simple and straightforward, since is a small device. The Cionni ring insertion is similar to that of CTR, except that it has to be inserted from the main port. There are a variety of techniques used for scleral suture fixation of Cionni ring and Ahmed segment, which are similar to the techniques used for a scleral fixated IOL such as the Hoffman pocket.[22] Our preferred technique is to make a partial thickness scleral groove about 1.5 mm posterior to the corneoscleral junction in the area of zonular weakness. Preplacement of a double armed 9-0 Prolene suture through the islet of the Cionni ring/Ahmed segment fixation hook is

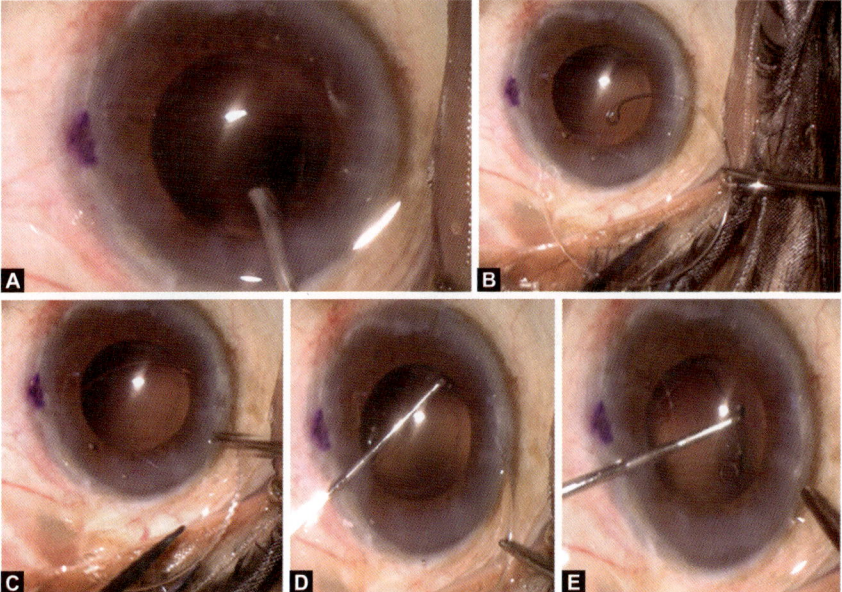

Figs. 8A to E: Capsular tension ring (CTR) insertion steps. (A) Capsular bag inflated with ophthalmic viscosurgical device (OVD); (B) CTR inserted through side port; (C) Forceps used to guide proximal islet of CTR into the bag; (D) Chopper is used from second side port to guide the distal part of CTR; (E) Chopper used to dial the distal islet of CTR into the bag.

done prior to its insertion. A 26-G needle is introduced ab externo through the base of the scleral groove such that it enters the eye between the iris base and anterior capsule. The straight needle of the Prolene suture is docked into the 26-G needle's lumen so that it can be backed out externally through the scleral groove. The other arm of the Prolene suture is externalized similarly through the same scleral groove about 1 mm away from the first needle. Once both ends of the suture are externalized, the device is inserted into the eye and dialed into position. The knots are tied, trimmed and tucked within the scleral groove. The knots should not be tied so tightly that the ring or segment peaks or distorts the capsule edge.

Intraocular Lens Insertion

Once the bag has been stabilized, the regular PCIOL can be inserted into the bag. Anterior vitrectomy is performed if required, and conjunctival wounds are closed.

Capsule tension rings and other devices aid in-the-bag placement of IOL even in the most challenging situations, with good postoperative visual recovery. However, in extreme cases, capsular bag may have to be abandoned along with thorough clean up using anterior vitrectomy followed by scleral fixated, iris clip IOL or other choice of implantation as per the surgeon's preference.

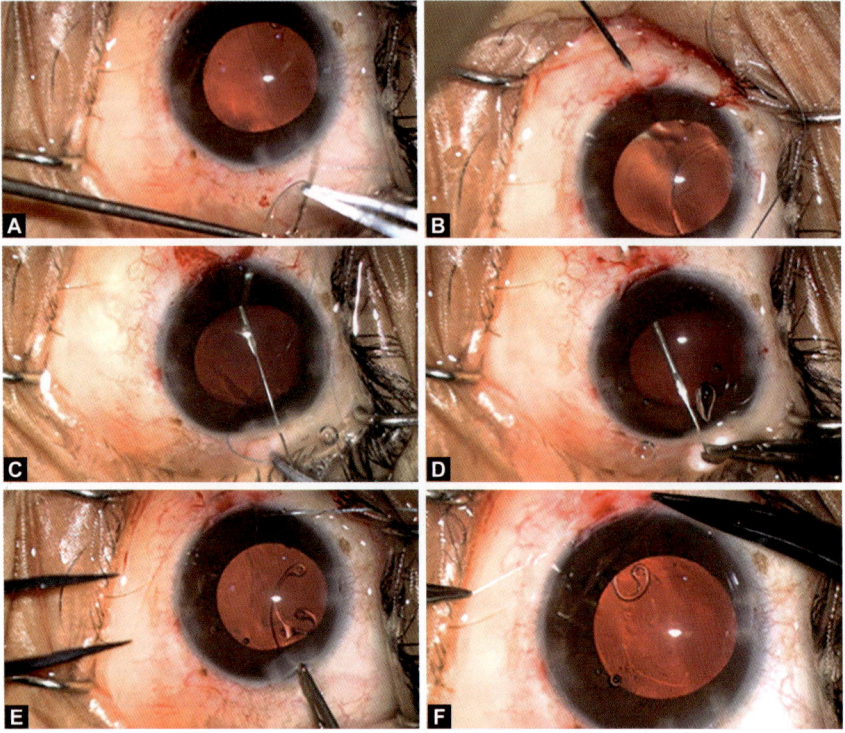

Figs. 9A to F: Steps of scleral fixation of Ahmed segment. (A) Double-armed 9-0 Prolene suture is passed through the fixation hook islet; (B) 26-G needle is inserted ab externo into the ciliary sulcus through a scleral groove 1.5 mm posterior to limbus; (C) One arm of the Prolene suture is rail-roaded through the needle and externalized; (D) The second arm of the suture is similarly externalized through the 26-G needle 1 mm away from the first suture arm; (E) With the sutures secure through the sclera, the Ahmed segment is introduced into the eye; (F) The Ahmed segment is positioned in the bag with the fixation hook above the rhexis, and the suture is tightened to anchor the bag to the sclera.

■ REFERENCES

1. Osher RH, Cionni RJ, Gimbel HV, et al. Cataract surgery in patients with pseudoexfoliation syndrome. Eur J Implant Ref Surg. 1993;5:46-50.
2. Fine IH, Hoffman RS. Phacoemulsification in the presence of pseudoexfoliation: challenges and options. J Cataract Refract Surg. 1997;23:160-5.
3. Avramides S, Traianidis P, Sakkias G. Cataract surgery and lens implantation in eyes with exfoliation syndrome. J Cataract Refract Surg. 1997;23:583-7.
4. Kuchle M, Viestenz A, Martus P, et al. Anterior chamber depth and complications during cataract surgery in eyes with pseudoexfoliation syndrome. Am J Ophthalmol. 2000;129:281-5.
5. Shingleton BJ, Heltzer J, O'Donoghue MW. Outcomes of phacoemulsification in patients with and without psuedoexfoliation syndrome. J Cataract Refract Surg. 2003;29:1080-6.
6. Jahan FS, Mamalis N, Crandall AS. Spontaneous late dislocation of intraocular lens within the capsular bag in psuedoexfoliation patients. Ophthalmology. 2001;108:1727-31.

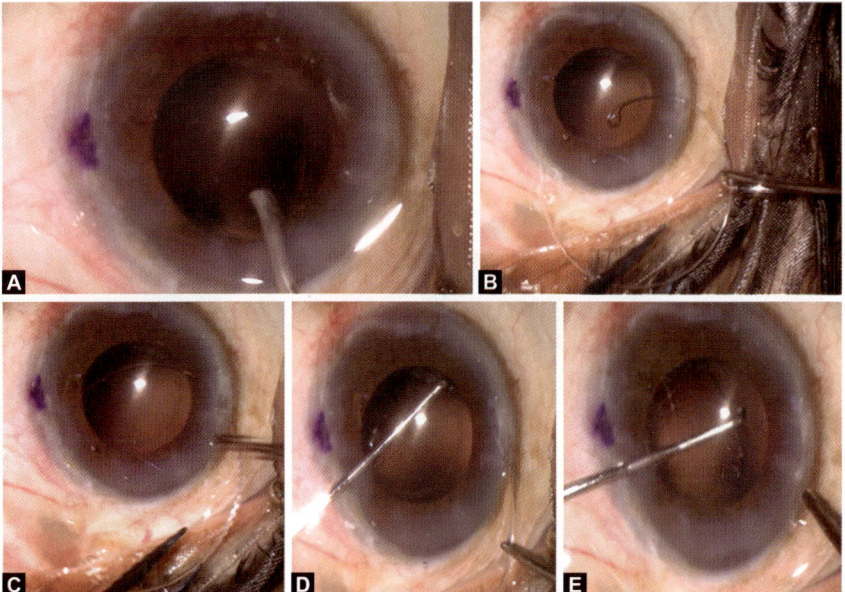

Figs. 8A to E: Capsular tension ring (CTR) insertion steps. (A) Capsular bag inflated with ophthalmic viscosurgical device (OVD); (B) CTR inserted through side port; (C) Forceps used to guide proximal islet of CTR into the bag; (D) Chopper is used from second side port to guide the distal part of CTR; (E) Chopper used to dial the distal islet of CTR into the bag.

done prior to its insertion. A 26-G needle is introduced ab externo through the base of the scleral groove such that it enters the eye between the iris base and anterior capsule. The straight needle of the Prolene suture is docked into the 26-G needle's lumen so that it can be backed out externally through the scleral groove. The other arm of the Prolene suture is externalized similarly through the same scleral groove about 1 mm away from the first needle. Once both ends of the suture are externalized, the device is inserted into the eye and dialed into position. The knots are tied, trimmed and tucked within the scleral groove. The knots should not be tied so tightly that the ring or segment peaks or distorts the capsule edge.

Intraocular Lens Insertion

Once the bag has been stabilized, the regular PCIOL can be inserted into the bag. Anterior vitrectomy is performed if required, and conjunctival wounds are closed.

Capsule tension rings and other devices aid in-the-bag placement of IOL even in the most challenging situations, with good postoperative visual recovery. However, in extreme cases, capsular bag may have to be abandoned along with thorough clean up using anterior vitrectomy followed by scleral fixated, iris clip IOL or other choice of implantation as per the surgeon's preference.

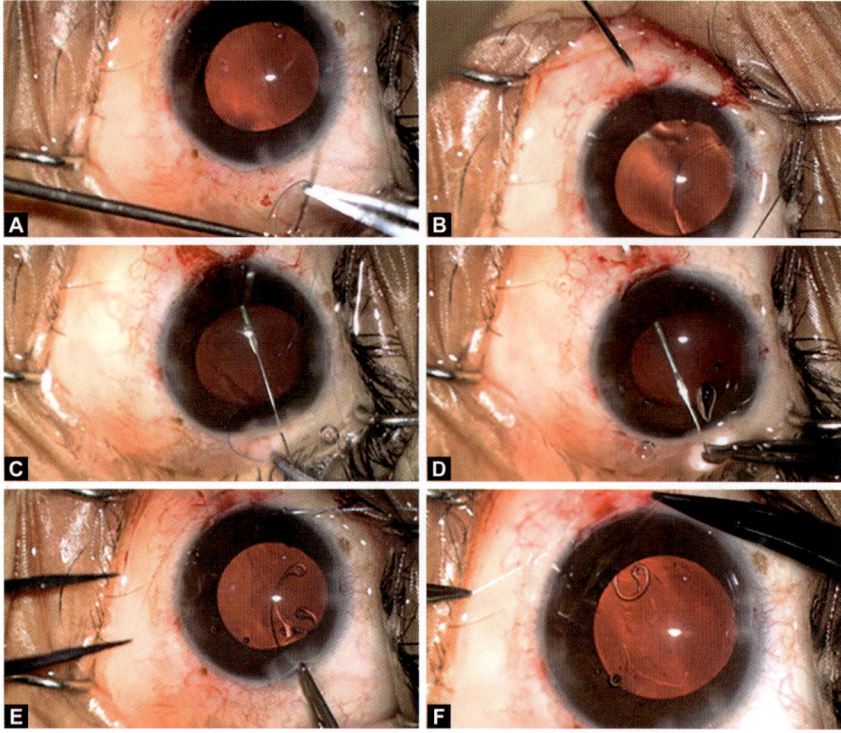

Figs. 9A to F: Steps of scleral fixation of Ahmed segment. (A) Double-armed 9-0 Prolene suture is passed through the fixation hook islet; (B) 26-G needle is inserted ab externo into the ciliary sulcus through a scleral groove 1.5 mm posterior to limbus; (C) One arm of the Prolene suture is rail-roaded through the needle and externalized; (D) The second arm of the suture is similarly externalized through the 26-G needle 1 mm away from the first suture arm; (E) With the sutures secure through the sclera, the Ahmed segment is introduced into the eye; (F) The Ahmed segment is positioned in the bag with the fixation hook above the rhexis, and the suture is tightened to anchor the bag to the sclera.

REFERENCES

1. Osher RH, Cionni RJ, Gimbel HV, et al. Cataract surgery in patients with pseudoexfoliation syndrome. Eur J Implant Ref Surg. 1993;5:46-50.
2. Fine IH, Hoffman RS. Phacoemulsification in the presence of pseudoexfoliation: challenges and options. J Cataract Refract Surg. 1997;23:160-5.
3. Avramides S, Traianidis P, Sakkias G. Cataract surgery and lens implantation in eyes with exfoliation syndrome. J Cataract Refract Surg. 1997;23:583-7.
4. Kuchle M, Viestenz A, Martus P, et al. Anterior chamber depth and complications during cataract surgery in eyes with pseudoexfoliation syndrome. Am J Ophthalmol. 2000;129:281-5.
5. Shingleton BJ, Heltzer J, O'Donoghue MW. Outcomes of phacoemulsification in patients with and without psuedoexfoliation syndrome. J Cataract Refract Surg. 2003;29:1080-6.
6. Jahan FS, Mamalis N, Crandall AS. Spontaneous late dislocation of intraocular lens within the capsular bag in psuedoexfoliation patients. Ophthalmology. 2001;108:1727-31.

7. Ahmed II, Cionni RJ, Kranemann C, et al. Optimal timing of capsular tension ring implantation: Miyake-Apple video analysis. J Cataract Refract Surg. 2005;31:1809-13.
8. Angunawela RI, Little B. Fish-tail technique for capsular tension ring insertion. J Cataract Refract Surg. 2007;33:767-9.
9. Nagamato T, Bissen-Miyajima H. A ring to support the capsular bag after continuous curvilinear capsulorhexis. J Cataract Refract Surg. 1994;20:417-20.
10. Legler UF, Witschel BM. The capsular ring: a new device for complicated cataract surgery. Ger J Ophthalmol. 1994;3:265.
11. Cionni RJ, Osher RH. Endocapsular ring approach to the subluxated cataractous lens. J Cataract Refract Surg. 1995;21:245-9.
12. Gimbel HV, Sun R, Heston JP. Management of zonular dialysis in phacoemulsification and IOL implantation using the capsular tension ring. Ophthalmic Surg Lasers. 1997;28:273-81.
13. Menapace R, Findl O, Georgopoulos M, et al. The capsular tension ring: designs, applications, and techniques. J Cataract Refract Surg. 2000;26:898-912.
14. Bayraktar S, Altan T, Küçüksümer Y, et al. Capsular tension ring implantation after capsulorhexis in phacoemulsification of cataracts associated with pseudo-exfoliation syndrome; intraoperative complications and early postoperative findings. J Cataract Refract Surg. 2001;27:1620-8.
15. Gimbel HV, Sun R. Clinical applications of capsular tension rings in cataract surgery. Ophthalmic Surg Lasers. 2002;33:44-53.
16. Henderson BA, Kim JY. Modified capsular tension ring for cortical removal after implantation. J Cataract Refract Surg. 2007;33:1688-90.
17. Hasanee K, Butler M, Ahmed II. Capsular tension rings and related devices: current concepts. Curr Opin Ophthalmol. 2006;17:31-41.
18. Hasanee K, Ahmed II. Capsular tension rings: update on endocapsular support devices. Ophthalmol Clin North Am. 2006;19:507-19.
19. Boomer JA, Jackson DW. Anatomic evaluation of the Morcher capsular tension ring by ultrasound biomicroscopy. J Cataract Refract Surg. 2006;32:846-8.
20. Marques DM, Marques FF, Osher RH. Subtle signs of zonular damage. J Cataract Refract Surg. 2004;30:1295-9.
21. Shingleton BJ, Marvin AC, Heier JS, et al. Pseudoexfoliation: high risk factors for zonule weakness and concurrent vitrectomy during phacoemulsification. J Cataract Refract Surg. 2010;36(8):1261-9.
22. Hoffman RS, Fine IH, Packer M. Scleral fixation without conjunctival dissection. J Cataract Refract Surg. 2006;32:1907-12.

CHAPTER
14

Scleral-Fixated Intraocular Lenses: A Review

Meena Chakrabarti, Arup Chakrabarti

■ INTRODUCTION

Phacoemulsification with implantation of an intraocular lens (IOL) into the capsular bag is accepted as the standard of care in the management of visually significant cataracts. Endocapsular placement ensured centration of the IOL in the pupillary axis and adequate support of the IOL-bag complex by the ciliary zonules. It also ensured the best possible surgical and refractive outcomes. However, in complicated cataract surgery where the integrity of the capsulozonular apparatus is compromised, alternative option of fixating the IOL is necessary. The surgical options for placing an IOL in an eye without adequate capsulozonular support include anterior chamber IOLs (ACIOLs), iris-fixated IOLs (IFIOLs) and scleral-fixated IOLs (SFIOLs).

A comprehensive review of literature on the various IOL options in the absence of adequate capsular support did not demonstrate a significant difference in the postoperative anatomic or functional outcomes between ACIOLs, IFIOLs and SFIOLs.[1-11] Each approach has its advantages as well an unique set of disadvantages which the surgeon should keep in mind while deciding on the surgical strategy in a given patient.

This review will focus on the use of both sutured and sutureless techniques of SFIOL implantation. The preoperative considerations, variations in the surgical techniques, complications and outcomes for both techniques will be discussed.

■ SUTURED SCLERAL FIXATION

In the event of a posterior capsular rent and inadequate capsular support, sutured scleral fixation is one of the most important surgical options that can be considered for visual rehabilitation of the patient.

Preoperative Considerations

Scleral-fixated IOLs are considered in eyes with no capsular or iris support. Patients who have adequate peripheral anterior or posterior capsular rim may be considered for sulcus-fixated IOLs while patients with normal iris and anterior chamber anatomy, and normal corneal endothelial integrity are suitable candidates for IFIOLs or ACIOLs. However, SFIOLs may be the only available option in eyes with Fuchs endothelial dystrophy, corneal edema, shallow AC, presence of peripheral anterior synechiae or loss of iris tissue.[12,13]

Scleral fixation of a posterior chamber IOL (PCIOL) is considered in one of the following three different scenarios:
1. In eyes with subluxated or dislocated PCIOL (three-piece IOL) where IOL rescue and repositioning has to be performed.[14-16]
2. In eyes where IOL repositioning may not be possible (single-piece IOL) and hence an IOL exchange is planned.
3. Aphakic patient for secondary IOL implantation.

Deciding on the Approach for Surgical Intervention

Scleral-fixated IOLs are performed both by the anterior and posterior segment surgeons. While SF-IOL with anterior vitrectomy (AV) is performed by the cataract surgeon, a three-port pars plana vitrectomy (PPV) is usually performed by the retinal surgeon prior to SFIOL implantation. The anterior approach is preferred for rescuing subluxated IOLs or subluxated capsular bag-IOL complex which is still visible in the pupillary area. The retinal surgeon takes over usually in situations where the patient has a dislocated IOL needing rescue and repositioning. The posterior approach also enables the surgeon to deal with unforeseen intraoperative problems, such as posterior IOL dislocation, retinal tear or retinal detachment.

Cho, et al. performed a retrospective analysis comparing the outcomes and complications in patients who underwent SFIOL implantation after AV and following PPV.[17] The SFIOL/AV group had a higher incidence of IOL dislocation (28% vs. 9%), while the SFIOL/PPV group had a higher incidence of IOL capture (23% vs. 3%). This group was more likely to experience a myopic shift postoperatively. However, the inherent bias in this retrospective study due to surgeon and patient factors prevent definitive conclusions from being drawn based on the available results.

Deciding on "Timing of Surgery"

Scleral-fixated IOL implantation following a complicated cataract surgery can be performed either as a primary or secondary procedure. Although there are no prospective randomized trials on the visual outcomes and long-term complications of SFIOLs performed as a primary or secondary procedure, data from retrospective studies report similar outcomes and complications.[17,18] Hence the decision to perform SFIOL implantation along with the primary cataract surgery or on a later date as a secondary procedure rests with the surgeon and also on the clinical circumstances.

Intraocular Lens Selection for Scleral Fixation

Intraocular Lens Type

Even though most PCIOLs can be sutured to the sclera via their haptics with square on slip knots, there are several specialized haptic designs that facilitate this maneuver. These include:

- Bulbous haptic ends to prevent suture slippage. This is available as part of the haptic design or an enlargement can be created by heating the haptic tip with a cautery to prevent suture slippage.
- Holes and eyelets for suture passage through the haptic have been developed to prevent suture slippage.

The commonly used PCIOLs are CZ70BD (Alcon) (one eyelet in each haptic), Opsia (Chauvin Opsia, France) (two eyelets in each haptic), and Akreos AO60 (Bausch and Lomb, California) (with a four-haptic design and an eyelet in each haptic).

The Aurolab scleral fixation IOL (Aurolab, India) is a single-piece rigid polymethyl methacrylate (PMMA) lens (with an eyelet at the point of maximum haptic spread) and is the most commonly used IOL for scleral fixation in India.

Intraocular Lens Power

As most IOL power calculations are based on in-the-bag location, power adjustment is necessary to account for a more anteriorly positioned lens in the ciliary sulcus. The postoperative spherical equivalent generally depends on the position of the implanted IOL. When the IOL is displaced in an anteriorly, the postoperative anterior chamber depth will be shallower than with endocapsular IOL location and hence a myopic shift in the refraction. Tatsuya Mimura, et al. reported on the refractive changes after transscleral fixation in 21 eyes with 12 years of follow-up.[19] The spherical refractive equivalent was -0.95±2.21D immediately after surgery, -1.16±2.28D after 2 years and -1.37±1.94D after 12 years. Thus, it is a general concept that sulcus-fixated IOL induces a myopic shift. Hayashi, et al. suggested at 0.50D reduction in IOL power for sulcus fixation, while Bayramlar, et al. advised that a 1.25D–1.50D reduction in the intended IOL power for PMMA lenses.[20,21] The effective lens position with sulcus fixation when compared with in-the-bag implantation was found to be 0.62–0.75 mm shorter.[22] Hence a reduction of at least 1.00 Diopter in the intended power is necessary for sulcus fixation.

How Can Ciliary Sulcus Fixation Be Achieved?

The ciliary sulcus is situated between the posterior surface of the iris root and the pars plicata on the inner surface of the eye. Duffey, et al. in an anatomic study on cadaver eyes reported that the external location of the ciliary sulcus is about 0.94 mm behind the surgical limbus in the vertical meridian and 0.5 mm in the horizontal meridian.[23] Therefore, in ab-externo methods, where the suture passes are made in these locations they are most likely to enter the ciliary sulcus. However, several studies demonstrated that the sulcus placement did not occur despite adhering to appropriate measurements as suggested by Duffey, et al. This could be explained by the fact that anatomical variations occur after cataract surgery.[24-26] Following intracapsular cataract extraction (ICCE), the ciliary processes are retracted and rotated anteriorly thereby limiting access to ciliary sulcus. So also when the eye has been opened and is hypotonus, the ciliary sulcus is collapsed and the ciliary processes lie in opposition with the posterior surface of iris. In this situation, the needle pass through the prescribed location will pass through the ciliary process or even the pars plana and not through the ciliary sulcus. In an ultrasound biomicroscopic study on 16 eyes with sutured SFIOLs, Bellucci et al. demonstrated that reducing the suture to limbus distance improved the chances of achieving ciliary sulcus fixation.[27] Performing an ultrasound biomicroscopy (UBM) examination of the anterior segment prior to surgery is necessary to identify anatomical variations that occur after cataract surgery.

Endoscopic visualization of the ciliary sulcus permits more accurate suture placement. However, it entails acquiring costly instrumentation and a more cumbersome procedure.[28-30] Another method of locating the ciliary sulcus is by transillumination, where in on the operation theater (OT) table, a light guide fiber is introduced into the eye through the cataract wound or through a separate pars plana sclerotomy. When the room is darkened, the ciliary sulcus is visible as a lighted band anterior to the dark ring of the ciliary body.[31]

Can, et al. described a novel technique of implanting a PCIOL in the absence of capsular support using a ciliary sulcus guide.[32] Based on the anatomical knowledge of the ciliary sulcus, Can, et al. devised an instrument which snugly fits into the ciliary sulcus and can hence guide the needle safely through the ciliary sulcus and sclera for ab-interno scleral fixation.

Surgical Techniques: Scleral-Sutured Intraocular Lenses

The surgical technique of securing the haptics of the IOL to the sclera evolved to its present stage through various significant modifications in the first published technique. A review of the various techniques beginning with the first published report in the 1986 by Malbran and colleagues[33] is described in Table 1.

The variations in technique can be grouped under:
- Method of introducing needles: Ab-externo and ab-interno
- Method of fixating haptic with fixation suture
- The number of points of PCIOL fixation
- Method of avoiding suture/knot erosion.

Malbran and colleagues (1986) published the first description of ab-externo two-point scleral fixation using lens guide sutures for fixation of a secondary IOL implant after ICCE. 10-0 polypropylene sutures were used to fixate the haptics of the rigid PMMA IOL at 3 o'clock and 9 o'clock positions, 2 mm posterior to the limbus. Using a 28-gauge needle, suture loops were introduced ab-externo to create two internal suture loops at 3 o'clock and 9 o'clock meridians.[33] Through a corneal incision the sutures were externalized at the limbus and secured by a hitch to the haptic of the IOL. The IOL was introduced into the posterior chamber and the suture loops were pulled out to position the implant. The suture was then tied on to the sclera achieving scleral fixation of the IOL.[33]

Ab-interno two-point fixation, where the needle pass was made from inside to outside was also performed by several groups of surgeons during the same period. The needle pass made from inside out was performed blindly in

Table 1: Comparison of various techniques of sutured scleral fixation.

Authors/Years	Scleral flaps	Points of fixation	Needle passes	AI/AE	Type of suture fixation	Eyelet
Malbran (1986)[33]	No	2 point	2	2 AE	Square knot	Nil
Lewis (1991)[34]	Yes	2 point	2	1 AE/1 AI	Square knot	Nil
Shapiro (1991)[35]	Yes	2 point	2	2 AE suture retrieved through corneosclera incision	Square knot	Nil
Basti (1994)[36]	Yes (direct introduction of suture using 26-gauge hollow needle. Suture eternized through section)	2 point	2	AE	Square knot	Nil
Ramocki (1999)[37]	Yes (small incision surgery/foldable Acrysof MA60BM IOL used)	2 point	2	1 AE/1 AI	Square knot	Nil
Eryildirim (1995)[38]	Yes (haptic looping/suture loop retrieved through the corneosclera section)	2 point	4 all AE 2 with needle port first 2 with reverse end of needle through original entry site	4 all AE	Girth hitch and suture loop over haptic	Yes
Lewis (1993)[34]	Ab-externo continuous loop fixation without scleral flaps	4 point	AE (2 with HN, 2 with SN)	AE continuous loop	Continuous loop	Yes
Rao (2000)[39]	Yes L-shaped	4 point	8 needle passes	AE	Continuous loop	Yes
Bergren (1994)[40]	Scleral groove	4 point	8 needle passes	4 AE 4 AI	Girth hitch	Yes
Smiddy (1990)[41]	No	2 point	2	AI	Square knot	No
Grigorian (2003)[42]	Yes (AI 4-point fixation with haptic looping)	4 point	6	Change to 3 per side 2 AE and AI	Continuous loop	Yes

(AI: ab-interno; AE: ab-externo)

an open soft globe and led to complications, such as hemorrhagic choroidal detachment, vitreous hemorrhage and unpredictable final placement of lens haptic. The procedure was performed blindly as the intraocular exit point of the needle was not visible. Subsequently several groups of surgeons refined the technique to include transillumination, UBM examination or endoscopic visualization of the ciliary sulcus.

Lewis, et al. (1991) refined the Malbran technique of ab-externo two-point scleral fixation by introducing the following modifications (ab-externo two-point scleral fixation with scleral flaps):[34]

- Lamellar scleral flaps were used to cover the suture knots and prevent long-term suture exposure.
- Railroading/docking a straight needle on a 10-0 polypropylene suture into a 26/28-gauge needle introduced 180° away.
- Ab-externo needle entry is 2 mm behind limbus thereby giving the IOL a final position in the ciliary sulcus that is reproducible.

The 10-0 polypropylene suture which traverses the eye was externalized, cut into two halves and tied to the haptic of the IOL. The IOL was introduced into the posterior chamber and the sutures were pulled out to center it. A scleral bite was taken near the point of entry of the suture and the suture was tied to itself.

Subsequent Variations in the Ab-Externo Technique

Direct Ab-Externo Insertion of Suture (Shapiro, et al. 1991)[35]

This method is similar to the Lewis technique except for a few modifications. It avoids the necessity to dock the straight needle of the 10-0 polypropylene suture into a hollow 26-gauge needle and railroading it out of the eye. This was achieved by passing the suture directly out of the eye through the superior corneoscleral incision. Passage of the needle through the corneoscleral wound may damage the intraocular structures and distort the already open globe.[35]

Direct Introduction of Suture by a 26-Gauge Hollow Needle (Basti, et al. 1994)[36]

Basti, et al. utilized a 26-gauge hollow needle through which the free end of the 10-0 polypropylene suture on a curved needle is passed. The hollow needle and the suture loops were passed ab-externo through the sclera and ciliary sulcus 0.50–0.75 mm from the limbus. The suture was withdrawn through the main incision using McPherson forceps. This method requires only routinely available material and has relatively lesser intraocular manipulations.[36]

Small Incision Technique (Ramocki, et al. 1999)[37]

Ramocki, et al. described a technique of two-point scleral fixation utilizing a small incision and foldable IOL. The 6 o'clock and 12 o'clock meridians are chosen for scleral fixation. Small incision technique by the Lewis method using foldable IOLs has been described by Regillo and Tidwell as well as by Tsai and Tseng, et al.[37,43,44]

Haptic Looping Method: (Eryildirim, et al. 1995)[38]
Eryildirim, et al. described a knotless haptic looping method for scleral fixation. In this method, each suture loop was inserted through the eyelet in the haptic of the rigid single-piece all-PMMA IOL. At one end the loop was passed over the IOL and at the other end the loop was passed over the haptic to lock the suture over the eyelets.[38]

Ab-Externo Continuous Loop Fixation (Lewis, et al.)[34]
This is a four-point fixation technique which allows burying the fixation knot. This technique was performed without a scleral flap and involves two needle passes. The sutures were retrieved through the corneoscleral wound, cut into two halves and both ends from each side were tied to itself after passing through the eyelet in the haptic. The initial knot was rotated out of the eye and the lens was placed in the sulcus. The long loops were cut shortened and tied. The final knot was rotated into the eye.[34]

Ab-Externo Continuous Loop Fixation with Scleral Flaps (Rao, et al. 2000)[39]
In this technique, the authors fashioned L-shaped sclera incision at 3 o'clock and 9 o'clock meridians and limbus based flaps were dissected. The 10-0 polypropylene suture with the long straight needle was passed through one scleral bed and guided out of the superior corneal incision with a 27-gauge needle. The suture was threaded through the eyelet from below upward and was passed back into the eye through the corneal incision and guided out of the eye by another 27-gauge needle inserted through the same sclera bed in an ab-externo fashion, 1 mm above the horizontal meridian. The same steps are repeated for the other haptic. The IOL in implanted into the eye and sutures were gently pulled to center the IOL and tied. The knot was rotated into the eye.[39]

Limbal Groove Incision and Double Suture Fixation to Haptic (Bergren, et al. 1994)[40]
In this technique, 3 mm long limbus parallel sclera grooves were placed 0.5–0.75 mm from the limbus at 3 o'clock and 9 o'clock positions. In this procedure, the suture passes were made through both ends of the limbal groove.[40]

Injectable Suture Device for Intraocular Ab-Externo Suture Fixation (Smith, et al. 2015)
The authors used a 24-gauge injector to deliver a preformed suture loop into the eye with the double-armed needles still outside the eye.[45]

Ab-Interno Scleral Fixation
Ab-Interno Two-Point Fixation (Smiddy, et al. 1990)
A double-armed 10-0 polypropylene suture was first bisected and each cut end is tied to the haptic of the IOL. The suture was exteriorized by an ab-interno needle pass. After IOL implantation, the suture was tied to itself after taking a lamellar sclera bite. The cut ends were left long (2 mm) and laid flat under the conjunctiva.[41,45]

Ab-Interno Four-Point Fixation with Haptic Looping (Grigorian, et al. 2003)[42]

This provides a very quick and efficient way of creating an intraocular loop with four-point fixation. Iris hooks were also used to facilitate visualization of the ciliary sulcus. Lamellar triangular scleral flaps were dissected at 3 o'clock and 9 o'clock positions. Flexible iris retractors were used to enlarge the pupil widely. After adequate AV, a long 27-gauge bent needle was inserted ab-externo at 3 o'clock and was pushed forward to exit the globe at 9.15 o'clock. The straight long needle on a 10-0 polypropylene suture was docked into the hollow of the 27-gauge needle, blunt end first. This device was withdrawn into the vitreous cavity and was redirected to exit the globe at 8.45 o'clock. The docked straight needle was drawn out and the bent 27-gauge needle was also taken out. The suture loop thus created was brought out through the limbal incision using a hook. Each loop was passed through the haptic eyelet and was looped over the haptic to form a knot.[42] The PCIOL was inserted and the sutures were tied. The ends were cut long enough to lie flat against the sclera under the scleral flap.

Endoscopy-Assisted Scleral-Fixated IOLs (Olsen, et al. 2011)

Intraocular endoscopy has been used for observing directly the needle penetration site for implanting the haptics of the PCIOL into the ciliary sulcus. It also aids in visualizing and trimming any areas of vitreous traction and also for scrutinizing the peripheral retina for breaks or detachment.[28-30] Sasahara, et al. compared endoscopy assisted versus routine technique of sutured SFIOLs and reported a dramatic reduction in the complication rate when an endoscope was used for visualization and suture placement.[46,47]

Pars Plana Phacoprosthesis

The IOL was introduced through the pars plana and was anchored to the sclera is that area. The optic was positioned in the posterior chamber allowing free movement of the iris and the best optical correction.[48] This technique however never gained popularity and is not used today. Ma, et al. in 2011 compared the clinical outcomes of transscleral fixation of PCIOLs in the ciliary sulcus and pars plana and reported comparable clinical outcomes and safety with both groups.[49] Fanger Han, et al. also evaluated the pars plana scleral fixation of PCIOL with the knot buried without scleral flaps and compared clinical outcomes and complications with transscleral fixation into ciliary sulcus. There was significant differences in clinical outcomes were observed between both groups. However, this technique did not gain popularity with the majority of surgeons. For pars plana fixation, a PCIOL must have a larger diameter of about 17 mm with an optic diameter of 7 mm, and a backward angulation of the haptics. The haptics are angled backward to allow the IOL optic to be in the position of the original lens. Therefore, the IOL power is estimated to be similar for in-the-bag placement. Because of the different location of IOL, the sclera entry is made 3.0–3.50 mm behind to the surgical limbus.

Modification in Materials for Scleral Fixation

Initially rigid IOLs were used for sutured scleral fixation. Presently newer IOLs, such as CZ70BD (Alcon) and Akreos A060 (B and L) are used. These lenses have suture eyelets to prevent suture slippage and IOL decentration. CZ70BD is a single-piece PMMA monofocal aspheric IOL with a suture eyelet at the point of maximum haptic spread and an overall diameter of 12.5 cm. The Akreos A060 is a hydrophilic acrylic monofocal aspheric lens with a four-haptic design and an eyelet in each of the four haptics for suture fixation.[48-50] Because of the concerns regarding suture breakage as well as long-term stability of 10-0 polypropylene suture, surgeons started using 9-0 polypropylene and Gore-Tex (CV-8 Gore-Tex) a nonabsorbable polytetrafluoroethylene (PTFE) monofilament sutures which is nonabsorbable and nonbiodegradable[51,52] (Figs. 1A to C).

Several needles are available for suturing PCIOLs. The Ethicon TG-160-2, Ethicon C1F-4, and Ethicon STC-6 (Ethicon, Somerville, New Jersey) can be used for ab-interno scleral fixation. The STC-6 straight needle is also used for ab-externo scleral fixation.

Suture-Related Modification

The trend toward usage of thicker and less biodegradable sutures was necessitated by multiple reports of late IOL dislocation in eyes where 10-0

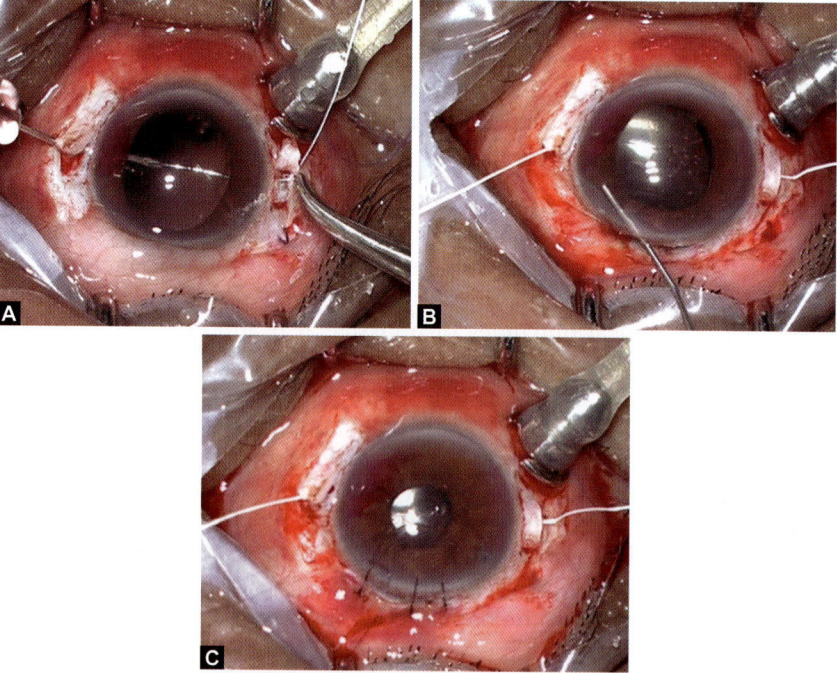

Figs. 1A to C: Two-point ab-externo scleral fixation using 8-0 Gore-Tex suture. (A) Ab-externo two-point needle pass; (B) The suture is retrieved through the corneoscleral section cut into two and tied to each haptic of an all polymethyl methacrylate (PMMA) intraocular lens (IOL) with haptic eyelet; (C) The sutures are pulled to center the IOL.

polypropylene sutures were used for scleral fixation.[53,54] The reported incidence of late IOL dislocation in various studies range from 2% to 15%.[53-55] Dislocation of SFIOLs have been reported as early as 15 months after surgery to as late as 10 years.[55-57] Buckley, et al. evaluated the long-term stability of SFIOLs secured with 10-0 polypropylene suture in children and reported an incidence of 15% (4/26 cases) late dislocation secondary to suture breakage at a mean 5.6 years after surgery.[53] Thicker sutures, such as 9-0 polypropylene or 7-0 Gore-Tex sutures have lesser incidence of intraoperative suture breakage. Although long-term follow-up studies in eyes where these sutures were used are not available, several small case series have reported excellent short-term stability. The longest reported follow-up is 33 months by Khan, et al. using Akreos or CZ70BD lens and 7-0 Gore-Tex suture in 83 eyes.[51]

Knot Erosion

Erosion of the suture knot through the conjunctiva following sutured scleral fixation is a serious complication and is a potential risk factor for endophthalmitis.[58-60] Knot erosion provides a direct open track into the eye through which exogenous pathogens can gain access to intraocular contents. Hence it became necessary to adopt any one of the modifications enumerated below to prevent this disastrous complication:

Use of Scleral Flaps

- Lewis, et al. used hinged triangular scleral flaps to cover the suture knots at the conclusions of the procedure.[34]
- Hoffman, et al. created sclera pockets or pouches to protect the suture knots. The lamellar scleral pouches open toward the limbus and is covered by the intact conjunctiva to afford effective protection for the suture knot and prevent erosion.[61] When the sutures are looped out of the pouch and tied, the knot gets buried within the pouch. Four-point ab-externo scleral fixation achieved by this technique required four-needle passes through the eye and was effective in achieving stable IOL fixation into the ciliary sulcus as well as in preventing knot erosion (Figs. 2A to K).

Use of Scleral Grooves

- Burying the knot into sclera can also prevent suture erosion.[25,62] However, burying the knot may prove difficult with short suture passes and when thicker sutures are used where the knot is too big to be buried.
- Passing the end of the externalized 10-0 polypropylene suture in a zigzag manner through the sclera in multiple locations. Favorable long-term results of this technique were reported by Szurman, et al. in 45 eyes.[63]

Intraocular Lens Tilt

Holladay, et al. reported that two-point scleral fixation was associated with IOL tilt greater than 15° causing higher order astigmatism which cannot be corrected with spectacles.[64] If the IOL tilt was significant it resulted in higher order aberrations and an additional refractive error.

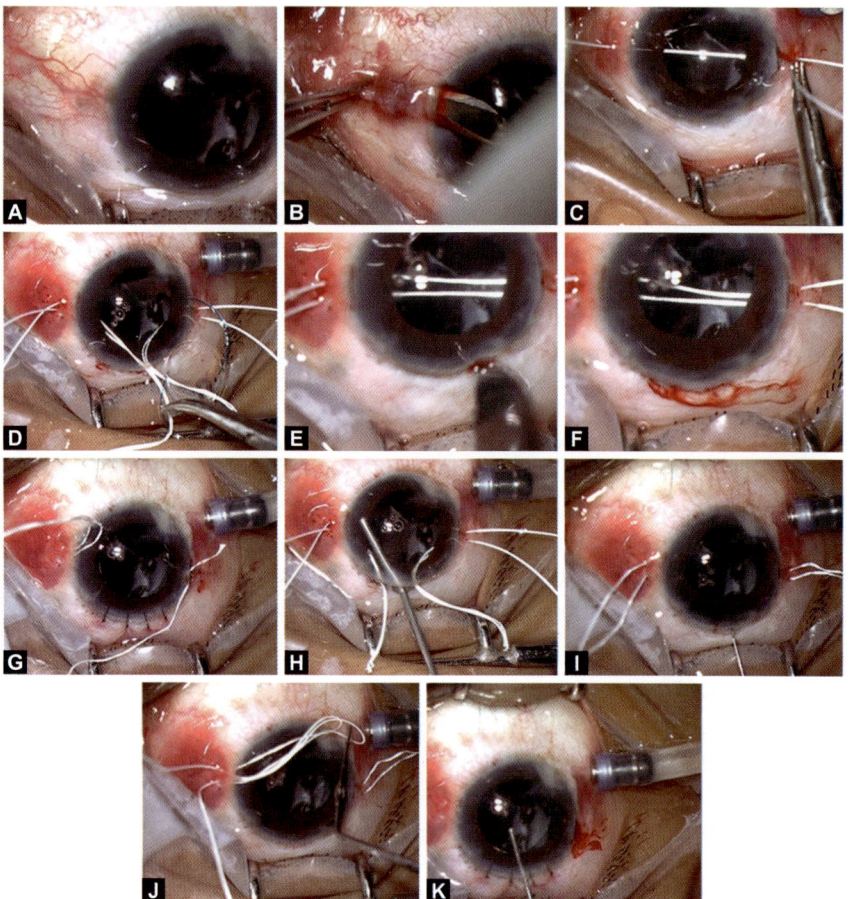

Figs. 2A to K: Hoffman's pouch and Gore-Tex suture for ab-externo four-point scleral fixation. (A) Remnants of the fibrosed posterior capsule with a large posterior capsular rent inferiorly. There is a corneal scar inferiorly due to a penetrating injury in childhood; (B) Dissection of Hoffman's pouch; (C and D) Ab-externo suture passes after cutting off the needle. The suture end is grasped using 23-gauge microvitreoretinal (MVR) forceps and introduced into the eye. By a handshake maneuver, the suture end is transferred to another 23-gauge forceps introduced through the Hoffman's pouch on the opposite site; (E to H) A limbal tunnel incision is fashioned, the sutures are pulled out and cut into two. Both suture ends on one side are anchored by square knot to the haptic of the IOL. The IOL is implanted into the eye and the sutures are pulled out to center the IOL; (I to K) Using a Sinskey hook, the suture is looped out of the Hoffman's pouch, shortened and tied to each other. The knot fits snugly into the pouch.

Teichmann, et al. in an in vitro experimental study demonstrated the occurrence of torque or tilt effect using the Alcon CZ70BD IOL. Hayashi, et al. compared the IOL tilt and decentration in transsclerally sutured IOLs and in-the-bag IOLs (6.35° vs. 3.18°, respectively).[65] Although there are no comparative studies comparing CZ70BD and Bausch and Lomb Akreos AO60, theoretically and logically, the four-point stabilization inherent to the Akreos IOL will reduce the incidence of lens decentration and tilt.

Khan, et al. described a technique combining 27-gauge PPV and scleral fixation of Akreos AO60 lens using CV-8 Gore-Tex sutures.[51] The sutures were cut into halves, and anchored to the two eyelets on each side of the Akreos lens. The nasal sutures were externalized first (before implanting the IOL) through the two 27-gauge sclerotomies. The same procedure was performed on the temporal side also. The two suture ends on each side are tied to each other and the knot was rotated into the sclerotomy. This type of four-point fixation will not produce any IOL tilt or decentration.

Complications associated with Sutured Scleral-Fixated Intraocular Lenses

The results of long-term follow-up studies in patients who have undergone transsclerally sutured PCIOLs are generally favorable. However, sutured SFIOL surgery is associated with certain unique complications.
- IOL dislocation
- IOL tilt
- Suprachoroidal hemorrhage
- Vitreous hemorrhage
- Retinal detachment
- Suture erosion
- Endophthalmitis.

The most commonly encountered intraoperative complication is suture breakage especially when 10-0 polypropylene sutures are used for sutured scleral fixation.

Suboptimal suture placement and use of thinner and less durable sutures for anchoring the haptic to the sclera are responsible for most of the postoperative complications.

One of the most important complications observed on long-term follow-up of SFIOLs is the presence of erosion of the suture knots through the scleral flaps and the conjunctiva. This creates a potential tract into intraocular tissues, and an increased risk of microbial contamination.[58-60] Initially when the fixation sutures were tied under the conjunctiva without using a lamellar scleral flap, the incidence of knot erosion was 24%.[66] In eyes where a scleral flap is used to cover the knot, the incidence of scleral flap atrophy and a visible knot under the conjunctiva is 15–27%.[67,68]

The stability of the IOL is initially dependent on the suture and later when the haptics become encased in fibrous tissue the suture integrity plays a minor role. IOL dislocation can result from suture breakage, slipping of knot, suture cheese wiring and also suture disintegration overtime. Suture removal should not be attempted when there is a knot erosion. Alternative methods to address this problem include trimming or cautery of the knot, surgical coverage with a corneal or sclera patch graft[69,70] (Figs. 3A and B).

Cystoid macular edema is the most common complication in most series with a higher incidence when compared to an uncomplicated cataract surgery with PCIOL implantation. An incidence of 5.5–6.1% has been reported in

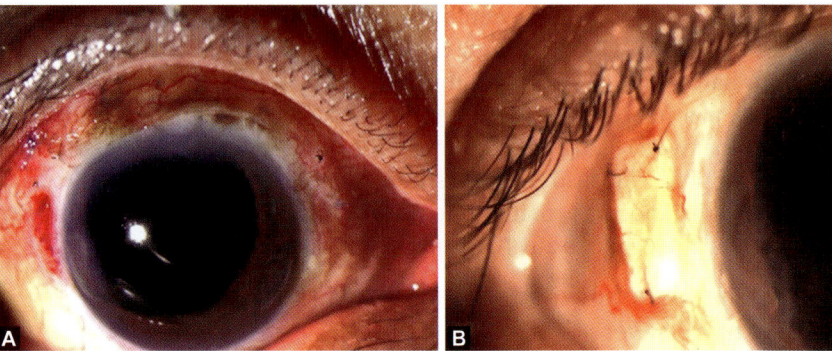

Figs. 3A and B: Suture knot erosion. (A) Showing erosion of suture knot through scleral flap; (B) Lamellar scleral graft is used to cover the exposed suture.

two studies.[71,72] Factors contributing to the development of cystoid macular edema are vitreous loss, prolonged operating time and light-induced toxicity.

Suturing PCIOLs to the ciliary sulcus entails needle passage through highly vascular uveal tissue and hence the occurrence of hyphema, vitreous hemorrhage and suprachoroidal hemorrhage. Positioning the suture placement 0.5–1 mm behind the surgical limbus, and avoiding the 3 o'clock and 9 o'clock meridians will prevent needle passage through the vascular ciliary body tissue or injury to the long posterior ciliary arteries.[68,73-75] Although intraocular hemorrhage in most cases is related to trauma during needle pass, it has also been reported to occur due to wicking of extraocular blood along the suture track.[76] Careful attention to hemostasis during extraocular dissection will avoid occurrence of this complications.

Sutured PCIOLs are anchored to the ciliary sulcus at one or more points in eyes without capsular support. This can result in IOL tilt and decentration leading to uncorrected astigmatism, higher order aberrations, myopic shift and a lateral shift of focus. A tilt less than 5° and decentration less than 2 mm do not cause significant astigmatism and is compatible with good visual function.[77] Significant lens tilt greater than 10° can be seen in (11.4–16.7%) of patients.[20,77]

Scleral-Fixated Intraocular Lens Implantation in Children

Children who have sustained ocular trauma or those who have undergone congenital cataract surgery form a subgroup of patients with inadequate capsular support in whom optimal management has not been standardized.

There are no prospective randomized studies comparing the outcomes of ACIOLs, IFIOLs and SFIOL in this age group and hence the surgical option considered for visual rehabilitation in this unique subgroup of patients is largely based on the surgeon's preference and patient-related clinical circumstances. The potential complications in this age group of patients for ACIOLs and SFIOLs are chronic iris chafing, iritis, and glaucoma. Short-term follow-up results for sutured SFIOL implantation in children (1–6 years follow-up) have yielded promising results but concerns regarding endophthalmitis,

IOL decentration or dislocation and suture-related complications prevent adoption of this option on a regular basis.[78-89] Presently short-term 6 months' follow-up result of sutureless scleral fixation in children is also available with promising results. However, long-term follow-up data is necessary to support the safety and efficacy of these techniques in children.[89]

Scleral fixation in small eyes is technically difficult for the following reasons:
- The pediatric eye is small with narrow palpebral aperture.
- There has been no anatomic study looking at the position of ciliary sulcus with respect to the limbus in children.
- The technique used should minimize the occurrence of suture erosion.
- The long-term effects and potential complications are unknown.
- Degradation of the suture overtime and IOL stability are matters of grave concern.

Other issues include the possibility of late-onset endophthalmitis, glaucoma, retinal detachment and haptic erosion through ciliary body.

A review and analysis of published literature on pediatric scleral fixation is tabulated in Table 2 which gives a comparative analysis of the surgical techniques employed, the final result as well as associated complications.

Sutured Scleral-Fixated Intraocular Lenses in Eyes Undergoing Penetrating Keratoplasty

During penetrating keratoplasty, SFIOLs are implanted by an open-sky method. A large Flieringa's ring is used to stabilize the globe as the manipulation occurs after removal of the recipient button. A large ring (≥18 mm) ensures that there is adequate space for peritomies at sites of scleral fixation.[90]

In-the-Bag Intraocular Lens Dislocation

In eyes with an in-the-bag dislocation or subluxation of the capsular bag-single-piece IOL complex, suture fixation to the sclera can be safety performed by technique described in Figures 4A to F.

■ SUTURELESS INTRASCLERAL HAPTIC FIXATED POSTERIOR CHAMBER INTRAOCULAR LENS

Introduction

In 2007, Gabor Scharioth, et al.[91,92] developed a technique of sutureless intrascleral haptic fixation for three-piece PCIOLs in eyes with absent capsular support. Later Agarwal, et al. presented a modification of this technique with dissection of lamellar scleral flap 180° apart and use of fibrin glue to reposition the scleral flaps and conjunctiva. Agarwal, et al. further refined their technique by an additional intrascleral tunnel into which the haptics of the IOL can be tucked in for increased stability.[93] Subsequently several modifications were introduced. In this review the various modifications in the sutureless scleral fixation technique, intraoperative problems, postoperative complications as well as functional outcomes will be covered in detail.

Table 2: Transscleral fixation in children.

	Follow-up	No. of eyes	Suture method	Scleral exit point	Complications
Kumar, et al. (1992)[81]	4–18 months	11 eyes (4–9 years)	AI; scleral flaps	0.75 mm posterior to limbus	IOL decentration suture erosion, glaucoma, CME marked AS reaction
Mittelviefhaus (2000)[88]	25–70 months	4 eyes (age 26–35 months)	AI, girth hitch knot rotated into eye and covered with Tenon's and conjunctiva	<1 mm	Nil
Zetterstorm (1999)[89]	9–33 months	21 eyes (1–11 years)	Ab-externo (Lewis) knot rotated into eye	1.5–2.00 mm behind limbus	IOL rotation Optic in AC
Sharpe (1996)[83]	3–38 months	7 years (1–19 years)	Ab-interno Scleral flaps	0.5 mm post to limbus	IOL decentration IOL tilting Suture erosion
Jacobi PC (2002)	6 months	26 eyes	MF IOL scleral flaps Ab-externo (Lewis)	0.75 mm posterior to limbus	↑IOP (11.5%), AS reaction 15.4%, IOL decentration 19.2%, suture erosion 7.4%, better stereopsis
Asadi, R et al (2008)	12–144 months	25 eyes	Scleral flaps Ab-externo (Lewis)	1 mm post to limbus	Transient intraocular hemorrhage 52%, transient choroidal effusion (8%), late endophthalmitis (4%), RD 4%, IOL dislocation (24%)
Caca I (2011)[85]	11–18 months	24 eyes	Scleral flaps Ab-interno 2 point		Transient ↑IOP, VH, RD
El Gendy HA (2016)	6 months	40 eyes	Endoscopy-assisted Ab-interno		↑IOP, decentration 5%, Vit 12.5%, RD
Byrd JM (2017)	46 months	70 eyes	Ab-externo 10-0 polypropylene 8.0 Gore-Tex		PCO 50%, UGH syndrome 2.8%, IOL dislocation 3%

(AI: ab-interno; AE: ab-externo; AS: anterior segment; VH: vitreous hemorrhage; RD: retinal detachment; AC: anterior chamber; CME: cystoid macular edema; UGH: uveitis-glaucoma-hyphema; PCO: posterior capsule opacification; RD: retinal detachment; MF: multifocal)

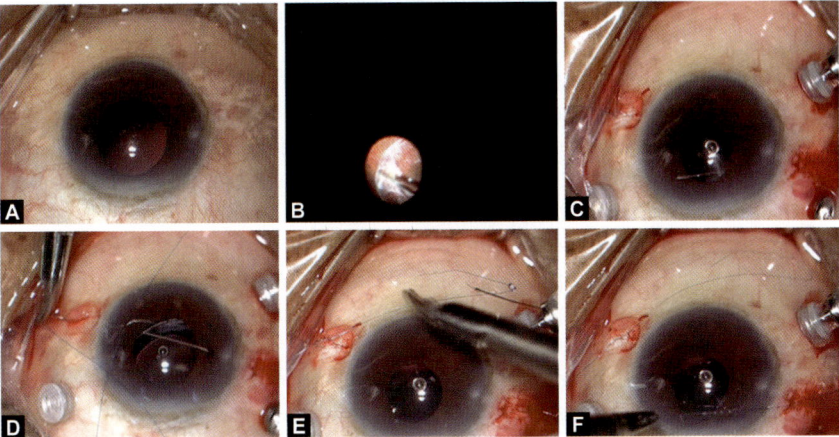

Figs. 4A to F: Late spontaneous dislocation of capsular bag-IOL complex in an elderly patient 7 years after the primary procedure. (A) The pupillary area is aphakic; (B) Dislocated capsular bag-IOL complex on the retinal surface. There is capsular bag fibrosis and contracture; (C) The dislocated capsular bag-IOL complex is brought to the pupil; (D) Limbal grooves are created after a local peritomy. 10-0 polypropylene suture on a straight ST6 needle is introduced ab-externo. The needle passes through the capsular bag and under the leading haptic of the IOL. The needle is brought out by puncturing the peripheral cornea. The needle is cut and the suture withdrawn through the second sclerotomy made in the groove thereby forming a suture loop around the haptic of the IOL. (E) The trailing haptic is also looped in a similar manner; (F) The suture is tied to itself so that the knot fits snugly into the scleral groove. The peritomy is closed.

Preoperative Workup

Adequate preoperative evaluation of the patient is necessary for planning the secondary IOL implantation. An assessment of the best corrected visual acuity, corneal endothelial cell count, intraocular pressure, fundus evaluation and optical coherence tomography (OCT) evaluation of the macula is necessary to prognosticate to the patient about the visual potential of the eye to be operated. Intrascleral tuck is contraindicated in patients with history of recurrent scleritis and scleromalacia.

Intraocular Lens Selection

The ideal IOL for sutureless scleral fixation is a three-piece IOL. Rigid PMMA single-piece IOLs are rarely used as the haptics tend to snap and break and hence all intraocular manipulations have to be performed very gently.

Surgical Technique of Intrascleral Sutureless Haptic Fixation of Posterior Chamber Intraocular Lens

Sutureless Intrascleral Haptic Fixation (Gabor Scharioth, et al. 2007)

The steps for successful intrascleral sutureless haptic fixation of a three-piece PCIOL as performed originally by Scharioth, et al. is as follows:[91,92]
1. Anterior chamber maintainer is used to maintain the IOP throughout the procedure. In patients with dislocated IOL, a three-port PPV is necessary.

Here a pars plana infusion cannula is used to ensure that the IOP is maintained.
2. Conjunctival peritomy is performed. Sclerotomies are made 180° apart, 1.5–2.0 mm posterior to the limbus with a sharp 23-gauge cannula.
3. Intrascleral tunnel is prepared starting from the ciliary sulcus sclerotomy using a 23-gauge bent sharp cannula. The intrascleral tunnel is directed counterclockwise like the haptic direction of a standard PCIOL.
4. A standard three-piece IOL with a haptic design similar to the diameter of the ciliary sulcus is implanted using an injector so that the leading haptic is on the iris surface and the trailing haptic is fixated and stabilized by the lips of the corneal incision.
5. The leading haptic is grasped at its tip with a straight 25-gauge Scharioth forceps and externalized through the 23-gauge sclerotomy.
6. The trailing haptic is grasped and introduced into the pupillary area and transferred to a 25-gauge Scharioth straight forceps introduced through the sclerotomy (Handshake technique).
7. Curved Scharioth forceps is used to implant the IOL haptic into the limbus parallel intrascleral tunnel.

The Scharioth technique was modified by Agarwal, et al. first by taking a lamellar scleral flap and use of fibrin glue. Later in 2008, they also added an intrascleral tunnel for haptic stabilization.

Glued Intrascleral Haptic Fixation of a Posterior Chamber IOL (Agarwal, et al. 2008)[93] (Figs. 5A to H)

1. Peritomy and dissection of lamellar scleral flaps 180° apart.
2. Sclerotomies are performed in the bed of the scleral flap with 20-gauge needle 1.5 mm behind the limbus.
3. An AC maintainer or a pars plana infusion helps to maintain the IOP.
4. A 23-gauge cutter is introduced through both the sclerotomy and a vitrectomy to clear any incarcerated vitreous is performed. Any residual cortical matter or capsular remnants present in the pupillary space is also cleared.
5. Corneal tunnel incision with 2.8 mm keratome. A side port incision is made midway between the left-sided sclerotomy and the corneal tunnel incision for manipulating the trailing haptic.
6. A three-piece hydrophobic acrylic PCIOL is loaded into its cartridge with the leading haptic protruding out. The IOL is implanted and simultaneously the tip of the leading haptic is grasped with a 23-gauge forceps introduced through the left-sided sclerotomy. Once the IOL is fully implanted with the trailing haptic stabilized at the section, the leading haptic is exteriorized. An assistant hold the leading haptic to prevent slippage into the eye.
7. The surgeon then grasps the trailing haptic and flexes it into the eye. The tip of the trailing haptic is grasped by a straight 23-gauge forceps introduced through the side port incision. A handshake maneuver is performed in transferring the trailing haptic to another 23-gauge forceps introduced through the right-sided sclerotomy. The trailing haptic is also exteriorized.

Scleral-Fixated IntraocularLenses: A Review

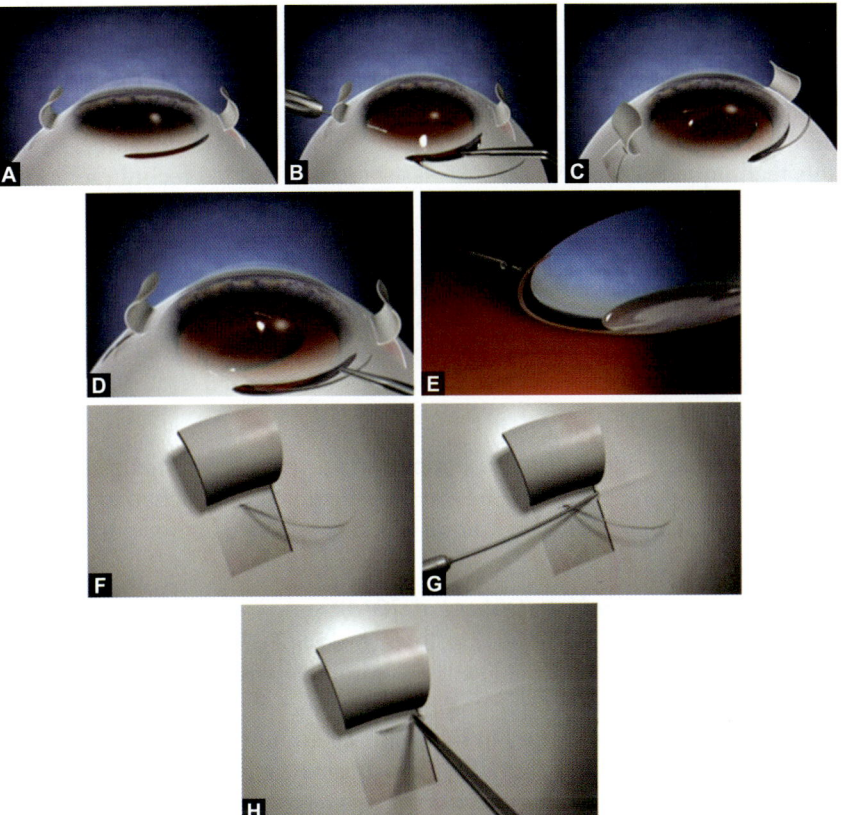

Figs. 5A to H: Sutureless glued IOL (Agarwal, et al.). (A) Dissection of lamellar scleral flaps. Limbal section is opened; (B) Three-piece IOL introduced through section and the leading haptic is grasped at its tip; (C) The leading haptic is exteriorized using a 23-gauge forceps through the sclerotomy on the bed of the flap on the left side; (D) The trailing haptic is grasped and introduced into the eye; (E) The tip of the trailing haptic is grasped and it is exteriorized; (F) Exteriorized haptic; (G) Fashioning of the tunnel; (H) Haptic tucked into the tunnel.

8. Both haptics are tucked into scleral tunnels made at the base of the flap using 23-gauge needle.
9. A drop of reconstituted fibrin glue is used to close the scleral flaps, peritomy and the corneal tunnel as well as the side port incisions.

Comprehending IOL signs[93] and its significance in sutureless intrascleral haptic fixation when foldable IOLs are used is necessary to ensure that the IOL has unfolded with proper orientation. When the foldable IOL is injected into the anterior chamber the unfolding of the IOL with a "lucky 7" sign for the leading haptic and an "upright C" for trailing haptic indicate that the IOL has unfolded into proper orientation.[93]

No-Assistant Technique/Two-Handed Technique

In the previously described technique by Agarwal, et al. after exteriorization of the leading haptic an assistant holds the haptic with a forceps to prevent its slippage back into the eye. The no-Assistant two-handed technique utilizes the reversal of vector forces when the trailing haptic crosses the mid pupillary plane. At this position more of the leading haptic is pushed out. Therefore, the trailing haptic is brought inferior to the mid pupillary plane, grasped at its tip and externalized, while the leading haptic is pushed out of the globe. Hence this technique is called NAT or No-Assistant two-handed technique[94] (Figs. 6A to F).

Suture-Assisted Sutureless Technique (Kora 2015)[95]

Suture-assisted sutureless technique also avoided the necessity of having an assistant hold the haptic to prevent slippage. The IOL haptics were tied to a looped 9-0 polypropylene suture. The suture needle is passed through the sclerotomy site and when pulled the haptic is exteriorized.[95]

Beiko and Steinert Technique[96]

The authors used silicone tires or stoppers to prevent the externalized leading haptic from slipping back into the eye. The silicone tires attached to iris hook was used as a stopper. This technique was very effective in preventing haptic slippage.[96]

Ohta Y-Fixation Technique (Ohta et al. 2014)[97]

The Y-fixation technique does not involve complicated intraocular manipulations and is able to achieve safe sutureless fixation. Two Y-shaped sutures are made 2 mm from the limbus and directed opposite to each other. A 23-gauge MVR knife is used to make the sclerotomy at the function of the limbs or along the stems of the Y. After externalizing the haptic, the scleral

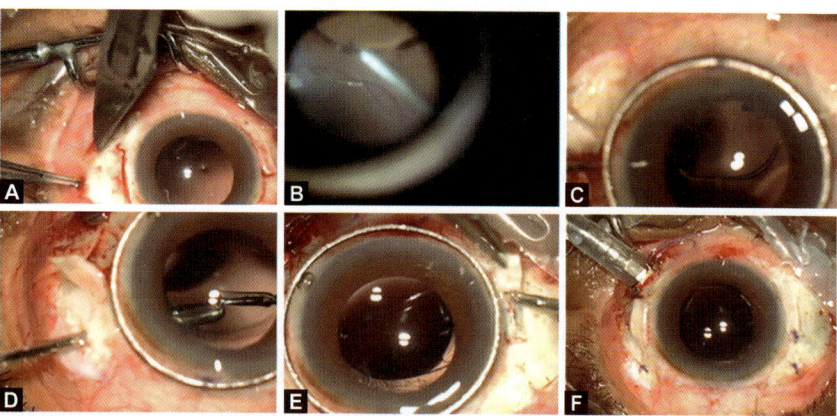

Figs. 6A to F: (A) Dissection of lamellar scleral flaps, 180° apart hinged in a counterclockwise manner; (B) Pars plana 20-gauge vitrectomy is performed all vitreous adhesions to the haptics of the IOL are removed and the IOL is mobilized 20-gauge MVR knife is used to make two sclerotomies 0.75-1 mm behind the limbus in the bed of the scleral flap; (C) The dislocated IOL is grasped using a 23-gauge forceps and brought up to the pupillary area. Using another 23-gauge intraocular MVR forceps the tip of the leading haptic is grasped and brought out through the left-sided sclerotomy; (D) Handshake technique for externalizing the trailing haptic using two 23-gauge MVR forceps; (E) Haptic tuck into a 23-gauge tunnel constructed along the base of the scleral flap; (F) Scleral flaps and sclerotomies are secured.

tunnel for tucking the exteriorized haptic is made at the base of a lamellar scleral flap made between the limbus of the Y incision.[97]

Cannula-Based Intrascleral Tuck[98]

Prenner and colleagues used a 23-gauge MVR blade and 23-gauge trocars to fashion the sclerotomies.[98,99] Abbey, et al. used 25-gauge trocars to create a 3 mm long scleral tunnel.[100] A conjunctival peritomy was not necessary. Externalization of the haptic is done through the cannula. The cannula is then removed from the sclera on to the shaft of the MVR force and the haptic gets pulled through the sclerotomy and scleral tunnel. At 12-month follow-up, there was no incidence of IOL decentration or dislocation. As the haptics are covered by conjunctiva and lamellar scleral tissue and are securely placed within the intrascleral tunnel, the chances of haptic exposure as well as the risk for endophthalmitis are minimized. Todorich B, et al. described a variation of this technique using 27-gauge trocar cannulas which forms a tighter tunnel around the haptics and reduce the risk of postoperative hypotomy.[101]

Yamane's Technique (Yamane, et al. 2014)[102]

Yamane and coworkers performed sutureless 27-gauge needle-assisted intrascleral haptic implantation. The authors used a 27-gauge needle to create a scleral tunnel 1.7 mm from the limbus. The haptics of the three-piece IOL are fed into the hollow of this 27-gauge needle. The needles introduced into the eye with the haptics in its hollow lumen are simultaneously withdrawn allowing intrascleral haptic fixation. Yamane, et al. reported the results of 10 months' follow-up. The complications encountered in this series of 35 cases were ocular hypertension (2/35 eyes) and optic capture (3/35 eyes).[102]

Extraocular Needle-Guided Haptic Insertion Technique (Baskaran, et al. 2017)[103]

Baskaran, et al. introduced a modification in Yamane's technique. Two scleral tunnels each 3 mm in length is fashioned 180° abort, parallel 2.5 mm behind the limbus and parallel to it. The tunnels are directed counterclockwise, a bent 26-gauge needle traverses each tunnel before puncturing the globe and entering the eye. The needle exits the eye through the corneoscleral section. The haptic of the three-piece IOL is threaded into the hollow of these two needles. When the needle is sequentially withdrawn along with insertion of the IOL into the posterior chamber. The authors used a silicone stoppers fashioned from 42 retinal band. The stoppers were threaded into the needle at the start of the procedure to prevent slippage of the haptic when the needle is withdrawn.[103]

Use of Microcatheters (Takayama, et al. 2015):[104] "The Lock-and-Lead" Technique

Transconjunctival sutureless intrascleral IOL fixation using intrascleral tunnels guided with two catheter needles and 30-gauge needles.[104]

Nitinol Flex Loop (Finesse Flex Loop)

Nitinol flex loop (Finesse flex loop)-assisted retrieval and sutureless intrascleral refixation of a dislocated IOL implant (Hsu J, 2018).[105]

Motorized Intraocular Lens Injector-Assisted Intrascleral Intraocular Lens Fixation (Hung, et al. 2017)

The authors used a foot-controlled motorized IOL injector to facilitate gentle and proper IOL implantation through a small incision. The steps of this procedure differ only in the technique of IOL implantation.[106]

Intraoperative Complications associated with Sutureless Scleral Fixation

As with any other procedure, a variety of intraoperative and postoperative complications are associated with sutureless scleral fixation.

The intraoperative complications encountered in this procedure include:

- *Haptic break or kink:* Undue pressure exerted on the haptics during externalization can cause Kinking of the haptics or a haptic breakage of a rigid IOL. Sometime due to excessive and uncontrolled manipulation the haptic can get dislodged from the optic. When haptic breakage occurs there is inadequate haptic length for scleral tuck. In this situation the surgeon is left with no other option than explantation of the IOL. Kinking of the haptic of the IOL usually does not pose serious problems and the haptic can be maneuvered into the scleral tunnel in majority of cases.
- *Inadequate "haptic tuck":* It occurs in three situations commonly:
  1. Haptic breakage
  2. When too long a scleral flap has been dissected
  3. In large diameter, eye where the limbal white-to-white distance is more than normal. In these eyes, a vertical scleral fixation at 6 o'clock to 12 o'clock meridians with shorter diameter is performed.
- *Intraoperative IOL decentration:* This is usually observed in eyes when the scleral flaps are not made exactly 180° apart. If the decentration is noticed intraoperatively, the surgeon can make another sclerotomy 180° from the one on the opposite side, internalize the haptic in the faulty location and re-externalize it through the new sclerotomy.

Another reason for intraoperative decentration is inadequate haptic tuck or improper tucking into a short scleral pocket.

POSTOPERATIVE COMPLICATIONS OF SUTURELESS SCLERAL FIXATION

- *Postoperative hypotony*: It can be managed by ensuring good wound integrity by closing the corneal incision as well as the sclerotomies. Injection of air bubble at the conclusion of surgery also ensures that the IOP is maintained.
- *IOL dislocation*: It is a rarely reported complication intraoperatively. Late IOL dislocation has been reported in 2/63 eyes of surgeons performed in four European centers in the European multicenter study.[92] Usually observed scenario is the dislocation of one of the haptics in the early postoperative period due to hypotony. Re-externalization and refixation of the haptic are possible in this situation.

Other complications that may be associated with this procedure are—endophthalmitis, retinal detachment, cystoid macular edema, transient elevation of IOP, transient vitreous hemorrhage, corneal edema and IOL optic capture.

SUTURED VERSUS SUTURELESS SCLERAL FIXATION

There are no comparison study on the long-term effects of sutured and sutureless scleral fixation. Studies reporting on the intermediate term comparisons have either not found any difference in the complication rate or final visual outcome. Ganekal, et al. reported a higher incidence of postoperative glaucoma and inflammation in the sutured group.[107] Haszcz, et al. compared sutured scleral fixation using Hoffman's pouch and Scharioth's intrascleral haptic tuck reported IOL dislocation in two eyes in the sutureless group.[108] No definitive conclusion on the superiority of one technique over the other can be drawn from the results of these short-term follow-up analysis.

CONCLUSION

Surgical techniques for scleral fixation are still evolving. Methods to reduce preoperative complications associated with incorrect position in the ciliary sulcus, improved suture material options, newer IOL designs as well as new and innovative techniques will definitely improve surgical outcomes and shorten the surgeon's learning curve. Larger case series with longer follow-up data and comparative studies are at present necessary to identify the optimum strategy in a given patient.

REFERENCES

1. Dubey R, Birchall W, Grigg J. Improved refractive outcome for ciliary sulcus-implanted intraocular lenses. Ophthalmology. 2012;119(2):261-5.
2. Banaee T, Sagheb S. Scleral fixation of intraocular lens in eyes with history of open globe injury. J Pediatr Ophthalmol Strabismus. 2011;48(5):292-7.
3. US Census Data 2011. [Accessed December, 2018].
4. Channa R, Zafar SN, Canner JK, et al. Epidemiology of eye-related emergency department visits. JAMA Ophthalmol. 2016;134(3):312-9.
5. Lyle WA, Jin JC. Secondary intraocular lens implantation: anterior chamber vs posterior chamber lenses. Ophthalmic Surg. 1993;24(6):375-81.
6. Gollogly HE, Hodge DO, St Sauver JL, et al. Increasing incidence of cataract surgery: population-based study. J Cataract Refract Surg. 2013;39(9):1383-9.
7. Wagoner MD, Cox TA, Ariyasu RG, et al. Intraocular lens implantation in the absence of capsular support: a report by the American Academy of Ophthalmology. Ophthalmology. 2003;110(4):840-59.
8. Yorston D. Cataract complications. Community Eye Health. 2008;21(65):1-3.
9. Ascaso FJ, Huerva V, Grzybowski A. Epidemiology, etiology, and prevention of late IOL-capsular bag complex dislocation: review of the literature. J Ophthalmol. 2015;2015:805706.
10. Karger RA, Jeng SM, Johnson DH, et al. Estimated incidence of pseudoexfoliation syndrome and pseudoexfoliation glaucoma in Olmsted County, Minnesota. J Glaucoma. 2003;12(3):193-7.

11. Sadiq MA, Vanderveen D. Genetics of ectopia lentis. Semin Ophthalmol. 2013;28(5-6):313-20.
12. Brunette I, Stulting RD, Rinne JR, et al. Penetrating keratoplasty with anterior or posterior chamber intraocular lens implantation. Arch Ophthalmol. 1994;112(10):1311-9.
13. Por YM, Lavin MJ. Techniques of intraocular lens suspension in the absence of capsular/zonular support. Surv Ophthalmol. 2005;50(5):429-62.
14. Gross JG, Kokame GT, Weinberg DV, et al. In-the-bag intraocular lens dislocation. Am J Ophthalmol. 2004;137(4):630-5.
15. Jehan FS, Mamalis N, Crandall AS. Spontaneous late dislocation of intraocular lens within the capsular bag in pseudoexfoliation patients. Ophthalmology. 2001;108(10):1727-31.
16. Fernandez-Buenaga R, Alio JL, Perez-Ardoy AL, et al. Late in-the-bag intraocular lens dislocation requiring explantation: risk factors and outcomes. Eye (Lond). 2013;27(7):795-801.
17. Lee VY, Yuen HK, Kwok AK. Comparison of outcomes of primary and secondary implantation of scleral-fixated posterior chamber intraocular lens. Br J Ophthalmol. 2003;87(12):1459-62.
18. Yalniz-Akkaya Z, Burcu A, Uney GO, et al. Primary and secondary implantation of scleral-fixated posterior chamber intraocular lenses in adult patients. Middle East Afr J Ophthalmol. 2014;21(1):44-9.
19. Mimura T, Amano S, et al. Refractive change after transscleral fixation of posterior chamber intraocular lenses in the absence of capsular support. Acta Ophthalmol Scand. 2004;82(5):544-6.
20. Hayashi K, Hayashi H, Nakao F, et al. Intraocular lens tilt and decentration, anterior chamber depth, and refractive error after trans-scleral suture fixation surgery. Ophthalmology. 1999;106(5):878-82.
21. Bayramlar H, Hepsen IF, Yilmaz H. Myopic shift from the predicted refraction after sulcus fixation of PMMA posterior chamber intraocular lenses. Can J Ophthalmol. 2006;41(1):78-82.
22. Suto C, Hori S, Fukuyama E, et al. Adjusting intraocular lens power for sulcus fixation. J Cataract Refract Surg. 2003;29(10):1913-7.
23. Duffey RJ, Holland EJ, Agapitos PJ, et al. Anatomic study of transsclerally sutured intraocular lens implantation. Am J Ophthalmol. 1989;108:300-9.
24. Apple DJ, Price FW, Gwin T, et al. Sutured retropupillary posterior chamber intraocular lenses for exchange or secondary implantation. The 12th annual Binkhorst lecture, 1988. American Academy of Ophthalmology. 1989;96(8):1241-7.
25. Lewis JS. Sulcus fixation without flaps. Ophthalmology. 1993;100(9):1346-50.
26. Tanzer DJ, Smith RE. Black iris-diaphragm intraocular lens for aniridia and aphakia. J Cataract Refract Surg. 1999;25(11):1548-51.
27. Bellucci R, Marchini G, Morselli S, et al. Scleral fixation re-examined by ultrasound biomicroscopy. J Cataract Refract Surg. 1995;7(6):326-30.
28. Althaus C, Sundmacher R. Intraoperative intraocular endoscopy in transscleral suture fixation of posterior chamber lenses: consequences for suture technique, implantation procedure, and choice of PCL design. Refract Corneal Surg. 1993;9(5):333-9.
29. Jürgens I, Lillo J, Buil JA, et al. Endoscope-assisted transscleral suture fixation of intraocular lenses. J Cataract Refract Surg. 1996;22(7):879-81.
30. Kozawa T, Osakabe Y. The endo-mirror, a new instrument for ophthalmic surgery requiring visualization of the ciliary sulcus. Ophthalmic Surg. 1994;25(6):397-400.

31. Horiguchi M, Hirose H, Koura T, et al. Identifying the ciliary sulcus for suturing a posterior chamber intraocular lens by transillumination. Arch Ophthalmol. 1993;111(12):1693-5.
32. Can E, Gul A, Birinci H. A safe method of ciliary sulcus fixation of foldable intraocular lens using a ciliary sulcus guide. Int Ophthalmol. 2016;36(4):463-8.
33. Malbran ES, Malbran E, Negri I. Lens guide suture for transport and fixation in secondary IOL implantation after intracapsular extraction. Int Ophthalmol. 1986;9(2-3):151-60.
34. Lewis JS. Ab externo sulcus fixation. Ophthalmic Surg. 1991;22(11):692-5.
35. Shapiro A, Leen MM. External transscleral posterior chamber lens fixation. Arch Ophthalmol. 1991;109(12):1759-60.
36. Basti S, Tejaswi PC, Singh SK, et al. Outside-in transscleral fixation for ciliary sulcus intraocular lens placement. J Cataract Refract Surg. 1994;20(1):89-92.
37. Ramocki JM, Shin DH, Glover BK, et al. Foldable posterior chamber intraocular lens implantation in the absence of capsular and zonular support. Am J Ophthalmol. 1999;127(2):213-6.
38. Eryildirim A. Knotless scleral fixation for implanting a posterior chamber intraocular lens. Ophthalmic Surg. 1995;26(1):82-4.
39. Rao SK, Gopal L, Fogla R, et al. Ab externo 4-point scleral fixation. J Cataract Refract Surg. 2000;26(1):9-10.
40. Bergren RL. Four-point fixation technique for sutured posterior chamber intraocular lenses. Arch Ophthalmol. 1994;112(11):1485-7.
41. Smiddy WE, Sawusch MR, O'Brien TP, et al. Implantation of scleral-fixated posterior chamber intraocular lenses. J Cataract Refract Surg. 1990;16(6):691-6.
42. Grigorian R, Chang J, Zarbin M, et al. A new technique for suture fixation of posterior chamber intraocular lenses that eliminates intraocular knots. Ophthalmology. 2003;110(7):1349-56.
43. Regillo CD, Tidwell J. A small-incision technique for suturing a posterior chamber intraocular lens. Ophthalmic Surg Lasers. 1996;27(6):473-5.
44. Tsai YY, Tseng SH. Transscleral fixation of foldable intraocular lens after pars plana lensectomy in eyes with a subluxated lens. J Cataract Refract Surg. 1999;25(8):722-4.
45. Smith JM, Erlanger M, Olson JL. Injectable suture device for intraocular lens fixation. J Cataract Refract Surg. 2015;4(12):2609-13.
46. Olsen TW, Pribila JT. Pars plana vitrectomy with endoscope-guided sutured posterior chamber intraocular lens implantation in children and adults. Am J Ophthalmol. 2011;151(2):287-96.
47. Sasahara M, Kiryu J, Yoshimura N. Endoscope-assisted transscleral suture fixation to reduce the incidence of intraocular lens dislocation. J Cataract Refract Surg. 2005;31(9):1777-80.
48. Girard LJ. Pars plana phacoprosthesis (aphakic intraocular implant): a preliminary report. Ophthalmic Surg. 1981;12(1):19-22.
49. Ma DJ, Choi HJ, Kim MK, et al. Clinical comparison of ciliary sulcus and pars plana locations for posterior chamber intraocular lens transscleral fixation. J Cataract Refract Surg. 2011;37(8):1439-46.
50. Cao D, Zhang H, Yang C, et al. Akreos Adapt AO intraocular lens opacification after vitrectomy in a diabetic patient: a case report and review of the literature. BMC Ophthalmol. 2016;16:82.
51. Khan MA, Gupta OP, Smith RG, et al. Scleral fixation of intraocular lenses using Gore-Tex suture: clinical outcomes and safety profile. Br J Ophthalmol. 2016;100(5):638-43.

52. Rasenberg K. Tips for fixating IOLs with Gore-Tex sutures: a step-by-step guide for suturing the Akreos and the CZ70BD intaocular lenses. Rev Ophthalmol. 2017.
53. Buckley EG. Safety of transscleral-sutured intraocular lenses in children. J AAPOS. 2008;12(5):431-9.
54. Price MO, Price FW Jr, Werner L, et al. Late dislocation of scleral-sutured posterior chamber intraocular lenses. J Cataract Refract Surg. 2005;31(7):1320-6.
55. Bading G, Hillenkamp J, Sachs HG, et al. Long-term safety and functional outcome of combined pars plana vitrectomy and scleral-fixated sutured posterior chamber lens implantation. Am J Ophthalmol. 2007;144(3):371-7.
56. Malta JB, Banitt M, Musch DC, et al. Long-term outcome of combined penetrating keratoplasty with scleral-sutured posterior chamber intraocular lens implantation. Cornea. 2009;28(7):741-6.
57. Assia EI, Nemet A, Sachs D. Bilateral spontaneous subluxation of scleral-fixated intraocular lenses. J Cataract Refract Surg. 2002;28(12):2214-6.
58. Kang HM, Chung EJ. Late-onset *Citrobacter koseri* endophthalmitis with suture exposure after secondary intraocular lens implantation. Korean J Ophthalmol. 2011;25(4):285-8.
59. Schechter RJ. Suture-wick endophthalmitis with sutured posterior chamber intraocular lenses. J Cataract Refract Surg. 1990;16(6):755-6.
60. Heilskov T, Joondeph BC, Olsen KR, et al. Late endophthalmitis after transscleral fixation of a posterior chamber intraocular lens. Arch Ophthalmol. 1989;107(10):1427.
61. Hoffman RS, Fine IH, Packer M. Scleral fixation without conjunctival dissection. J Cataract Refract Surg. 2006;32(11):1907-12.
62. Kir E, Kocaturk T, Dayanir V, et al. Prevention of suture exposure in transscleral intraocular lens fixation: an original technique. Can J Ophthalmol. 2008;43(6):707-11.
63. Szurman P, Petermeier K, Aisenbrey S, et al. Z-suture: a new knotless technique for transscleral suture fixation of intraocular implants. Br J Ophthalmol. 2010;94(2):167-9.
64. Holladay JT. Evaluating the intraocular lens optic. Surv Ophthalmol. 1986;30(6):385-90.
65. Teichmann KD, Teichmann IA. The torque and tilt gamble. J Cataract Refract Surg. 1997;23(3):413-8.
66. Holland EJ, Daya SM, Evangelista A, et al. Penetrating keratoplasty and transscleral fixation of posterior chamber lens. Am J Ophthalmol. 1992;114:182-7.
67. Epstein E. Suture problems. J Cataract Refract Surg. 1989;15:116.
68. Bellucci R, Pucci V, Morselli S, et al. Secondary implantation of angle-supported anterior chamber and scleral-fixated posterior chamber intraocular lenses. J Cataract Refract Surg. 1996;22:247-52.
69. Bucci FA, Holland EJ, Lindstrom RL. Corneal autografts for external knots in transsclerally sutured posterior chamber lenses. Am J Ophthalmol. 1991;112:353-4.
70. Schein OD, Kenyon KR, Steinert RF, et al. A randomized trial of intraocular lens fixation techniques with penetrating keratoplasty. Ophthalmology. 1993;100:1437-43.
71. Stark WJ, Gottsch JD, Goodman DF, et al. Posterior chamber intraocular lens implantation in the absence of capsular support. Arch Ophthalmol. 1989;107:1078-83.

72. Mackool RJ, Sirota MA. Intracapsular foldable posterior chamber lens implantation in eyes with posterior capsule tears or zonular fiber instability. J Cataract Refract Surg. 1998;24:739-40.
73. Chang JH, Lee JH. Long-term results of implantation of posterior chamber intraocular lens by suture fixation. Korean J Ophthalmol. 1991;5:42-6.
74. Solomon K, Gussler JR, Gussler C, et al. Incidence and management of complications of transsclerally sutured posterior chamber lenses. J Cataract Refract Surg. 1993;19:488-93.
75. Sundmacher R, Reinhard T, Althaus C. Black-diaphragm intraocular lens for correction of aniridia. Ophthalmic Surg. 1994;25:180-5.
76. Lane SS, Lubniewski AJ, Holland EJ. Transsclerally sutured posterior chamber lenses: improved lens designs and techniques to maximize lens stability and minimize suture erosion. Semin Ophthalmol. 1992;7:245-52.
77. Durak A, Oner HF, Kocͺak N, et al. Tilt and decentration after primary and secondary transsclerally sutured posterior chamber intraocular lens implantation. J Cataract Refract Surg. 2001;27:227-32.
78. Buckley EG. Scleral fixated (sutured) posterior chamber intraocular lens implantation in children. J AAPOS. 1999;3(5):289-94.
79. Burcu A, Yalniz-Akkaya Z, Abay I, et al. Scleral-fixated posterior chamber intraocular lens implantation in pediatric and adult patients. Semin Ophthalmol. 2014;29(1):39-44.
80. Hsu HY, Edelstein SL, Lind JT. Surgical management of non-traumatic pediatric ectopia lentis: a case series and review of the literature. Saudi J Ophthalmol. 2012;26(3):315-21.
81. Kumar M, Arora R, Sanga L, et al. Scleral-fixated intraocular lens implantation in unilateral aphakic children. Ophthalmology. 1999;106(11):2184-9.
82. Ozmen AT, Dogru M, Erturk H, et al. Transsclerally fixated intraocular lenses in children. Ophthalmic Surg Lasers. 2002;33(5):394-9.
83. Sharpe MR, Biglan AW, Gerontis CC. Scleral fixation of posterior chamber intraocular lenses in children. Ophthalmic Surg Lasers. 1996;27(5):337-41.
84. Bardorf CM, Epley KD, Lueder GT, et al. Pediatric transscleral-sutured intraocular lenses: efficacy and safety in 43 eyes followed an average of 3 years. J AAPOS. 2004;8(4):318-24.
85. Caca I, Sahin A, Ari S, et al. Posterior chamber lens implantation with scleral fixation in children with traumatic cataract. J Pediatr Ophthalmol Strabismus. 2011;48(4):226-31.
86. Hyun DW, Lee TG, Cho SW. Unilateral scleral fixation of posterior chamber intraocular lenses in pediatric complicated traumatic cataracts. Korean J Ophthalmol. 2009;23(3):148-52.
87. Lam DS, Ng JS, Fan DS, et al. Short-term results of scleral intraocular lens fixation in children. J Cataract Refract Surg. 1998;24(11):1474-9.
88. Mittelviefhaus H, Mittelviefhaus K, Gerling J. Transscleral suture fixation of posterior chamber intraocular lenses in children under 3 years. Graefes Arch Clin Exp Ophthalmol. 2000;238(2):143-8.
89. Zetterstrom C, Lundvall A, Weeber H Jr, et al. Sulcus fixation without capsular support in children. J Cataract Refract Surg. 1999;25(6):776-81.
90. Mannarino AP, Hannush SB. A new technique for transscleral fixation of a posterior chamber intraocular lens in the absence of capsular support during penetrating keratoplasty. Refract Corneal Surg. 1990;6:353-6.
91. Gabor SG, Pavlidis MM. Sutureless intrascleral posterior chamber intraocular lens fixation. J Cataract Refract Surg. 2007;33(11):1851-4.

92. Scharioth GB, Prasad S, Georgalas I, et al. Intermediate results of sutureless intrascleral posterior chamber intraocular lens fixation. J Cataract Refract Surg. 2010;36(2):254-9.
93. Agarwal A, Kumar DA, Jacob S, et al. Fibrin glue-assisted sutureless posterior chamber intraocular lens implantation in eyes with deficient posterior capsules. J Cataract Refract Surg. 2008;34(9):1433-8.
94. Narang P, Narang S. Glue-assisted intrascleral fixation of posterior chamber intraocular lens. Indian J Ophthalmol. 2013;61(4):163-7.
95. Kara N. A modified glued transscleral intraocular lens implantation: suture-assisted sutureless technique. J Refract Surg. 2015;31(7):488-91.
96. Beiko G, Steinert R. Modification of externalized haptic support of glued intraocular lens technique. J Cataract Refract Surg. 2013;39:323-5.
97. Ohta T, Toshida H, Murakami A. Simplified and safe method of suture less intrascleral posterior chamber intraocular lens fixation: Y-fixation technique. J Cataract Refract Surg. 2014;40:2-7.
98. Prenner JL, Feiner L, Wheatley HM, et al. A novel approach for posterior chamber intraocular lens placement or rescue via a sutureless scleral fixation technique. Retina. 2012;32(4):853-5.
99. Wilgucki JD, Wheatley HM, Feiner L, et al. One-year outcomes of eyes treated with a sutureless scleral fixation technique for intraocular lens placement or rescue. Retina. 2015;35(5):1036-40.
100. Abbey AM, Hussain RM, Shah AR, et al. Suture less scleral fixation of intraocular lenses: outcomes of two approaches. Graefes Arch Clin Exp Ophthalmol. 2015;253(1):1-5.
101. Todorich B, Thanos A, Woodward MA, et al. Sutureless intrascleral fixation of secondary intraocular lens using 27-gauge vitrectomy system. Ophthalmic Surg Lasers Imaging Retina. 2016;47(4):376-9.
102. Yamane S, Inoue M, Arakawa A, et al. Sutureless 27-gauge needle-guided intrascleral intraocular lens implantation with lamellar scleral dissection. Ophthalmology. 2014;121(1):61-6.
103. Baskaran P, Ganne P, Bhandari S, et al. Extraocular needle-guided haptic insertion technique of scleral fixation of intraocular lenses (X-NIT). Indian J Ophthalmol. 2017;65(8):747-50.
104. Takayama K, Akimoto M, Taguchi H, et al. Transconjunctival sutureless intra-scleral intraocular lens fixation using intrascleral tunnels guided with catheter and 30-gauge needles. Br J Ophthalmol. 2015;99:1457-9.
105. Hsu J. Nitinol flex loop-assisted retrieval and sutureless intrascleral refixation of a dislocated intraocular lens implant. Retina Cases Brief Rep. 2018.
106. Hung JH, Wang SH, Teng YT, et al. Motorized injector-assisted intraocular lens fixation. Kaohsiung J Med Sci. 2017;33:137-43.
107. Ganekal S, Venkataratnam S, Dorairaj S, et al. Comparative evaluation of suture-assisted and fibrin glue-assisted scleral fixated intraocular lens implantation. J Cataract Refract Surg. 2012;28(4):249-52.
108. Haszcz D, Nowomiejska K, Oleszczuk A, et al. Visual outcomes of posterior chamber intraocular lens intrascleral fixation in the setting of postoperative and post-traumatic aphakia. BMC Ophthalmol. 2016;16(1):50.

CHAPTER
15

Message from Clinical Trials and How to Adopt them for Real Life Situations in Management of Retinal Vascular Disorders

Lingam Gopal

■ INTRODUCTION

With so many clinical trials being performed and sometimes contradictory results coming out of the trials, the clinician is genuinely confused as to what is the right step and what is not. This chapter covers only the most important and currently relevant of the trials that dictate treatment plan. Most trials that were included were multicentric randomized clinical trials. It is not a compendium on all possible trials performed on these disorders. The real-life situation described under each disorder is not only a summary of important outcomes of the trials but also the author's perception of the current practices.

The following common vascular conditions will be discussed: diabetic retinopathy (DR), diabetic macular edema (DME), retinal vein occlusions (RVO), central retinal vein occlusion (CRVO), branch retinal vein occlusion (BRVO), age-related macular degeneration (AMD), neovascular age-related macular degeneration (nAMD), and retinopathy of prematurity (ROP). The chapter summarizes the results of important studies pertaining to these entities and provides a guidance in real life situation as to how to adopt these results in daily care of patients.

■ EFFICACY VERSUS EFFECTIVENESS

Randomized controlled trials (RCT) are the gold standard to establish efficacy of a drug or treatment protocol. Effectiveness in contrast is the impact of the treatment protocol in real life situation.

Why is Efficacy Different from Effectiveness?

The RCTs are conducted under strict controlled conditions. Bias is almost eliminated at every stage—(selection of patients, selection of treatment to be given, evaluation of treatment outcome, etc.) but for random bias. They have a high internal validity. However, they have a number of inclusion and exclusion criteria; rigid schedule for follow-up and investigations; rigid criteria for treatment administration, etc. Hence, they have low generalizability to society at large.

Factors that influence the effectiveness of a medication would depend on several factors that may be unique to the individual/geographic location/society, etc.

These include:
- Presence or absence of screening programs to detect disease early
- Presence or absence of robust health network that makes it easy for a patient to seek early evaluation and treatment
- Economics of going through the periodic evaluation and treatment schedule
- Family support, especially in case of the elderly.

Diabetic Retinopathy and Control of Systemic Factors

Clinical trials regarding systemic factors and occurrence/progression of diabetic retinopathy are shown in Table 1.

Real-life Situation

There is strong evidence to suggest that strict control of blood glucose levels, along with blood pressure have significant effect on occurrence and progression of diabetic retinopathy, including diabetic maculopathy.

The kind of control of blood glucose that is possible in studies may not be practicable in real life due to several reasons.
- Risk of hypoglycemia will make the patients err on the side of less rigid control
- Frequency of estimation of blood glucose may not be enough to guide a rigid control
- Modification of progression of back ground DR changes may not be evident since the end-point is more of comparative evaluation of fundus photos rather than nonoccurrence of an event.
- From the patient perspective, ocular symptoms wise, there may not be much to appreciate effect of the rigid control of blood glucose or blood pressure
- The onus is on the clinician (diabetologist) to drive home the positive benefits of good control of diabetes mellitus (DM) and blood pressure (BP) (even if not intensive control). Repeated emphasis of this message is beneficial in the long run.
- Considering the above discussion, real-life impact of control of systemic factors remains difficult to assess.

Table 1: Summary of clinical trials regarding systemic factors and occurrence/progression of diabetic retinopathy.

Title	Intervention	Results
DCCT[1]	Intensive vs usual control of blood glucose in type 1 DM	• 10% reduction in HbA_{1C} reduces progression of retinopathy by 43%
UKPDS group[2]	Intensive vs usual control of blood glucose in type 2 DM	• 25% reduction in microvascular end-points
Action to control cardiovascular risk in diabetes and ACCORD eye study group[3]	Intensive control of blood glucose, blood pressure and dyslipidemia in type 2 DM	• *Glycemic control:* 33% reduction in rate of progression of DR • *Fenofibrate use:* 6.5% progression of DR vs 10.4% with placebo • *BP control:* 10.4% progression of DR vs 8.8% with standard treatment
HDS (part of UKPDS dealing with hypertension)[4]	Additional tight control of BP	• At 9 years follow-up 47% reduction in risk of >3 line loss of VA
ADVANCE trial (action in diabetes and vascular disease: Preterax and diamicron MR controlled evaluation)[5]	BP lowering and intensive glucose control in type 2 DM	• Only mild effect on DR progression • Better effect on DME
EUCLID trial[6]	Lisinopril in insulin dependent DM	• Significant reduction in progression of DR even in non-hypertensive patients
DIRECT[7]	Candesartan in DM	• Significant reduction in 3 step progression of DR; No effect on DME or PDR
FIELD study[8]	Fenofibrate and lipid lowering agents in type 2 DM	• Reduction in 2 step progression of DR • Requirement for first laser lowered
RASS[9]	Enalapril or losartan in normotensive type 1 DM	• DR progression reduced by 2 step
Steno-2 study[10]	Multifactorial target driven intervention against BP, HbA_{1C}, LDL cholesterol, triglycerides	• 50% reduction in risk of retinopathy, nephropathy and cardiovascular risk

(DCCT: diabetes control and complications trial; HbA_{1C}: hemoglobin A_{1C}; UKPDS: The United Kingdom prospective diabetes study; DIRECT: diabetic retinopathy Candesartan trials; FIELD: fenofibrate intervention and event lowering in diabetes; ACCORD: the action to control cardiovascular risk in type 2 diabetes; DME: diabetic macular edema; DR: diabetic retinopathy; EUCLID: effects of ticagrelor and clopidogrel in patients with peripheral artery disease; HDS: hypertension in diabetes study; LDL: low-density lipoprotein; PDR: proliferative diabetic retinopathy; RASS: the renin angiotensin system study; VA: visual acuity)

Diabetic Maculopathy

In the management of DME, several trials took place evaluating the role of lasers, anti-vascular endothelial growth factor (VEGF) drugs, steroids, and surgery. Table 2 summarizes the clinical trials involving lasers in DME trials. Table 3 summarizes the clinical trials involving anti-VEGF in DME. Table 4 summarizes the clinical trials involving corticosteroids in DME.

Logistic issues in real life:
- Cost factor
- Patient compliance
- Availability of Doctor
- Convenience
- Need to come periodically for follow-up.

Treatment issues in real life:
- When to initiate active treatment
- When to call for follow-up

Table 2: Summary of trials involving lasers in diabetic macular edema (DME).

Study	Intervention	Results
Early treatment for diabetic retinopathy study (ETDRS)[11]	Focal/grid laser in eyes with DME	• At 3 years, risk of moderate visual loss reduced by 50%
DRCR net protocol A[12]	Focal/grid laser vs mild macular grid in eyes with DME	• Standard ETDRS protocol better than minimal macular grid
DRCR net protocol B[13]	Focal/grid laser vs IVTA for DME	• Laser better than IVTA
Meta-analysis of 6 RCTs[14]	Subthreshold laser vs conventional laser	• Two types have similar anatomical outcome although vision is perhaps better in subthreshold group in the short term (up to 1 year)

(ETDRS: early treatment for diabetic retinopathy study; DME: diabetic macular edema; DRCR: Diabetic Retinopathy Clinical Research; IVTA: intravitreal triamcinolone acetonide; RCT: randomized controlled trial)

Table 3: Summary of trials involving antivascular endothelial growth factor (anti-VEGF drugs) in diabetic macular edema (DME).

Title	Intervention	Results
RBZ (Ranibizumab) for edema of macula in diabetes-2 (READ-2 study)[15]	RBZ or laser or both in 1:1:1 randomization	• 7.4 letter gain with RBZ vs 0.5 letter gain with laser at month 3 • Combining laser with RBZ can reduce number of injections at 2 years
READ-3 study[16]	High dose RBZ (2 mg) vs usual 0.5 mg dose	• High dose had no additional benefit

Contd...

Contd...

Title	Intervention	Results
RESOLVE study[17]	0.3 and 0.5 mg RBZ vs sham	• RBZ had 10 line gain vs 1.4 line loss in sham
DRCR net protocol[18]	0.5 mg RBZ with prompt or deferred laser vs intravitreal triamcinolone acetonide (IVTA) with prompt laser	• RBZ with deferred laser better than prompt laser • Laser may reduce number of injections • RBZ with laser superior to IVTA with laser
RESTORE and REVEAL studies[19,20]	To demonstrate superiority of RBZ over laser	• Combining laser with RBZ did not have additional benefit • Over 3 years, there is decreasing need for injections using PRN approach
RISE and RIDE studies[21]	RBZ monthly vs sham with sham control receiving RBZ in 3rd year	• RBZ superior to sham • Late initiation of RBZ also shows improvement but less than early initiation • Less likely to develop PDR
DRCR net study[22]	PRN dosing over long run and its affect	• Good benefits despite reducing need for injections (8–9 in 1st year; 2–3 in 2nd year; 1–2 in 3rd and 0–1 in 4th year)
RESTORE extension study[23]	PRN dosing over long run and its affect	• Good improvement in vision with 3.9 injections in 2nd year and 2.9 injections in 3rd year
DA VINCI study[24]	Aflibercept (AFL) vs laser	• >10 letters improvement with AFL vs 1.3 letter loss with laser
VIVID and VISTA studies[25]	AFL vs Laser 5 monthly doses followed by 8 weekly	• 8 weekly follow-up injections had same result as PRN. So follow-up frequency can be reduced
Study by Ahmadieh[26]	Bevacizumab (BCZ) vs placebo	• Significant central macular subfield thickness (CMT) reduction with BCZ. Additional Triamcinolone had no value
BOLT study[27]	BCZ vs laser	• 31% had >10 letter improvement with BCZ vs 7.9% with laser
DRCR net protocol T[28]	Head to head comparison with BCZ, AFL and RBZ for DME	• All three had similar improvement at 1 year if initial BCVA > 20/50 • For initial BCVA < 20/50 AFL did better than RBZ or BCZ • Smaller percentage of AFL group needed additional laser

(DME: diabetic macular edema; DRCR: Diabetic Retinopathy Clinical Research; PRN: pro re nata; REVEAL: randomized evaluation of the effects of anacetrapib through lipid-modification; RISE and RIDE: ranibizumab for diabetic macular edema)

Table 4: Summary of trials with corticosteroids in diabetic macular edema (DME).

Study	Intervention	Results
DRCR net protocol B[13]	Focal/Grid laser vs IVTA	• Laser better than steroid
DRCR net protocol I[18]	0.5 mg RBZ with prompt or deferred laser vs IVTA with prompt laser	• IVTA + laser had 1.5 letters worse vision than sham + laser group
MEAD study[29]	Dexamethasone implant (OZURDEX) for DME	• 22.4% had >15 letter gain and 106 µ reduction in CMT • Glaucoma occurred in 41.5% but only one case needed filtering surgery • No cumulative raise in IOP with sequential implants
Ozurdex PLACID study[30]	Ozurdex + laser compared to laser	• Laser + Ozurdex did better
BEVORDEX study	Ozurdex vs BCZ	• Similar results; more cataract with Ozurdex
Ozurdex Champlain study[31]	Ozurdex in vitrectomized eye	• Single injection resulted in reduced CMT
FAME A and B studies[32,33]	Iluvien (flucinolone acetonide) vs sham	• 28.7% gained >15 letters at 3 years • Chronic DME also responded • Effect lasts for one year

(CMT: central macular subfield thickness; DME: diabetic macular edema; DRCR: Diabetic Retinopathy Clinical Research; IVTA: intravitreal triamcinolone acetonide; MEAD: macular edema: assessment of implantable dexamethasone in diabetes; FAME: the fluocinolone acetonide intravitreal implant for diabetic macular edema)

- When to switch drug
- When to terminate treatment
- Cataract surgery in presence of DME
- Approach in bilateral DME
- Systemic factors that influence management.

Cost Factor

In general, the treatment costs over a period are more for diabetics having DME than it is for AMD.[34] This increased cost is more due to the treatment of nonophthalmic issues.

Cost of treat and extend versus Pro Re Nata (PRN) philosophy: Treat and extend philosophy enables increasing the interval between visits but initial costs are high since injection is administered each visit.

Pro Re Nata needs the patient to come every month for follow-up. In practice, many follow 'observe and extend' policy where in injection is given only if there is an indication of activity. If serial visits at 4 weeks are OK, the interval of follow-up is extended although injection is not given each visit. This is less than ideal but perhaps acceptable under circumstances of cost considerations.

When to Initiate Treatment?

According to most studies, treatment was initiated only if the central subfield macular thickness was more than 300 µ on spectral domain optical coherence tomography (OCT). The visual acuity cut-off point to initiate treatment was 20/40 for most studies and 20/50 for Ozurdex study.

However, in real-life situation, the absolute values of visual acuity and central subfield thickness are not always taken into consideration. Patients with 20/30 vision but with the central subfield thickness of more than 300 µ are fairly common. Patients with central subfield thickness of around 300 µ but having gross intraretinal edema may be treated since there may be retinal thinning due to ischemia.

In borderline indications, one may postpone the decision to treat under the following circumstances:
- Recent change in medication for DM
- Recent introduction of glitazones for DM control
- Poor control of systemic parameters.

Choice of Drug the First Time Around

The choice between steroids and anti-VEGF drugs as the first line is not always straight forward.
- One would intuitively opt for anti-VEGF drugs first time considering the risk of glaucoma and cataract formation with steroids.
- However, in situations such as pregnancy, recent stroke or myocardial infarction, one may opt for steroid as first choice.

Among the anti-VEGF drugs, the choice in general is based on individual surgeon's preference and cost considerations. Cost factor can act both ways. On one hand we have patients who cannot afford the frequent injections and hence choose the cheapest option (Bevacizumab) and on the other we have patients whose perception is costlier the better.

If one were to go by the Diabetic Retinopathy Clinical Research (DRCR) Net protocol T results, one would have the choice of bevacizumab or ranibizumab if the visual acuity is better than 20/50 while if visual acuity is worse than 20/50 aflibercept would be preferred.

Loading Dosage

Although most studies recommend three loading doses, recommendations by the company marketing aflibercept is to administer monthly injection for 5 months; followed by 2 monthly injections till 1 year; and then only switch to treat and extend. While this may be the ideal, there may be several cases that may be amenable to treat and extend even before 1 year.

Frequency of Follow-up

According to study recommendations, even under treat and extend philosophy, one would not be able to extend the interval beyond 12 weeks. However, there may be situations where we are justified in extending the interval of visits beyond 12 weeks.

- Stable situation with dry macula noted for over 12 months of follow-up
- Persistent DME despite maximum treatment with little scope for visual impairment
- Patient unwilling for intervention despite indication.

When to Switch to Alternative Drug?
It is often that we are faced with the dilemma of whether we should try an alternative drug. There are however, no strict guidelines from studies. The following indications may be acceptable to consider switch in medication.
- If there is no improvement even after 5–6 months of monthly injections
- If one cannot prolong the inter injection interval beyond 1 month even after 6 months.
- Fresh stroke or heart attack when usually one switches to steroid from anti-VEGF drugs.

When to Stop Treatment?
Typically
- If the vision has improved to the maximum and the foveal contour is normal
- No further improvement—defined as less than 10% reduction in central subfield thickness or <5 letter improvement in visual acuity after last injection and if in the judgment of the treating physician, no further improvement is expected.

In Real-life Situation
- There is usually some tolerance to para foveal residual fluid.
- Grossly ischemic macula with no improvement expected (observed) even with dry macula.

Identifying Lack of Response
Typically
Lack of reduction in central subfield thickness/no improvement in visual acuity after at least 2 injections.

Caveats
- Improvement in vision that has gone unnoticed: This can happen when patients are not that sensitive to change in visual acuity (illiterate subjects). It can also happen that there is response initially but edema recurred by the time of follow-up.
- Systemic status at the time of injection: This factor has been studied but not understood fully. Several studies have shown that high HbA_{1C} levels may be associated with poor response to injection.

■ BILATERAL DIABETIC MACULAR EDEMA
Study protocols usually involve one eye. In practice, there are many patients who would need treatment in both eyes. The advisability of administering bilateral simultaneous injections is not clear. There has been one report by

Nakhleh et al. wherein endophthalmitis occurred in one out of 334 injections. However, the endophthalmitis occurred in one eye although injection was bilateral.

Where feasible one can inject the two eyes one day apart. If both eyes are injected same time, precautions should be taken using separate povidone Iodine preparation, separate set of needles, speculum, etc. for the two eyes.

Patient Compliance

Although patient compliance is a universal issue, the problem is more acute in developing countries like India where facilities for advanced medical care are concentrated in specific locations.

Each review entails:
- Travel to and fro
- Time spent in the hospital:
  - For consultation
  - For optical coherence tomography
  - For injection
  - For postinjection review
  - For other systemic problems.

Patient compliance would depend on individual patient's outlook, their socioeconomic status, the access to medical care and how much the visual handicap caused by the disease is affecting their livelihood.

In a study by Wecker et al.[35] of a 5-year follow-up data of PRN treatment for various conditions, DME patients had a 62% vision stabilization at year 5. About 19% had significant increase and another 19% had significant fall in vision. This clearly indicates that despite initial improvement in vision in a majority of cases, over long term, with PRN treatment, the visual acuity returns to base line (stabilization).

The injection frequencies reduced from six in first year to between 1 and 6 in consecutive years.

PROLIFERATIVE DIABETIC RETINOPATHY

Proliferative diabetic retinopathy is traditionally treated with laser pan-retinal photocoagulation (PRP). PRP has been the main modality of treatment for last three decades or more. The treatment is destructive in nature and aims to preserve central retinal function at the expense of peripheral retina. The expected side effects of PRP are the loss of peripheral field of vision, decreased night vision, and exacerbation of DME. Anti-VEGF agents used for DME have been shown to retard the progression of diabetic retinopathy (Table 5). This lead to an exploratory trial of its use in proliferative disease as well.

Real life situation:
- PRP still remains the most common mode of management of proliferative diabetic retinopathy in view of the low cost, lack of need for frequent follow-up, and good efficacy in resolution of the proliferative disease. PRP is however associated with significant peripheral field loss.
- In the presence of DME and proliferative diabetic retinopathy, one may resort to anti-VEGF drug alone without PRP.

Table 5: Summary of clinical trials on proliferative diabetic retinopathy (PDR).

Study	Intervention	Results
DRS[36]	PRP as treatment for PDR	• Risk of severe visual loss reduced by 50% in eyes with high risk characteristics
DRCR net Protocol S[37]	PRP vs intravitreal RBZ for proliferative diabetic retinopathy	• At 2 years the visual outcome is better with RBZ • 19% more frequent occurrence of DME with PRP in the eyes with no DME to start with • Vitrectomy was needed in 4% of RBZ group vs 15% of PRP group • RBZ noninferior to PRP in treatment of PDR • PRP cost-effective • In eyes with PDR and DME, RBZ better option
Meta-analysis[38]	Anti-VEGF in PDR	• Reduced risk of vitreous hemorrhage

(DME: diabetic macular edema; DRCR: Diabetic Retinopathy Clinical Research; DRS: diabetic retinopathy study; PRP: pan-retinal photocoagulation; RBZ: ranibizumab; VEGF: vascular endothelial growth factor)

Table 6 summarizes the clinical trials on vitrectomy for DR-related vitreous hemorrhage.

Real life situation:
- Injecting anti-VEGF is not an option to treat vitreous hemorrhage
- Preoperative anti-VEGF is useful to reduce the risk of intraoperative and postoperative hemorrhage
- While deciding on preoperative anti-VEGF, injecting it 5–10 days before surgery appears to be optimal time
- In some cases, with recurrent vitreous hemorrhage following vitrectomy, anti-VEGF injection may help and avoid repeat surgery.

RETINAL VEIN OCCLUSIONS

Retinal vein occlusions can affect branch, trunk, and central retinal veins. Table 7 summarizes treatment trials on RVO.
- No role of laser photocoagulation for macular edema secondary to CRVO
- Anti-VEGF or steroid implant is treatment of choice for vein occlusion-related macular edema
- Not all visual gains were maintained beyond 1 year
- Steroid if chosen should be either ozurdex or iluvien implant rather than triamcinolone acetonide.
- Significant variability in response among patients.
- Patient responding poorly to anti-VEGF did so early in course of treatment
- Minimal difference between PRN and monthly treatment once initial treatment has resolved the edema.

Table 6: Summary of trials on vitrectomy for diabetic retinopathy-related vitreous hemorrhage.

Study	Intervention	Results
DRVS study[39]	Early vs deferred vitrectomy in severe vitreous hemorrhage in diabetic retinopathy	• At 4 years, proportion of 10/20 or better result more in early vitrectomy group in type 1 DM • No advantage of early vitrectomy in type II DM
DRCR net[40]	Intravitreal RBZ vs saline for vitreous hemorrhage	• Over 1/3rd of eyes in each group needed vitrectomy by 1 year • No difference between saline and RBZ
Radivit trial[41]	RBZ pretreatment in diabetic vitrectomy—a pilot RCT	• At 12 weeks vitreous cavity hemorrhage persisted in 2 of control group vs none in RBZ group
IBe Tra study[42]	Preoperative use of BCZ vs reduction in intraoperative bleeding- RCT	• Reduced intraoperative bleeding observed with preoperative use of BCZ
RCT on timing of preoperative BCZ[43]	Comparison of preoperative BCZ given 1–3 days before surgery vs 5–10 days before surgery	• Better final vision at 6 months if preoperative BCZ is given 5–10 days before surgery rather than 1–3 days before

(DRCR: Diabetic Retinopathy Clinical Research; DRVS: diabetic retinopathy vitrectomy study; RBZ: ranibizumab; RCT: randomized controlled trial)

Table 7: Summary of trials on retinal vein occlusions.

Study	Intervention	Results
CVOS study[44]	Laser grid vs observation in CRVO	• Reduction in angiographic evidence of edema with no visual benefit
RELATE study[45]	RBZ 0.5 mg/2 mg with additional PRP or alone	• Additional PRP had no benefit either in reduction of edema or reducing the number of injections
CRUISE study[46]	0.3 or 0.5 mg RBZ or sham for CRVO monthly for 6 months	• >15 letter gain at 6 months seen in 46.2% with 0.3 mg; 47.7% with 0.5 mg vs 16.9% with sham.
BRAVO study[47]	0.3 or 0.5 mg RBZ or sham for BRVO monthly for 6 months	• >15 letter gain at 6 months seen in 55.2% with 0.3 mg; 61.1% with 0.5 mg vs 28.8% with sham • Reduction in central foveal thickness and >20/40 vision was significantly more often seen in treated group
HORIZON study[48]—open label extension study of CRUISE and BRAVO subjects for long term safety	PRN RBZ for all subjects	• No new safety events observed • Reduced follow-up and fewer injections in second year associated with decline in vision in CRVO but not in BRVO

Contd...

Contd...

Study	Intervention	Results
RETAIN[49] study, long-term outcomes of subset of patients from CRUISE and BRAVO	Patients seen every month in year 1 and at least every 3 months in year 2—treated with ranibizumab when intra-retinal fluid was present; Additional laser if injections needed in two consecutive visits	• 50% of BRVO and 44% of CRVO subjects had edema resolution for 6 months after last injection. Mean number of injections in unresolved group was 3.2 in year 4 in BRVO subjects and 5.9 in CRVO subjects
GALILEO study[50]	AFL 2 mg vs sham for CRVO	• >15 letters gain in 60.2% with AFL vs 22.1% sham at week 24
COPERNICUS study[51]	AFL 2 mg vs sham for CRVO	• >15 letters gain in 56.1% with AFL vs 12.3% sham at week 24
SCORE2 study[52]	AFL vs BCZ for macular edema due to CRVO	• BCZ was not inferior to Aflibercept
SCORE study[53]	IVTA 1 and 4 mg	• At 12 months no difference noted between standard care and IVTA 1 mg as well as 4 mg
GENEVA study[54]	Ozurdex implant for BRVO and CRVO	• 41% (0.7 mg) and 40% (0.35 mg) improvement vs 23% in sham group • More recent onset edema did better
SHORE study[55]	After initial 7 monthly injections, PRN vs monthly 0.5 mg ranibizumab for CRVO	• After edema regression by 7th month, subsequent monthly or PRN injection had equal effect on maintenance

(BCZ: bevacizumab; BRAVO: ranibizumab for the treatment of macular edema after branch retinal vein occlusion: evaluation of efficacy and safety; BRVO: branch retinal vein occlusion; CRUISE: central retinal vein occlusion study; CRVO: central retinal vein occlusion; CVOS: central vein occlusion study; HORIZON: an open-label extension trial of ranibizumab for choroidal neovascularization secondary to age-related macular degeneration; IVTA: intravitreal triamcinolone acetonide; PRN: pro re nata; PRP: panretinal photocoagulation; RBZ: ranibizumab; RETAIN: extended follow-up of patients with macular edema due to retinal vein occlusion; SCORE: the standard care vs corticosteroid for retinal vein occlusion)

- Recommend switching to aflibercept or ozurdex if 3 monthly injections do not show significant response (<10% decrease in central foveal thickness) with ranibizumab.
- Beyond 3 months if good response, follow-up can be increased beyond 1 month. If partial or nonresponder, monthly follow-up would still be needed.
- Need to investigate for the cause of occlusions: No investigations are required in patients who are known diabetics, hypertensives or cases of dyslipidemia. In bilateral cases and those occurring in young people with no diabetes, hypertension or dyslipidemia investigations are usually considered. In addition to excluding above mentioned disorders, they are also tested for complete blood cell count (CBC), serum protein

electrophoresis, hemotological tests, syphilis serology, thromobophilic screening, activated protein C resistance, lupus anticoagulant, anticardiolipin antibodies, protein C and protein S estimation, and antithrombin III.

RETINOPATHY OF PREMATURITY

Interventional trials conducted on ROP and their results are shown in Table 8.
Real life situation:
- Type 1 ROP defined as zone 1 plus disease of any stage; zone 1 stage 3 without plus disease; zone 2 stage 2 or 3 with plus disease is an indication for treatment within 48 hours
- Type 2 ROP defined as zone 1 stage 1 or 2 without plus disease; zone 2 any stage without plus disease can be reviewed weekly till they normalize or progress to type 1 and need treatment.
- Cryo has been replaced by laser photocoagulation as preferred modality of treatment despite the cryo ROP study having used cryotherapy. This switch took place in view of the tremendous advantages of laser over cryo.
- Injection of anti-VEGF as monotherapy (without laser) has not found uniform support despite the BEAT ROP (Bevacizumab Eliminates the Angiogenic Threat of Retinopathy of Prematurity) study reports.
- Most surgeons use anti-VEGF as primary modality for zone 1 or posterior severe zone 2—more as a temporizing measure to permit vascularization to proceed to some extent into the periphery before subjecting them to laser photocoagulation. Anti-VEGF is also commonly resorted to when the response to laser is not optimal.

NEOVASCULAR AGE RELATED MACULAR DEGENERATION

Results of interventional trials in patients with neovascular age-related macular degeneration (AMD) are summarized in Table 9.

DRY AGE RELATED MACULAR DEGENERATION

Results of interventional trials in patients with dry age-related macular degeneration are summarized in Table 10.
Real life situation:
- Considering the increased frequency of polypoidal choroidal vasculopathy (PCV) in Asian population, investigations with indocyanine green (ICG) has become mandatory in most cases of suspected AMD.
- With the advent of anti-VEGF drugs, direct thermal laser to choroidal neovascular membrane is given up entirely-even for extra-foveal membranes.
- Radiation has not been found useful – both as monotherapy (as was done in the pre-anti-VEGF era with external beam) or with anti-VEGF drugs (delivered as premacular radiation)
- Photodynamic therapy (PDT) is currently restricted to PCV and not the usual AMD.

Table 8: Summary of trials on retinopathy of prematurity.

Study	Intervention	Results
Cryo ROP study[56-69]	Treatment of threshold ROP with cryo vs natural course	• Onset of ROP correlates better with post menstrual age (PMT) • At one year unfavorable outcome seen in 25.7% of treated vs 47.4% of untreated • Most unfavorable outcome in untreated eyes occurred in zone 1 and severe posterior zone 2 ROP • Visual fields in treated eyes smaller by 6.4° • Functional disability in multiple domains more likely in children with threshold ROP (19.7% vs 3.7%) • Based on results type 1 and 2 ROP have been identified. These define relative risk of progression and thereby the need for immediate intervention. Type 1 ROP needs immediate treatment, while type 2 ROP can be watched weekly.
BEAT ROP study[70,71]	BCZ as monotherapy vs laser for stage 3 + ROP	• Primary outcome was recurrence of ROP • BCZ found advantageous for zone 1 but not zone 2 ROP • More high myopia seen with laser treatment

(BCZ: bevacizumab; BEAT: bevacizumab eliminates the angiogenic threat; ROP: retinopathy of prematurity)

Table 9: Summary of trials on neovascular AMD.

Study	Intervention	Results
Macular photocoagulation study[72]	Laser photocoagulation of subfoveal neovascularization with argon or krypton laser	• Precipitous drop in vision in treated eyes but later stability. After 2 years treated eyes lost 3 lines and untreated eyes 4 lines
RAD study[73]	Double masked RCT of radiation therapy vs sham in subfoveal CNV due to AMD	• No benefit seen with application of 16Gy radiation
TAP study[74]	Placebo controlled, double masked RCT of 3 monthly photodynamic therapy (PDT) for subfoveal CNV due to AMD	• At 1 year, 61% of treated eyes lost less than 3 lines vision vs 46% of untreated eyes • Benefit maximal with predominantly classic CNV
VIP study[75]	Placebo controlled double masked RCT using PDT for pure occult CNV (with no classic component) in AMD	• At 2 years, both groups were similar in terms of loss of 3 lines or more vision • *Subgroup analysis:* Eyes with smaller lesion size or lower levels of baseline vision fared better with treatment compared to no treatment

Contd...

Contd...

Study	Intervention	Results
Pegpatanib for AMD[76]	RCT of intravitreal injection of pegaptanib sodium 6 weekly vs placebo	• 33% of treated eyes retained vision vs 23% of untreated • 70% of treated eye lost less than 3 lines vision vs 55% in controls
Anchor study[77]	RBZ vs PDT-randomized trial for predominantly classic CNVM	• 3 line improvement in 35.7% of RBZ 0.3 mg group and 40.3% of RBZ 0.5 mg group vs 5.6% of PDT
Marina study[78]	RBZ monthly injections for 24 months vs placebo for minimally classic/occult CNVM	• 3 line improvement in 33.8% vs in 5% of control group • Mean improvement in vision was 6.5 letters in RBZ 0.3 mg group and 7.2 letters in RBZ 0.5 mg group vs loss of 10.4 letters in sham group • Recovery maintained at 24 months
Pier study[79]	RBZ monthly for 3 injections followed by quarterly treatments	• 4.5 letter decline between 3–12 months with quarterly treatment
Excite study[80]	Following initial monthly 3 injections of RBZ, comparison of quarterly fixed dose regimen vs continuation of monthly regimen	• With RBZ, higher visual gain with monthly regimen over quarterly
Pronto study[81,82]	• OCT based pro re nata (PRN) regime after initial 3 injections of RBZ. PRN dosing if persistent fluid or increase in thickness by >100 μ • In year 2 PRN dosing given for any qualitative change seen on OCT	• At 1 year, 9.3 letter gain with 5.6 injections • At 2 years, 11.1 letter gain with 9.9 injections
Sailor and Sustain study[83,84]	Evaluated further the role of PRN dosing of RBZ after 3 monthly injections. Open label	• PRN dosing not found to maintain the gains of initial improvement
Horizon study[85]	Extension study of patients from Marina and Anchor studies. Open label RBZ on PRN basis	• Patients who had monthly injections now lost 5.3 letters from baseline
Salute study[86]	RCT of Treat and extend vs PRN for RBZ	• Visual results similar in both groups with reduced clinic visits for Treat and extend regime
Montblanc[87] and Denali[88]	RCT of combination of PDT and RBZ vs sham and RBZ	• Did not support use of combination therapy
Harbor study[89]	Trial of 2.0 mg of RBZ	• No advantage found

Contd...

Contd...

Study	Intervention	Results
View 1 and 2 studies[90,91]	• RCT of comparison of AFL and RBZ • In second year PRN dosing is given based on criteria but definite injection at least once in 3 months	• AFL found noninferior to RBZ. BCVA maintained (<3 line drop) in 95% or more. • By 2nd year, AFL needed less injections
ARI 2 study[92]	Switch to AFL (3 monthly injections followed by 6 weekly) in eyes that had at least 6 RBZ injections and had persistent PED and fluid	• Switch to AFL beneficial in reducing size of PED and improving vision
BRAMD study[93]	BCZ vs RBZ for AMD	• BCZ not inferior to RBZ • BCZ had more variable responses and more residual fluid
CATT study[94]	5-year outcome of BCZ vs RBZ for neovascular AMD	• No difference in visual result or morphological outcome
Ivan study[95]	RCT comparing BCZ and RBZ in monthly and PRN dosing	• No difference between the two drugs • No difference between the two regimens (continuous and discontinuous) in final distance VA at 2 years. Near vision and contrast sensitivity worse with PRN dosing
MERITAGE trial[96]	Epimacular radiation using Strontium 90/Yttrium 90 source along with Ranibizumab	• Radiation did not reduce the need for RBZ injections over 2 years, although appeared safe
EVEREST 2 study[97]	RBZ alone vs with PDT for idiopathic choroidal polypoidal vasculopathy	• At 1 year, combination therapy superior to monotherapy in both polyp regression as well as final visual acuity. 69.3% in combination group and 34.7% in RBZ group achieved polyp regression
PLANET study (unpublished data)	AFL as monotherapy vs AFL with PDT given as rescue therapy	• Polyp regression rate similar with or without PDT (81.7% vs 88.9%)

(AMD: age-related macular degeneration; ARI2: aflibercept after ranibizumab intravitreal injections 2; CATT: comparison of age-related macular degeneration treatments trial; CNV: choroidal neovascularization; CNVM: choroidal neovascular membranes; OCT: optical coherence tomography; RAD: radiation therapy for age-related macular degeneration; RBZ: ranibizumab; RCT: randomized controlled trial; TAP: treatment of age-related macular degeneration with photodynamic therapy; VIP: verteporfin in photodynamic therapy)

- In view of the Everest 2 results, PCV is treated with combination of PDT and anti-VEGF drugs rather than monotherapy. However, recurrences are mostly treated with anti-VEGF drugs alone. Repeat PDT was administered not earlier than 3 months and only if angiography showed active polyps

Table 10: Summary of trials on dry AMD.

Study	Intervention	Results
AREDS study[98]	Double masked trial of use of antioxidants/zinc and copper/antioxidants plus zinc/placebo in eyes with large drusen, noncentral geographic atrophy in both eyes or advanced AMD in one eye	• In high risk group risk of advanced AMD was reduced with use of antioxidants and zinc
Drusen laser study[99,100]	Prophylactic laser to drusen to reduce risk of CNVM	• Green laser increased the risk of CNV in eyes with drusen
Veterans LAST trial[101]	Lutein antioxidant supplementation trial in eyes with atrophic AMD	• Macular pigment optical density and visual acuity improved with lutein alone and with other nutrients
TREX-AMD trial[102]	Choroidal thickness and risk of macular atrophy (MA)	• Eyes with MA have thinner choroids. Thin choroid at baseline increases risk of MA in 18 months
AREDS 2 study[103]	Beta-carotene of AREDS was replaced with Lutein and zeaxanthine. Omega-3 polyunsaturated fatty acids, docosahexaenoic acid (DHA) and eicosapentaenoic acid (EPA) were also added	• Had no positive affect on progression to advanced AMD • Sub-group analysis showed compared to betacarotene, those that took lutein and zeaxanthin had 18% reduced risk of progression to advanced AMD • Risk of lung cancer is also reduced with this switch from betacarotene to lutein and zeoxanthine

(AMD: age-related macular degeneration; AREDS: the age-related eye disease study; CNV: choroidal neovascularization; CNVM: choroid neovascular membranes; LAST: lutein antioxidant supplementation trial; TREX: treat-and-extend)

that leak (along with OCT evidence of activity in the form of intra and subretinal fluid). However, in real-life situation, PDT is perhaps less often repeated than what was done in the protocol. This could be due to reluctance to repeat the angiography too often and also support from other studies that show monotherapy with aflibercept may induce regression of polyps.

- Although the initial anti-VEGF studies were with pegaptanib sodium, this drug did not stand the test of time and has been almost totally replaced by the other options--ranibizumab, bevacizumab and aflibercept.
- Bevacizumab has been shown to be as effective as ranibizumab. Hence, where cost considerations are important, bevacizumab remained the main stay of treatment. Where cost is not the most important factor, the clinicians chose ranibizumab or aflibercept.

- As initiation, between ranibizumab and aflibercept, the option of one versus other is mostly choice of the surgeon. Some surgeons opt to use aflibercept as the first line of treatment in specific situations—presence of significant pigment epithelial detachment and in cases of PCV—due to the perceived advantage of aflibercept in these two circumstances.
- As follow-up treatment, switch to different drug is usually advocated if no response is seen on 2-3 consecutive injections.
- In a developing country like India, treat and extend policy is difficult to implement in a majority of cases despite its proven value. Most patients opt for observe and extend—although not ideal.
- Dry AMD has remained without specific treatment but for low vision aid trial.
- Most patients with dry AMD are given nutrient supplements with lutein and zeaxanthin.
- Considering the plethora of these supplements available in the market and the fierce advertisement that goes with it, one finds most patients consuming multiple medications with the mistaken belief that more is better. They sometimes add on top of the formulated drugs, nonformulated ones such as bilberry extract, fish oil, etc.
- One also sees patients demanding and consuming these supplements even if there is no risk factor (such as drusen, fellow eye with nAMD, geographic atrophy, etc.), just because they are in that vulnerable age group. The prophylactic value in these patients is questionable.
- Several drugs are in the pipeline to try and halt the dry AMD—both as oral drugs or eye drops. However, most studies are in phase 1 or 2 trials and none that has shown conclusive results.
    - Trimetazidine, a drug that is used in angina pectoris to prevent ischemia and improve glucose utilization, did not slow the conversion of dry to wet AMD.
    - Alpostadil, a prostaglandin E1 used for its vasodilatory effect. Preliminary studies show very marginal benefit.
    - MC-1101, a topically instilled drug aimed at dilating choroidal blood vessels. Trial under way.
    - Moxaverine, a phosphodiesterase inhibitor—showed contradictory results.
    - Sildenafil did not cause any significant improvement
    - Fenretinide,[104] a retinol analog—some benefit seen in reducing lesion growth rates of geographic atrophy. There was also reduced incidence of choroidal neovascular membrane (CNVM) noted.
    - ACU-4429 (emixustat), a modulator of isomerase needed for conversion of all—a trans retinol to 11 cis retinal—no positive result
    - Tandospirone, a neuroprotector, CNTF (ciliary neurotrophic factor), appears to slow progress in of geographic atrophy.
    - Others that have been tried include brimonidine, RN6G, GSK 933776, lampalizumab, copaxone, iluvien acetonide, rapamycin, etc.

REFERENCES

1. The relationship of glycemic exposure (HbA1C) to the risk of development and progression of retinopathy in the Diabetes Control and Complications Trial. Diabetes. 1995;44:968-83.
2. Intensive blood-glucose control with sulphonylureas or insulin compared with conventional treatment and risk of complications in patients with type 2 diabetes (UKPDS 33). UK Prospective Diabetes Study (UKPDS) Group. Lancet 1998;352:837-53.
3. Chew EY, Ambrosius WT, Davis MD, et al. Effects of medical therapies on retinopathy progression in type 2 diabetes. N Engl J Med. 2010;363:233-44.
4. Tight blood pressure control and risk of macrovascular and microvascular complications in type 2 diabetes: UKPDS 38. UK Prospective Diabetes Study Group. BMJ. 1998;317:703-13.
5. Beulens JW, Patel A, Vingerling JR, et al. Effects of blood pressure lowering and intensive glucose control on the incidence and progression of retinopathy in patients with type 2 diabetes mellitus: A randomized controlled trial. Diabetologia. 2009;52:2027-36.
6. Chaturvedi N, Sjolie AK, Stephenson JM, et al. Effect of lisinopril on progression of retinopathy in normotensive people with type 1 diabetes. The EUCLID Study Group. Lancet. 1998;351:28-31.
7. Sjølie AK, Klein R, Porta M, et al. Effect of candesartan on progression and regression of retinopathy in type 2 diabetes (DIRECT-Protect 2): A randomised placebo-controlled trial. Lancet. 2008;372:1385-93.
8. Keech AC, Mitchell P, Summanen PA, et al. Effect of fenofibrate on the need for laser treatment for diabetic retinopathy (FIELD study): A randomised controlled trial. Lancet. 2007;370:1687-97.
9. Klein R, Moss SE, Sinaiko AR, et al. The relation of ambulatory blood pressure and pulse rate to retinopathy in type 1 diabetes mellitus. The renin angiotensin system study. Ophthalmology. 2006;113:2231-6.
10. Gaede P, Vedel P, Larsen N, et al. Multifactorial intervention and cardiovascular disease in patients with type 2 diabetes. N Engl J Med. 2003;30:383-93.
11. Photocoagulation for diabetic macular edema. Early treatment diabetic retinopathy study report number 1. Early treatment diabetic retinopathy study research group. Arch Ophthalmol. 1985;103:1796-806.
12. Fong DS, Strauber SF, Aiello LP, et al. Comparison of the modified early treatment diabetic retinopathy study and mild macular grid laser photocoagulation strategies for diabetic macular edema. Arch Ophthalmol. 2007;125:469-80.
13. Diabetic Retinopathy Clinical Research Network. A randomized trial comparing intravitreal triamcinolone acetonide and focal/grid photocoagulation for diabetic macular edema. Ophthalmology. 2008;115:1447-9.
14. Chen G, Tzekov R, Li W, et al. Sub-threshold micropulse diode laser versus conventional laser photocoagulation for diabetic macular edema: A meta-analysis of randomized controlled trials. Retina. 2016;36:2059-65.
15. Do DV, Nguyen QD, Khwaja AA, et al. Ranibizumab for edema of the macula in diabetes study: 3 years outcomes and the need for prolonged frequent treatment. JAMA Ophthalmol. 2013;131:139-45.
16. Do DV, Sepah YJ, Boyer D, et al. Month 6 primary outcomes of the READ 3 study (Ranibizumab for Edema of the macula in DiabetesProtocol 3 with high dose). Eye (Lond). 2015;29:1538-44.

17. Massin P, Bandelllo F, Garweg JG, et al. Safety and efficacy of ranibizumab in diabetic macular edema (RESOLVE study). Diabetes Care. 2010;33:2399-2405.
18. Bressler SB, Glassman A, Almukhtar T, et al. Five-year outcomes of ranibizumab with prompt or deferred laser versus laser or triamcinolone plus deferred ranibizumab for diabetic macular edema. Am J Ophthalmol. 2016;164:57-68.
19. Mitchell P, Bandello F, SchmidtErfurth U, et al. The RESTORE study: Ranibizumab monotherapy or combined with laser versus laser monotherapy for diabetic macular edema. Ophthalmology. 2011;118:615-25.
20. Ishibashi T, Li X, Koh A, et al. The REVEAL Study: Ranibizumab monotherapy or combined with laser versus laser monotherapy in Asian patients with diabetic macular edema. Ophthalmology. 2015;122:1402-15.
21. Nguyen QD, Brown DM, Marcus DM, et al. Ranibizumab for diabetic macular edema: Results from 2 phase III randomized trials: RISE and RIDE. Ophthalmology. 2012;119:789-801.
22. Elman MJ, Ayala A, Bressler NM, et al. Intravitreal ranibizumab for diabetic macular edema with prompt versus deferred laser treatment: 5 year randomized trial results. Ophthalmology. 2015;122:375-81.
23. SchmidtErfurth U, Lang GE, Holz FG, et al. Three year outcomes of individualized ranibizumab treatment in patients with diabetic macular edema: The RESTORE extension study. Ophthalmology. 2014;121:1045-53.
24. Do DV, Nguyen QD, Boyer D, et al. One year outcomes of the da Vinci study of VEGF trap- eye in eyes with diabetic macular edema. Ophthalmology. 2012;119:1658-65.
25. Ziemassen F, Schlottman PG, Lim JI, et al. Initiation of intravitreal aflibercept injection treatment in patients with diabetic macular edema: A review of VIVID-DME and VISTA-DME data. Int J Retina Vitreous. 2016;2:16.
26. Ahmadieh H, Ramezani A, Shoeibi N, et al. Intravitreal bevacizumab with or without triamcinolone for refractory diabetic macular edema; a placebo-controlled, randomized clinical trial. Graefes Arch Clin Exp Ophthalmol. 2008;246:483-9.
27. Michaelides M, Kaines A, Hamilton RD, et al. A prospective randomized trial of intravitreal bevacizumab or laser therapy in the management of diabetic macular edema (BOLT study) 12 month data: Report 2. Ophthalmology. 2010;117:1078-86.e2.
28. Wells JA, Glassman AR, Ayala AR, et al. Aflibercept, bevacizumab, or ranibizumab for diabetic macular edema. N Engl J Med. 2015;372:1193-203.
29. Maturi RK, Pollack A, Uy HS, et al. Intra ocular pressure in patients with diabetic macular edema treated with dexamethasone intravitreal implant in the 3-year MEAD study. Retina. 2016;36:1143-52.
30. Callanan DG, Gupta S, Boyer DS, et al. Dexamethasone intravitreal implant in combination with laser photocoagulation for the treatment of diffuse diabetic macular edema. Ophthalmology. 2013;120:1843-51.
31. Boyer DS, Faber D, Gupta S, et al. Dexamethasone intravitreal implant for treatment of diabetic macular edema in vitrectomized patients. Retina. 2011;31(5):915-23.
32. Campochiaro PA, Brown DM, Pearson A, et al. Long term benefit of sustained-delivery fluocinolone acetonide vitreous inserts for diabetic macular edema. Ophthalmology. 2011;118:626-35.
33. Campochiaro PA, Brown DM, Pearson A, et al. Sustained delivery fluocinolone acetonide vitreous inserts provide benefit for at least 3 years in patients with diabetic macular edema. Ophthalmology. 2012;119:2125-32.

34. Schmid MK, Reich O, Boehni SC, et al. Comparison of outcomes and costs of ranibizumab and aflibercept treatment in real life. PLoS One. 2015;10(8):e0135050.
35. Wecker T, Ehlken C, Buhler A, et al. Five-year visual acuity outcomes and injections patterns in patients with pro-re-nata treatments for AMD, DME, RVO and myopic CNV. Br J Ophthalmol. 2017;101:353-9.
36. The diabetic retinopathy study research group. Photocoagulation treatment of proliferative diabetic retinopathy. Clinical application of diabetic retinopathy study (DRS) findings. DRS report number 8. Ophthalmology. 1981;88:583-600.
37. Gross JG, Glassman AR, Lee M, et al. Pan retinal photocoagulation vs intra vitreal Ranibizumab for Proliferative diabetic retinopathy: A randomized clinical trial. JAMA. 2015;24:2137-46.
38. Martinez-Zapata MJ, Martí-Carvajal AJ, Solà I, et al. Anti-vascular endothelial growth factor for proliferative diabetic retinopathy. Cochrane Database Syst Rev. 2014;(11):CD008721.
39. DRVS study group. Early vitrectomy for severe vitreous hemorrhage in diabetic retinopathy. Four-year results of a randomized trial: Diabetic Retinopathy Vitrectomy Study Report. Arch Ophthalmol. 1990;108(7):958-64.
40. Bhavsar AR, Torres K, Glassman AR, et al. Evaluation of results 1 year following short-term use of ranibizumab for vitreous hemorrhage due to proliferative diabetic retinopathy. JAMA Ophthalmol. 2014;132(7):889-90.
41. Comyn O, Wickham L, Charteris DG, et al. Ranibizumab pretreatment in diabetic vitrectomy: A pilot randomised controlled trial (the RaDiVit study). Eye (Lond). 2017;31(9):1253-8.
42. da R Lucena D, Ribeiro JA, Costa RA, et al. Intraoperative bleeding during vitrectomy for diabetic tractional retinal detachment with versus without preoperative intravitreal bevacizumab (IBeTra study). Br J Ophthalmol. 2009;93(5):688-91.
43. Castillo J, Aleman I, Rush SW, et al. Preoperative bevacizumab administration in proliferative diabetic retinopathy patients undergoing vitrectomy: A randomized and controlled trial comparing interval variation. Am J Ophthalmol. 2017;183:1-10.
44. Brown DM, Campochiaro PA, Singh RP, et al. Ranibizumab for macular edema following central retinal vein occlusion: Six month primary end point results of a phase III study. Ophthalmology. 2010;117:1124-33.
45. CVOS study group. Evaluation of grid pattern photocoagulation for macular edema in central vein occlusion. Ophthalmology. 1995;102:1425-33.
46. Campochiaro PA, Hafiz G, Mir TA, et al. Scatter laser does not reduce macular edema or treatment burden in the patients with vein occlusion: The RELATE trial. Ophthalmology. 2015;122:1426-37.
47. Campochiaro PA, Heier JS, Feiner L, et al. Ranibizumab for macular edema following branch retinal vein occlusion: Six month primary end point results of a phase III study. Ophthalmology. 2010;117:1102-12.
48. Heier Js, Campochiaro PA, Yau L, et al. Ranibizumab for macular edema due to retinal vein occlusions: long-term follow-up in the HORIZON trial. Ophthalmology. 2012;119:802-9.
49. Campochiaro PA, Sophie R, Pearlman J, et al. Long-term outcomes in patients with retinal vein occlusion treated with ranibizumab: The RETAIN study. Ophthalmology. 2014;121(1):209-19.
50. Ogura Y, Roider J, Korobelnik JF, et al. Intravitreal aflibercept for macular edema secondary to central retinal vein occlusion: 18-month results of the phase 3 GALILEO study. Am J Ophthalmol. 2014;158(5):1032-8.

51. Heier JS, Clark WL, Boyer DS, et al. Intravitreal aflibercept injection for macular edema due to central retinal vein occlusion: Two-year results from the COPERNICUS study. Ophthalmology. 2014;121(7):1414-20.e1.
52. Scott IU, VanVeldhuisen PC, Ip MS, et al. Effect of bevacizumab vs aflibercept on visual acuity among patients with macular edema due to central retinal vein occlusion: The SCORE 2 randomized clinical trial. JAMA. 2017;317(20):2072-87.
53. Scott IU, Ip MS, VanVeldhuisen PC, et al. A randomized trial comparing the efficacy and safety of intravitreal triamcinolone with standard care to treat vision loss associated with macular Edema secondary to branch retinal vein occlusion: The Standard Care vs Corticosteroid for Retinal Vein Occlusion (SCORE) study report 6. Arch Ophthalmol. 2009;127(9):1115-28.
54. Haller JA, Bandello F, Belfort R Jr, et al. Dexamethasone intravitreal implant in patients with macular edema related to branch or central retinal vein occlusion twelve-month study results. Ophthalmology. 2011;118(12):2453-60.
55. Campochiaro PA, Wykoff CC, Singer M, et al. Monthly versus as-needed ranibizumab injections in patients with retinal vein occlusion: The SHORE study. Ophthalmology. 2014;121(12):2432-42.
56. Cryotherapy for retinopathy of prematurity cooperative group. Multicenter trial of cryotherapy for retinopathy of prematurity, one year outcome-structure and function. Arch Ophthalmol. 1990;108:1408-16.
57. Cryotherapy for Retinopathy of Prematurity Cooperative Group. Multicenter trial of cryotherapy for retinopathy of prematurity: Natural history ROP: Ocular outcome at 5(1/2) years in premature infants with birth weights less than 1251 g. Arch Ophthalmol. 2002;120(5):595-9.
58. Cryotherapy for Retinopathy of Prematurity Cooperative Group. Contrast sensitivity at age 10 years in children who had threshold retinopathy of prematurity. Arch Ophthalmol. 2001;119(8):1129-33.
59. Cryotherapy for Retinopathy of Prematurity Cooperative Group. Effect of retinal ablative therapy for threshold retinopathy of prematurity: results of Goldmann perimetry at the age of 10 years. Arch Ophthalmol. 2001;119(8):1120-5.
60. Cryotherapy for Retinopathy of Prematurity Cooperative Group. Multicenter trial of cryotherapy for retinopathy of prematurity: Ophthalmological outcomes at 10 years. Arch Ophthalmol. 2001;119(8):1110-8.
61. Quinn GE, Dobson V, Siatkowski R, et al. Does cryotherapy affect refractive error? Results from treated versus control eyes in the cryotherapy for retinopathy of prematurity trial. Ophthalmology. 2001;108(2):343-7.
62. Cryotherapy for Retinopathy of Prematurity Cooperative Group. Involution of retinopathy of prematurity. Arch Ophthalmol. 2000;118(5):645-9.
63. Msall ME, Phelps DL, DiGaudio KM, et al. Behalf of the Cryotherapy for Retinopathy of Prematurity Cooperative Group. Severity of neonatal retinopathy of prematurity is predictive of neurodevelopment functional outcome at age 5.5 years. Pediatrics. 2000;106(5):998-1005.
64. Repka MX, Summers CG, Palmer EA, et al. The incidence of ophthalmologic interventions in children with birth weights less than 1251 grams. Results through 5 1/2 years. Ophthalmology. 1998;105(9):1621-7.
65. Saunders RA, Donahue ML, Christmann LM, et al. The Cryotherapy for Retinopathy of Prematurity Cooperative Group. Racial variation in retinopathy of prematurity. Arch Ophthalmol. 1997;115(5):604-8.
66. Dobson V, Quinn GE, Abramov I, et al. Colour vision measured with pseudo isochromatic plates at five-and-a-half years in eyes of children from the CRYO-ROP study. Invest Ophthalmol Vis Sci. 1996;37(12):2467-74.

67. Quinn GE, Dobson V, Hardy RJ, et al. The CRYO-Retinopathy of Prematurity Cooperative Group. Visual fields measured with double-arc perimetry in eyes with threshold retinopathy of prematurity from the cryotherapy for retinopathy of prematurity trial. Ophthalmology. 1996;103(9):1432-7.
68. Quinn GE, Dobson V, Barr CC, et al. The Cryotherapy for Retinopathy of Prematurity Cooperative Group. Visual acuity of eyes after vitrectomy for retinopathy of prematurity: Follow-up at 5 1/2 years. Ophthalmology. 1996;103(4):595-600.
69. Good WV, Early Treatment for Retinopathy of Prematurity Cooperative Group. Final results of the Early Treatment for Retinopathy of Prematurity (ETROP) randomized trial. Trans Am Ophthalmol Soc. 2004;102:233-48.
70. Mintz-Hittner HA, Kennedy KA, Chuang AZ, et al. Efficacy of intravitreal bevacizumab for stage 3+ retinopathy of prematurity. N Engl J Med. 2011;364(7):603-15.
71. Geloneck MM, Chuang AZ, Clark WL, et al. Refractive outcomes following bevacizumab monotherapy compared with conventional laser treatment: a randomized clinical trial. JAMA Ophthalmol. 2014;132(11):1327-33.
72. Macular Photocoagulation Study Group Laser photocoagulation of subfoveal neovascular lesions in age-related macular degeneration. Results of a randomized clinical trial. Arch Ophthalmol. 1991;109(9):1220-31.
73. RAD study group. A prospective randomized double masked trial on radiation therapy for neovascular age related macular degeneration (RAD study). Ophthalmology. 1999;106:2239-47.
74. Treatment of age-related macular degeneration with photodynamic therapy (TAP) Study Group. Photodynamic therapy of subfoveal choroidal neovascularization in age-related macular degeneration with verteporfin: One-year results of 2 randomized clinical trials—TAP report. Arch Ophthalmol. 1999;117(10):1329-45.
75. Verteporfin In Photodynamic Therapy Study Group. Verteporfin therapy of subfoveal choroidal neovascularization in age-related macular degeneration: Two-year results of a randomized clinical trial including lesions with occult with no classic choroidal neovascularization—verteporfin in photodynamic therapy report 2. Am J Ophthalmol. 2001;131(5):541-60.
76. Gragoudas ES, Adamis AP, Cunningham ET Jr, et al. Pegaptanib for neovascular age-related macular degeneration. N Engl J Med. 2004;351(27):2805-16.
77. Brown DM, Kaiser PK, Michels M, et al. Ranibizumab versus verteporfin for neovascular age-related macular degeneration. N Engl J Med. 2006;355(14):1432-44.
78. Rosenfeld PJ, Brown DM, Heier JS, et al. Ranibizumab for neovascular age-related macular degeneration. N Engl J Med. 2006;355(14):1419-31.
79. Regillo CD, Brown DM, Abraham P, et al. Randomized, double-masked, sham-controlled trial of ranibizumab for neovascular age-related macular degeneration: PIER Study year 1. Am J Ophthalmol. 2008;145:239-48.
80. Schmidt-Erfurth U, Eldem B, Guymer R, et al. Efficacy and safety of monthly versus quarterly ranibizumab treatment in neovascular age-related macular degeneration: The EXCITE study. Ophthalmology. 2011;118:831-9.
81. Fung AE, Lalwani GA, Rosenfeld PJ, et al. An optical coherence tomography-guided, variable dosing regimen with intravitreal ranibizumab (Lucentis) for neovascular age-related macular degeneration. Am J Ophthalmol. 2007;143:566-83.

82. Lalwani GA, Rosenfeld PJ, Fung AE, et al. A variable-dosing regimen with intravitreal ranibizumab for neovascular age-related macular degeneration: Year 2 of the PrONTO Study. Am J Ophthalmol. 2009;148:43-58.e1.
83. Boyer DS, Heier JS, Brown DM, et al. A Phase IIIb study to evaluate the safety of ranibizumab in subjects with neovascular age-related macular degeneration. Ophthalmology. 2009;116:1731-9.
84. Holz FG, Amoaku W, Donate J, et al. Safety and efficacy of a flexible dosing regimen of ranibizumab in neovascular age-related macular degeneration: The SUSTAIN study. Ophthalmology. 2011;118:663-71.
85. Singer MA, Awh CC, Sadda S, et al. HORIZON: An open-label extension trial of ranibizumab for choroidal neovascularization secondary to age-related macular degeneration. Ophthalmology. 2012;119:1175-83.
86. Eldem BM, Muftuoglu G, Topbas S, et al. A randomized trial to compare the safety and efficacy of two ranibizumab dosing regimens in a Turkish cohort of patients with choroidal neovascularization secondary to AMD. Acta Ophthalmol. 2015;93:e458-64.
87. Larsen M, Schmidt-Erfurth U, Lanzetta P, et al. Verteporfin plus ranibizumab for choroidal neovascularization in age-related macular degeneration: Twelve-month MONT BLANC study results. Ophthalmology. 2012;119:992-1000.
88. Kaiser PK, Boyer DS, Cruess AF, et at. Verteporfin plus ranibizumab for choroidal neovascularization in age-related macular degeneration: Twelve-month results of the DENALI study. Ophthalmology. 2012;119:1001-10.
89. Busbee BG, Ho AC, Brown DM, et al. Twelve-month efficacy and safety of 0.5 mg or 2.0 mg ranibizumab in patients with subfoveal neovascular age-related macular degeneration. Ophthalmology. 2013;120:1046-56.
90. Heier JS, Brown DM, Chong V, et al. Intravitreal aflibercept (VEGF trap-eye) in wet age-related macular degeneration. Ophthalmology. 2012;119:2537-48.
91. Schmidt-Erfurth U, Kaiser PK, Korobelnik JF, et al. Intravitreal aflibercept injection for neovascular age-related macular degeneration: Ninety-six-week results of the VIEW studies. Ophthalmology. 2014;121:193-201.
92. Blanco-Garavito R, Jung C, Uzzan J, et al. Aflibercept after Ranibizumab intravitreal injections in exudative age related macular degeneration. The ARI2 study. Retina. 2017;21.
93. Schauwvlieghe AM, Dijkman G, Hooymans JM, et al. Comparing the effectiveness of bevacizumab to ranbizumab in patients with exudative age related macular degeneration. The BRAMD study. PloS One. 2016;11(5):e0153052.
94. Maguire MG, Martin DF, Ying GS, et al. Five year outcomes with antivascular endothelial growth factor treatment of neovascular age-related macular degeneration: The comparison of age-related macular degeneration treatment trials. Ophthalmology. 2016;123(8):1751-61.
95. Chakravarthy U, Harding SP, Rogers CA, et al. Alternative treatments to inhibit VEGF in age-related choroidal neovascularisation: 2-year findings of the IVAN randomised controlled trial. Lancet. 2013;382:1258-67.
96. Patrarca R, Dugel PU, Bennet M, et al. Macular epiretinal brachytherapy in treated age-related macular degeneration (MERITAGE) month 24 safety and efficacy results. Retina. 2014;34(5):874-9.
97. Koh A, Lai TYY, Takahashi K, et al. Efficacy and Safety of ranibizumab with or without verteporfin photodynamic therapy for polypoidal choroidal vasculopathy: A randomized clinical trial. JAMA Ophthalmol. 2017;135(11):1206-13.

98. Age-related Eye Disease Study Research Group. A randomized, placebo-controlled, clinical trial of high-dose supplementation with vitamins C and E, beta carotene, and zinc for age-related macular degeneration and vision loss: AREDS report no. 8. Arch ophthalmol. 2001;119(10):1417-36.
99. Owen SL, Bunce C, Brannon AJ, et al. Prophylactic laser treatment hastens choroidal neovascularization in unilateral age-related maculopathy: Final results of the drusen laser study. Am J Ophthalmol. 2006;141(2):276-81.
100. Owens SL, Bunce C, Brannon AJ, et al. Prophylactic laser treatment appears to promote choroidal neovascularisation in high-risk ARM: Results of an interim analysis. Eye (Lond). 2003;17(5):623-7.
101. Richer S, Stiles W, Statkute L, et al. Double-masked, placebo-controlled, randomized trial of lutein and antioxidant supplementation in the intervention of atrophic age-related macular degeneration: The Veterans LAST study (Lutein Antioxidant Supplementation Trial). J Optometry. 2004;75(4):216-30.
102. Fan W, Abdelfattah NS, Uji A, et al. Subfoveal choroidal thickness predicts macular atrophy in age-related macular degeneration: Results from the TREX-AMD trial. Graefes Arch Clin Exp Ophthalmol. 2018;256(3):511-8.
103. Age-related Eye Disease Study Research Group. Lutein + zeaxanthin and omega-3 fatty acids for age related macular degeneration: The Age-related eye disease study 2 (AREDS 2) randomized clinical trial. JAMA. 2013;309:2005-15.
104. Mata NL, Lichter JB, Vogel R, et al. Investigation of oral fenretinide for treatment of geographic atrophy in age related macular degeneration. Retina. 2013;33:498-507.

CHAPTER
16

Optical Coherence Tomography—Angiography in Retinal Diseases

Chaitra Jayadev, Arpitha Pereira, Santosh GK Gadde

■ INTRODUCTION

Optical coherence tomography (OCT) is a noninvasive, depth-resolved imaging technique based on low-coherence interferometry. It is capable of generating structural images of ocular anatomy based on back-reflected light. Although conventional structural OCT helps in visualizing pathologic changes that impact vision, it offers poor contrast between small blood vessels and static tissue in most retinal layers. In order to visualize vascular changes, fluorescein (FA) or indocyanine green angiography (ICGA) would have to be used. While useful, they require intravenous dye injection, which is time consuming and can have adverse side effects. Finally, these techniques provide little information in terms of depth information due to the two-dimensional (2D) nature of the acquired images.

Thus, in order to develop a dye-free method for visualizing ocular vasculature, a number of functional extensions of OCT have been explored—one among them being OCT angiography. Optical coherence tomography angiography (OCTA) is a new, noninvasive imaging technique that generates volumetric angiography images in a matter of seconds thus producing high-resolution, 3D angiograms of the retinal and choroidal vascular networks.

■ PRINCIPLE

Optical coherence tomography angiography is based on the concept that in a static eye, the only moving structures in the fundus are red blood cells that circulate in the retinal and choroidal vasculature. OCTA utilizes the flowing red blood cells as an intrinsic contrast agent to generate flow signals allowing for visualization of vascular networks without the need of dye injection.[1,2]

Optical coherence tomography angiography acquires repeated OCT B scans at the same location to detect motion. The development of OCTA was not possible during the era of slower speed time-domain systems. With the introduction of Fourier-domain OCT systems, the scanning speed of OCT improved by a factor of 50, opening the door for more advanced OCT applications. The OCT signal backscattered from tissue components remains steady for there is no movement in the tissue while the OCT signal backscattered from the vessel changes over time as the RBCs tumble and move through the vessel. By calculating the differences in OCT signals acquired at the same location at different time points, OCTA distinguishes the moving particles from static tissue and therefore is able to generate flow signals and allows the visualization of microvascular networks in biologicals tissues.[3]

Multiple approaches have been described for quantifying this change through assessment of the phase, intensity, or both of the OCT signal and accordingly classified as phase-signal-based OCTA techniques, intensity-signal-based OCTA techniques, and complex-signal-based OCTA techniques (Table 1).

PHASE-BASED OPTICAL COHERENCE TOMOGRAPHY ANGIOGRAPHY

Phase-based OCTA uses the phase information from backscattered OCT signals. Moving erythrocytes induce a Doppler shift (change in frequency or wavelength of a wave for an observer who is moving relative to the wave source) in backscattered OCT signals and this shift can be used to perform blood flow measurements. The first Doppler OCT displayed flow information by evaluating phase changes between the two adjacent A-scan lines.[4]

However, Doppler OCT can measure only axial flow and, with dedicated scanning protocols and hardware modifications, transverse flow can be measured.[5]

With continued improvement of OCT systems speeds due to hardware advancements, methods for achieving OCTA shifted from using a comparison between adjacent A-scans to a comparison between sequential cross-sectional B-scans. This approach has made possible the detection of slower

Table 1: Commercially available OCTA machines

OCTA	OCT platform	Algorithm
AngioVue	Optovue	SSDA
AngioPlex	Zeiss CIRRUS™ OCT	OMAG
SS-OCT Angio™	Swept Source OCT DRI OCT Triton series system (TOPCON)	OCTARA™
Spectralis® OCT Angiography	Heidelberg	Amplitude decorrelation
AngioScan	Nidek RS-3000	Modified OMAG

(OCTA: optical coherence tomography angiography; SSDA: split-spectrum amplitude-decorrelation; OMAG: optical microangiography; OCTARA: optical coherence tomography angiography ratio analysis)

flow. A phase variance technique for vascular imaging has also been demonstrated by using repeated B-scans at the same location.[6]

■ AMPLITUDE-BASED OPTICAL COHERENCE TOMOGRAPHY ANGIOGRAPHY

Amplitude-based OCTA method, also known as magnitude based, uses intensity and speckle information of OCT signals. Compared to phase-based approaches, amplitude-based strategies are less susceptible to the phase noise. Speckle is a random pattern of noise that is generated as a result of OCT signal backscattering from the tissue. There exists a difference in speckle patterns generated by moving and static scatterers.[7] Other intensity-based approaches include differential logarithmic intensity variance, the intensity difference between successive B-scans, and comparison of vessel reflectivity characteristics from nonvascular areas.[8]

An alternative method, known as Split-spectrum amplitude-decorrelation (SSADA), using an algorithm based on the time-varying speckle phenomenon has also been used.[9] Unlike correlation mapping, SSADA computes a decorrelation signal between two adjacent B-scans to detect flow. The full OCT spectrum is split into narrower bands and each band is processed separately to generate several flow signals for same B-scan. SSADA has an improved signal-to-noise ratio (SNR), but the axial resolution is reduced. Therefore, it is less susceptible to axial bulk motion. This property makes SSADA particularly suitable for imaging of ocular blood flow.[10]

■ COMPLEX SIGNAL-BASED OPTICAL COHERENCE TOMOGRAPHY ANGIOGRAPHY

Complex signal-based methods utilize both phase and intensity information from OCT signals. The approaches based solely on phase are less sensitive to perpendicular flow; while the strategies relying on intensity alone suffer from difficulty in detecting slower flow, if it induces changes in phase only. Complex methods can provide better results by combining information both from the phase and amplitude of OCT signals.

Optical microangiography (OMAG) is a complex signal-based method, first reported in 2007, which has subsequently evolved. It provides excellent imaging of the retinal and choroidal vasculatures up to a capillary-level resolution.[11,12] The most recently developed algorithm split-spectrum amplitude and phase gradient analysis (SSAPGA) combines the phase gradient analysis method with split spectrum amplitude information. SSAPGA has demonstrated superior results compared to other methods.[13] All of the above-mentioned OCTA techniques provide useful information about retinal vasculature. Multiple investigator groups have compared these methods. Complex approaches seem to provide better imaging of retinal flow in terms of vessel connectivity, contrast, and SNR.[3]

IMAGE PROCESSING

Optical coherence tomography angiography allows for construction of 3D dataset representing the vascular portion of the scanned tissue by virtue of its depth-resolved property. Accurate segmentation of the structural image is essential for optimal evaluation of retinal and choroidal vasculature. Fully automated segmentation algorithms are highly efficient and accurate when it comes to the healthy retina. However, in the diseased eye, anatomical features are usually distorted and may require manual segmentation. The more commonly used segmentation boundaries include internal limiting membrane (ILM), outer boundary of the nerve fiber layer (NFL), outer boundary of the inner plexiform layer, outer boundary of the inner nuclear layer (INL), outer boundary of the outer plexiform layer (OPL), retinal pigmented epithelium (RPE), and Bruch's membrane (BM).

The 3D flow data are usually presented as 2D images, comparable to conventional angiography. The flow signal in specific tissue layers or slabs could be compressed into one 2D *en face* image. These slabs are defined by two relevant segmentation boundaries. For instance, the inner retinal circulation is the flow signal between the ILM and outer boundary of OPL, while the normally avascular outer retinal slab is defined between the outer boundary of OPL and BM. Another method for presenting OCT angiograms is to use the conventional cross-sectional approach. Flow signal is color coded and overlaid on the structural OCT image. Displaying structural data along with the flow data in the same B-scan can be useful in providing detailed information on the depth of vascular abnormalities such as retinal or choroidal neovascularization (CNV).

Quantification

Quantification of OCTA is important for objective evaluation of retinal abnormalities. The following are various indices that have been used:
- *Vessel density*: It is the percentage area occupied by the blood vessels from en face angiogram. Vessel density is more useful for the diagnosis and monitoring of vascular pathology.[14]
- *Flow index*: It is the average flow signal in the area of interest in an *en face* angiogram. Flow index has been found to be more sensitive in detecting the metabolic and physiologic changes in retinal tissue.[15,16]
- Capillary dropout or nonperfusion area refers to the significant area (larger than the normal gap between capillaries) devoid of flow signal that would normally be vascular. Measurement of avascular area can serve as a valuable metric for objective evaluation of diseases characterized by capillary loss such as diabetic retinopathy (DR) and glaucoma.[17]
- Neovascularization area is the sum of pixel areas in a pathologic neovascular net identified on the *en face* OCT angiogram.[18,19]
- Perfusion density mapping is another approach to assess abnormal flow regions.[20] It is a color-coded map demonstrating the vascular density in different areas of the scanned region.

- Quantitative parameters have the potential to provide new objective biomarkers for eye diseases, facilitating diagnosis, monitoring, and treatment. However, further investigations are needed for validation and reliability assessment of the new metrics.

OPTICAL COHERENCE TOMOGRAPHY ANGIOGRAPHY OF NORMAL EYES

The most widely available prototype OCTA system is the AngioVue software of the RTVue XR Avanti spectral-domain OCT (SD-OCT) (Optovue, Inc, Fremont, CA), which uses a SSADA algorithm (Figs. 1A to F). This device is capable of obtaining volumetric scans of 304 × 304 A-scans at 70,000 A-scans per second in approximately 3.0 seconds. The software offers the option of 2 × 2 mm, 3 × 3 mm, 6 × 6 mm, and 8 × 8 mm OCT angiograms.[1] The scan quality decreases significantly with larger fields of view. The 3 × 3 mm scans provide a very high resolution; however, 6 × 6 mm scans provide a wider field of view with an excellent scan resolution. Additionally, montaging multiple images of the smaller area can generate high-resolution angiograms without compromising the final resolution.[21-23]

The device makes use of automated segmentation to provide full-thickness retinal scans of the "superficial" and "deep" inner retinal vascular plexuses,

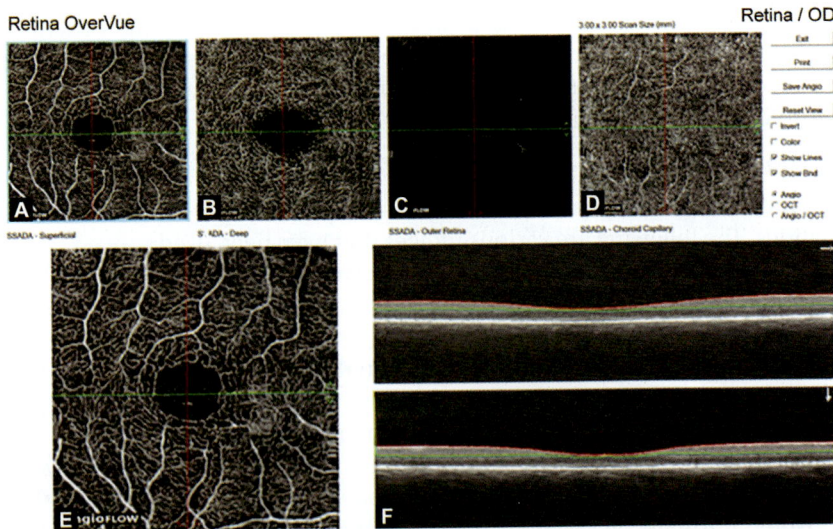

Figs. 1A to F: Optical coherence tomography (OCT) angiogram fields of view and segmentation layers on AngioVue. The normal right eye of a 30-year-old Indian man using the AngioVue optical coherence tomography angiography (OCTA) software of the RTVue XR Avanti (Optovue Inc., Fremont, CA). (A) 3 × 3 mm OCT angiogram of the "superficial" inner retina; (B) 3 × 3 mm OCT angiogram of the "deep" inner retina; (C) 3 × 3 mm OCT angiogram of the outer retina shows absence of vasculature. The white represents noise; (D) 3 × 3 mm OCT angiogram of the choriocapillaries is generally homogenous. There is back shadowing from retinal vessels; (E) Enlarged view of selected slab; (F) OCT B-scan image.

outer retina, and choriocapillaries (CC). The OCT angiogram segmentation of the superficial inner retina contains a projection of the vasculature in the retinal nerve fiber layer (RNFL) and ganglion cell layer (GCL). The deep inner retina OCT angiogram segmentation shows a composite of the vascular plexuses at the border of the inner plexiform layer (IPL) and inner nuclear layer (INL) and the border of the INL and outer plexiform layer (OPL).[1,23]

The superficial vascular plexus (SVP) appears as a homogeneous web of white lines representing vasculature against a dark background in a regular, centripetal fashion converging toward the foveal avascular zone (FAZ). Deep capillary plexus (DCP) of a normal retina is displayed as a fine, homogenous, close-knit pattern of horizontal and radial capillaries, spread evenly and centered on FAZ. The outer retina normally does not show any vascular plexus. It appears dark on OCTA.

Optical coherence tomography angiogram of the choriocapillaries is generally homogenous. There is black shadowing from retinal vessels.[24] Visualization of choroidal circulation by OCTA is more difficult than that of retinal circulation because of the light scattering property of the retinal layers, particularly the RPE. While commercially available SD-OCTA systems with 840 nm light sources are able to provide visualization at the level of the choriocapillaries,[24] OCTA systems at longer wavelengths can achieve deeper penetration and theoretically improve choroidal imaging.[25]

ARTIFACTS

Weak Optical Coherence Tomography Signal

The generation of structural OCT images depends on the backscattering of light from tissue structures. The OCT signal can be reduced globally by media opacity, pupil vignetting, and defocusing of the light beam. In such cases, low-quality images will be generated, obscuring inner eye components and producing unreliable flow information. Using light sources with longer wavelengths (SS-OCT) can theoretically overcome mild media opacities.

Motion Artifacts

Optical coherence tomography angiography relies on intrinsic motion contrast as the basis for detecting flow. Bulk tissue and saccadic eye movements can produce noise and motion artifacts, resulting in overestimation of the flow signal. Multiple approaches have been introduced to overcome motion artifacts. Motion correction technology is a technique that has been used in commercial OCT systems. In this method, two OCT volumes are acquired with perpendicular scanning directions and then registered and merged.[26] Variants of eye tracking have also been adopted on commercial OCTA systems.[23] Eye tracking systems work by detecting eye movement for real-time correction of motion artifacts. These methods can significantly reduce motion artifacts and improve the reliability of OCTA scans (Figs. 2A and B). However, residual defects can still be present as motion lines vessel duplication, or vessel discontinuity.

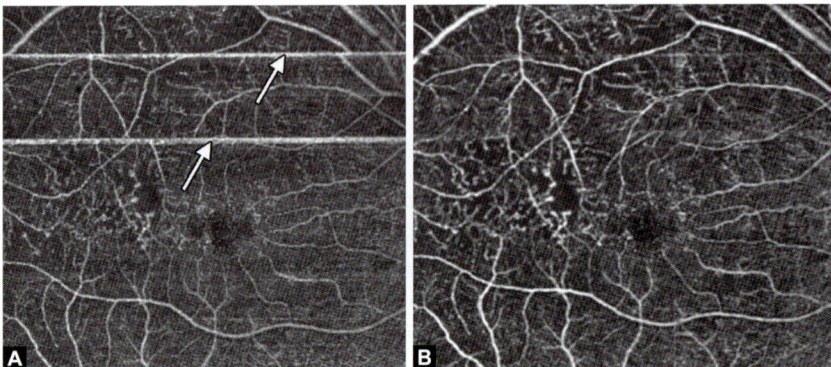

Figs. 2A and B: Movements artifacts. (A) White line artifacts (white arrows). With eye movements during an image frame, one region is imaged and is then juxtaposed with a noncontiguous region because of the movements; (B) Artifact corrected by the software (OptoVue RTVue XR AVANTI Inc., Fremont, CA).

Projection Artifacts

Flowing red blood cells in more superficial vasculature cast time-varying shadows on the deeper retinal layers.[24] These flow projection artifacts lead to duplication of the superficial vascular pattern on deeper microcirculation, as well as the normally avascular outer retinal slab. OCTA projection artifacts can lead to inaccurate measurement of flow index and vessel density of deeper retinal vasculature.[27] Several solutions have been proposed to overcome OCTA projection artifacts. One method is to subtract the more superficial flow signal from the deeper *en face* angiograms, called the "slab-subtraction" method. This approach can disrupt the continuity of vessels in the deeper vascular plexuses and potentially underestimate their vessel density. More recently, an algorithm called "projection-resolved" OCTA (PR-OCTA) was developed to suppress the projected flow signal while preserving the natural continuity of ocular microvasculature, allowing for improved visualization and quantification of different retinal vascular layers in normal and diseased eyes.[28,29]

AngioAnalytics

Optovue's quantification tool is called AngioAnalytics and it provides numerical data on flow and nonflow areas. It can also generate flow density maps. This tool can be used to track disease progression and treatment response.[30]

- **Flow area:** This parameter is particularly useful in cases of neovascularization (Figs. 3A and B). The operator marks the area of new vessels and the software computes the vessel area in mm^2.
- **Nonflow areas:** These are regions where there is no flow detected by SSADA. This is useful in cases of ischemic retinopathies. Ischemic areas are color coded in yellow by the software. Flow density map, this tool is able to measure the percentage of vascular *en face* angiograms.

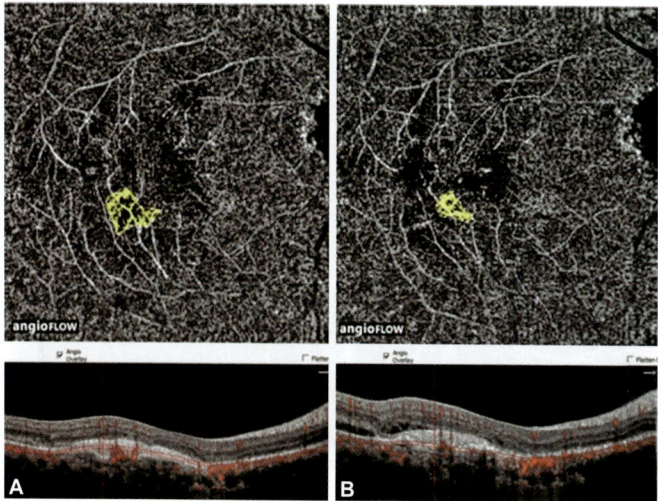

Figs. 3A and B: (A) Use of AngioAnalytics (OptoVue RTVue XR AVANTI Inc, Fremont, CA) software to measure flow area. Neovascular complex (yellow network) at first presentation; (B) Neovascular complex 1 month post anti-VEGF demonstrating decreased flow area.

OPTICAL COHERENCE TOMOGRAPHY ANGIOGRAPHY OF RETINAL DISORDERS

Diabetic Retinopathy

Optical coherence tomography angiography can demonstrate qualitatively similar results to FA in displaying classic findings of diabetic retinopathy including microaneurysms, capillary dropout, vascular looping/beading, and vascular proliferation.[31] Nonproliferative diabetic retinopathy (NPDR) is characterized by several changes in retinal microvasculature such as loss of pericytes, basement membrane thickening, and smooth muscle cell loss, all of which leads to the development of microaneurysms—the first visible sign of NPDR.[32]

Microaneurysms are described as focally dilated capillaries with a round, saccular, or fusiform shape. OCTA allows the visualization of microaneurysms in either superficial capillary plexus (SCP) or DCP layers. The detection rate of microaneurysms by OCTA is significant lower than by FA.[33] It is believed that some microaneurysms cannot be detected by OCTA because their blood flow is too slow (Figs. 4A and B).

Optical coherence tomography angiography has been used to study vessel tortuosity, an indicator of the severity of NPDR.[34] In NPDR, vessel tortuosity increases with the progression of the diabetic disease either in superficial retinal layers or in deep retinal layers. It can also detect venous beading as contiguous focal dilations of retinal vessels, which sometimes are not homogeneously perfused, causing a partial visualization of vascular dilations.[35] Cotton–wool spots, on both fluorescein angiography and OCTA, may correspond to areas of decreased perfusion.[31]

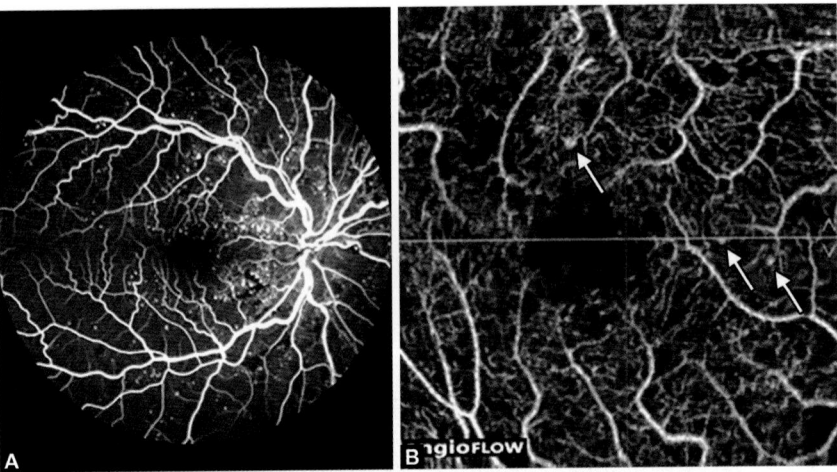

Figs. 4A and B: (A) FA of a 65-year-old female patient with moderate NPDR showing multiple pin point hyperfluorscent areas indicating microaneuryms and vascular beading; (B) OCTA (OptoVue RTVue XR AVANTI Inc, Fremont, CA) image of SCP of the same eye showing microaneuryms (white arrows), lesser in number compared to FA.

(FA: fluorescein angiography; NPDR: nonproliferative diabetic retinopathy; OCTA: optical coherence tomography angiography; SCP: superficial capillary plexus)

Projection-resolved OCTA allows the identification of dilated vessels forming hairpin loops in the deeper plexus of ischemic areas. These lesions are consistent with intraretinal microvascular abnormalities (IRMA), which are difficult to detect by conventional imaging but can easily be seen with PR-OCTA.

Finally, intraretinal hemorrhages may stop or attenuate the signal coming from decorrelated structures resulting in blocking of signal from perfused vessels.

Many studies have demonstrated a significant widening of FAZ before the clinical manifestation of diabetic retinopathy. Similarly, the FAZ enlargement is also well documented in patients with clinical diabetic retinopathy. FAZ enlargement has been noted in both superior vascular plexus and deep vascular plexus; the finding being more pronounced in DCP (Figs. 5A and B).[36] Thus, OCTA could serve as a predictor of diabetic retinopathy even before a systemic diagnosis has been established.

Unlike FA, OCTA does not assess leakage. This is advantageous over FA especially during quantification as leakage can blur boundaries. It can help the clinician better differentiate between small neovascular tufts from microaneurysms, which are seen on FA as smaller areas of focal leakage (Figs. 6A to C).[35]

Capillary nonperfusion/ischemia is a major driver and a vital prognostic factor in the disease process. Venous beading and looping seen in the superficial plexus has been seen to correspond to FA. Likewise, CNP areas can also be correlated.[37]

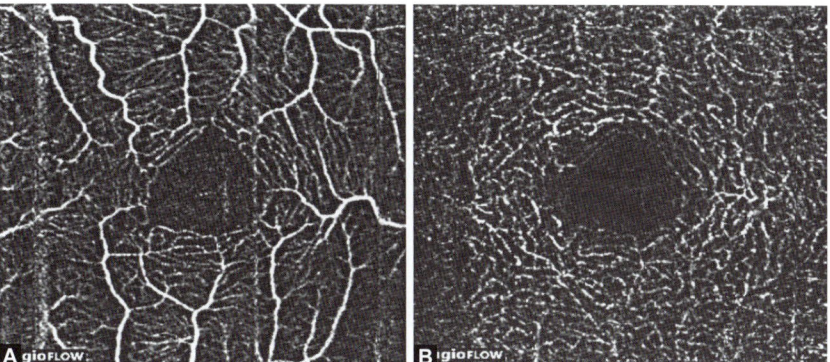

Figs. 5A and B: (A) A 3 × 3 mm OCTA (OptoVue RTVue XR AVANTI Inc., Fremont, CA) scan of a 50-year-old, male, diabetic patient with moderate NPDR demonstrating FAZ enlargement. The findings are less marked in SVP; (B) Compared to DCP.

(FAZ: foveal avascular zone; NPDR: nonproliferative diabetic retinopathy; OCTA: optical coherence tomography angiography; SVP: superficial vascular plexus)

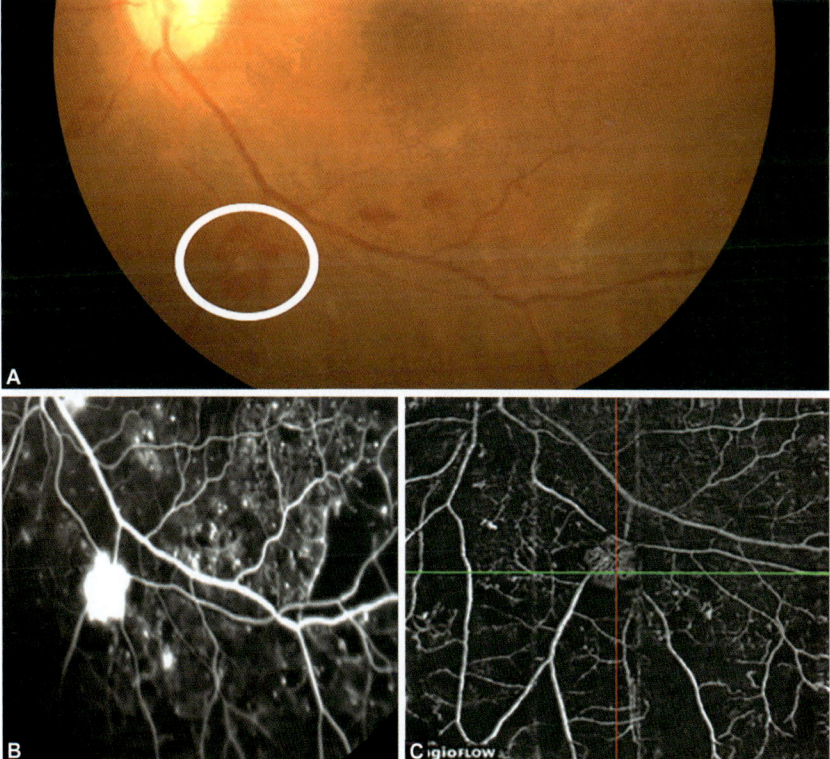

Figs. 6A to C: (A) Color fundus photograph of the left eye of 52-year-old male affected by proliferative diabetic retinopathy showing neovascular tuft (white circle); (B) OCTA (6 × 6 mm) of the SCP allows a better delineation of new vessels when compared to (C) Fluorescein angiography.

(SCP: superficial capillary plexus)

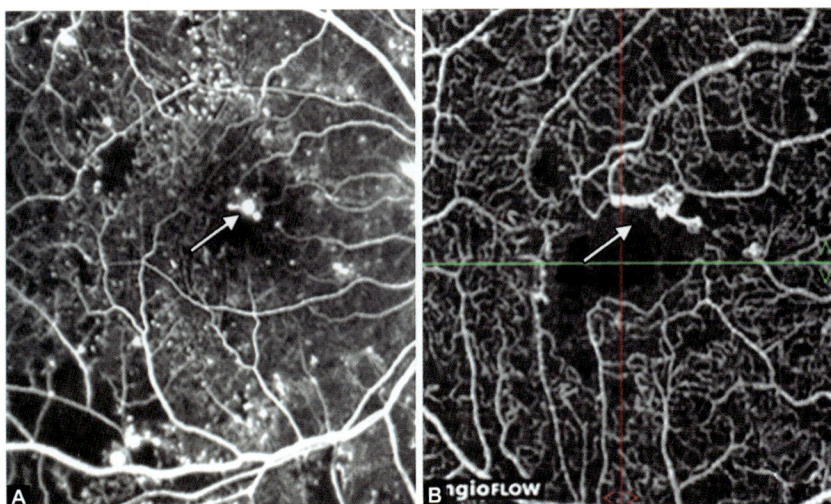

Figs. 7A and B: (A) FA showing venous looping (arrow) and distorted FAZ; (B) OCTA (OptoVue RTVue XR AVANTI Inc, Fremont, CA) image of same eye showing well-delineated venous looping (arrow) and distorted FAZ.

(FA: fluorescein angiography; FAZ: foveal avascular zone; OCTA: optical coherence tomography angiography)

Optical coherence tomography angiograms of patients affected by PDR showed lower retinal capillary density, higher capillary tortuosity, dilated capillary segments, capillary dropouts, capillary loops, and enlarged FAZ with asymmetric contour (Figs. 7A and B).[38]

Two different morphologic features of new vessels are identifiable with OCTA: exuberant vascular proliferation (EVP), which consists of fine vessels with irregular proliferation, and pruned vascular loops. EVP is present in treatment-naïve eyes with PDR and it is associated with high degree of leakage on fluorescein angiography, representing active proliferation. It has been shown that EVP may convert to pruned new vessels after PRP.[39]

Optical coherence tomography angiography may also be used to assess response post-treatment. Post-PRP, change in caliber of new vessels has been noted.

Thus, OCTA is capable of detecting vascular changes in diabetic population; it may be used as an adjunct with structural OCT and FA to better study the retinal changes caused by diabetes.

Retinal Vein Occlusion

Retinal vein occlusion (RVO) is the most common vascular disorder next to the diabetic retinopathy. The severity of visual symptoms due to the RVO depends on the presence of macular edema and the extent of the area with vascular nonperfusion (Figs. 8A to F). Both central retinal vein occlusion (CRVO) and branch retinal vein occlusion (BRVO) have been studied with OCTA. The features include FAZ enlargement in both SCP and DCP, capillary nonperfusion corresponding to the area involved, microvascular abnormalities, vascular congestion, telangiectasia, collateral formation, and neovascularization.[40,41]

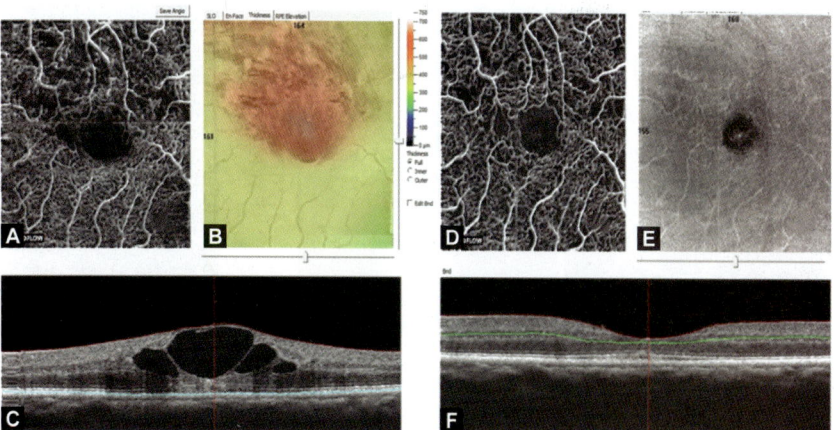

Figs. 8A to F: (A) OCTA (OptoVue RTVue XR AVANTI Inc, Fremont, CA) superficial layer; (B) en face OCT; (C) corresponding OCT B scan in a case of branched retinal vein occlusion with macular edema; (D) Resolution of macular edema post anti-VEGF; (E) OCTA superficial layer E en face OCT; (F) corresponding OCT B scan.
(OCTA: optical coherence tomography angiography; VEGF: vascular endothelial growth factor)

Optical coherence tomography angiography has demonstrated a similar or superior ability to FA in detecting vascular changes, particularly using 3 × 3 mm scans. However, the narrower field limits precludes its use as a modality for detecting peripheral ischemia, an important parameter in course of RVO.[42,43]

Compared to FA, OCTA has shown a superior capability of delineating and measuring FAZ diameter. FAZ diameter is always increased, both in SVP and DCP, in eyes with vein occlusion. However, FAZ diameter in DCP has been documented to be larger than FAZ diameter in SVP.[41,44] OCTA parameters that correlate with peripheral ischemia include disruption of the perifoveal capillary arcade in SVP, capillary network disruption in DCP, and deep capillary bed nonperfusion (Figs. 9A to C).[45]

The DCP of retina appears to be the most affected vascular network in RVO. OCTA, with its ability to study each vascular bed separately, offers an opportunity to detect changes in each bed individually.

Retinal Artery Occlusion

A limited number of case reports and smaller studies have described the features of retinal artery occlusion, using OCTA. A good agreement between FA and OCTA has been shown. OCTA may show reduced flow in the area next to arterial embolus. More marked capillary ischemia is noted in SVP than the adjacent DCP.[46]

Optical coherence tomography angiography of patients with central retinal artery occlusion (CRAO) and branched retinal artery occlusion (BRAO) have demonstrated a severe capillary nonperfusion in both superficial and deep plexuses in areas that show delayed filling on FA (Figs. 10A to I). Distinct differences in the distribution of zones of decreased vascular perfusion

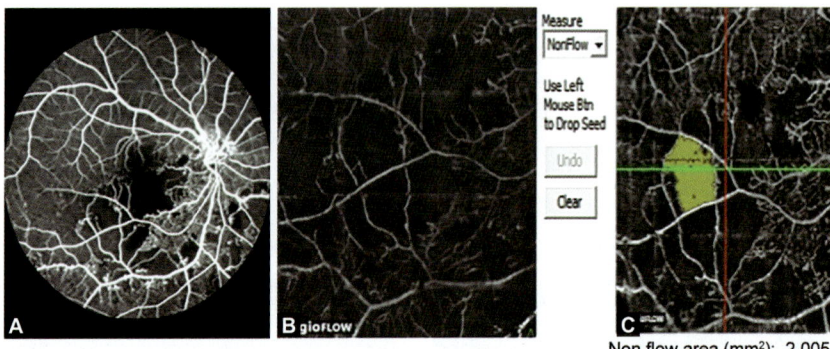

Non flow area (mm²): 2.005

Figs. 9A to C: (A) FA in a case of inferotemporal BRVO demonstrating capillary nonperfusion areas; (B) OCTA demonstaring capillary nonperfusion areas that correlate well with FA; (C) Use of AngioAnalytics to quantify nonperfusion areas.

(BRVO: branch retinal vein occlusion; FA: fluorescein angiography; OCTA: optical coherence tomography angiography)

between the superficial and deep retinal capillary plexus corresponding to areas of delayed dye perfusion on FA have been demonstrated.[47] In acute phases, both CRAO and BRAO may show an equivalent perfusion defect in both superficial and deep plexus. However, in chronic phases, reorganization of vascular interconnections may contribute to the substantial restoration of DCP flow.[46,48]

Macular Telangiectasia Type 2

MacTel type 2 is a bilateral disease characterized by changes in the capillary network and neurosensory atrophy. Slit lamp biomicroscopy reveals reduced retinal transparency, crystalline deposits, ectatic capillaries, and blunted venules. Complications of this disorder include proliferation of pigment plaques, photoreceptor loss, foveal atrophy, and retinal neovascularization that may result in visual loss.[49] FA has remained a mainstay for the diagnosis of MacTel 2.[50]

Several authors have described OCTA findings of MacTel 2, showing a great concordance between FA and OCTA in the detection of associated vascular changes (Figs. 11 to 13).[51-53]

Superficial layer: Stages 1-3 show enlargement of the FAZ, beginning temporally with a progressive horizontal increase in the FAZ diameter in the later stages. An increase in the intervascular space with progressive capillary rarefaction has been shown. These changes are accompanied by abnormal anastomoses between the capillary networks of the superficial and deeper layers. The finer vascular anastomoses could be appreciated as discrete bunches at multiple areas, more in the temporal aspect of the macula. The changes in larger blood vessels are more pronounced in the later stages with an abrupt ending and posterior dipping which can be traced into the deeper layers with adjustment of segmentation. Stages 4 and 5 demonstrate a gross decrease in retinal thickness and extensive empty spaces showing prominent larger blood vessels with radiating branches and widespread dark gray empty areas.

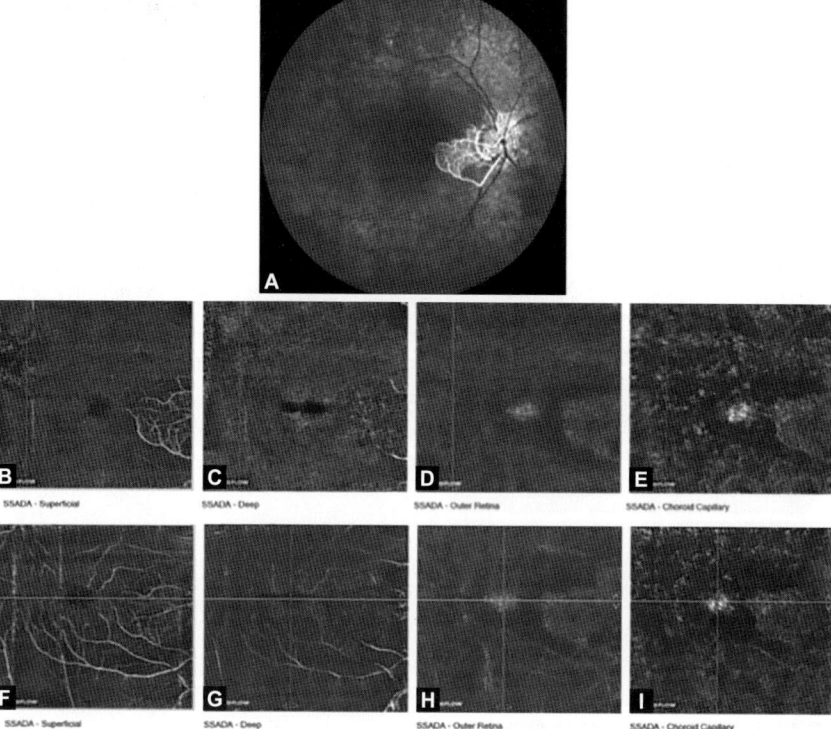

Figs. 10A to I: (A) FFA at 20 seconds showing filling of the cilioretinal artery with retrograde flow into the veins. The area perfused by the cilioretinal artery does not involve the fovea. OCTA [OptoVue RTVue XR AVANTI Inc, Fremont, CA (SSADA algorithm)] done pre and immediately postparacentesis. OCTA done before paracentesis (B to E) showing no perfusion in the superficial plexus; (B) except a localized area supplied by the cilioretinal artery that is perfused; deep plexus; (C) shows disruption in the vascular areas with coarse texture and the outer retina; (D) is not affected. An altered area on choroidal level; (E) can be noticed which may be reduced back signals due to the retinal edema due to CRAO. The OCTA changes correspond very precisely to the early frames of FFA. The brighter areas on choroid capillary layer correspond to the better contrast of the fovea and perfused cilioretinal artery in comparison with the dark arc like area seen in outer retina and choroid as this dark area is the representation of the retinal edema due to CRAO itself. OCTA done postparacentesis. (F to I) reveals increased perfusion of the retinal vasculature in both superficial and deep layers. The superficial layer. (F) shows reperfusion quite clearly with an established centripetal pattern. The deep layer (G and H) shows artifacts of the vessels of superficial plexus. The choroidal layer (I) shows no alteration.
(CRAO: central retinal artery occlusion; FFA: fundus fluorescein angiography; OCTA: optical coherence tomography angiography; SSADA: split-spectrum amplitude-decorrelation)

Deep layer: The deeper layer showed similar changes as in the superficial layer with few pathognomonic alterations. The deeper layer demonstrated changes earlier than the superficial layer in the initial stages. The normal close-knit ring of perifoveal capillaries decreases in density, appears more pronounced and brighter. There is a patchy loss of the network temporally to begin with and progressive loss of the entire ring leading to an increase in

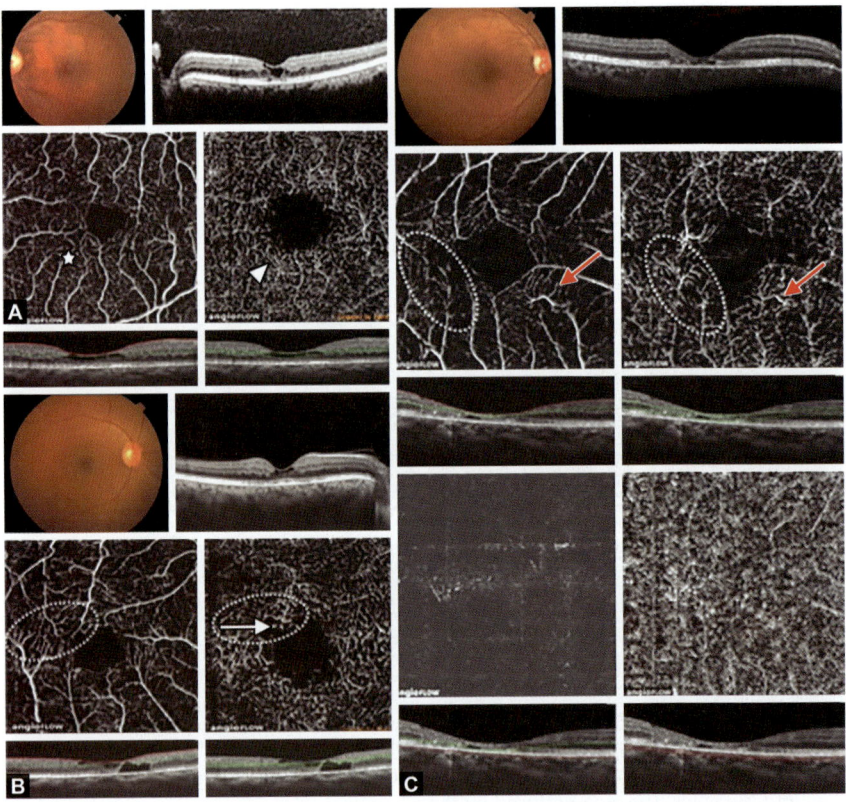

Figs. 11A to C: (A) Stage1: Color fundus photo showing dull foveal reflex and optical coherence tomography (OCT) reveals intraretinal hyporeflective spaces with changes in photoreceptor layer. OCTA-macular telangiectasia type 2 (MacTel2) showing mild irregularity of the foveal avascular zone (FAZ) and minimally increased intervascular spaces more in the superficial plexus (★) and broken regular network of FAZ with broken twig like capillaries at deep plexus (arrowhead); (B) Stage 2: Color fundus photo showing altered fovea with slight graying of perifoveal area with OCT showing intraretinal hyporeflective spaces and internal limiting membrane drape at the fovea. On OCTA, besides stage 1 changes, there is progressive temporal enlargement and capillary rarefaction of FAZ in superficial layers (dotted circled area). Deep layer shows decrease in perifoveal capillary density but more pronounced and brighter capillary twigs, lost FAZ ring (dotted circle) and few aneurysmal dilatations (arrow). Outer retina and choroid are uninvolved; (C) Stage 3: Color fundus image showing vascular telangiectasia with graying of perifoveal retina. OCT shows decreased central foveal thickness, intraretinal hyporeflective spaces and photoreceptor loss. OCTA shows gross segmental loss of perifoveal capillary network, more temporally in both superficial and deep layers with increase in the FAZ and also noticeable distortion, more in the deeper plexus (dotted circled area). The right-angled vessel dipping can be appreciated and traced from superficial to deep plexus (red arrows). Outer retina and choroid is uninvolved.

the FAZ diameter in the later stages. Brush-like branching pattern of smaller vessels secondary to capillary barring can be seen. Prominent larger vessel segments with blunt ends suggestive of vessel dipping and gross capillary rarefaction can be appreciated.

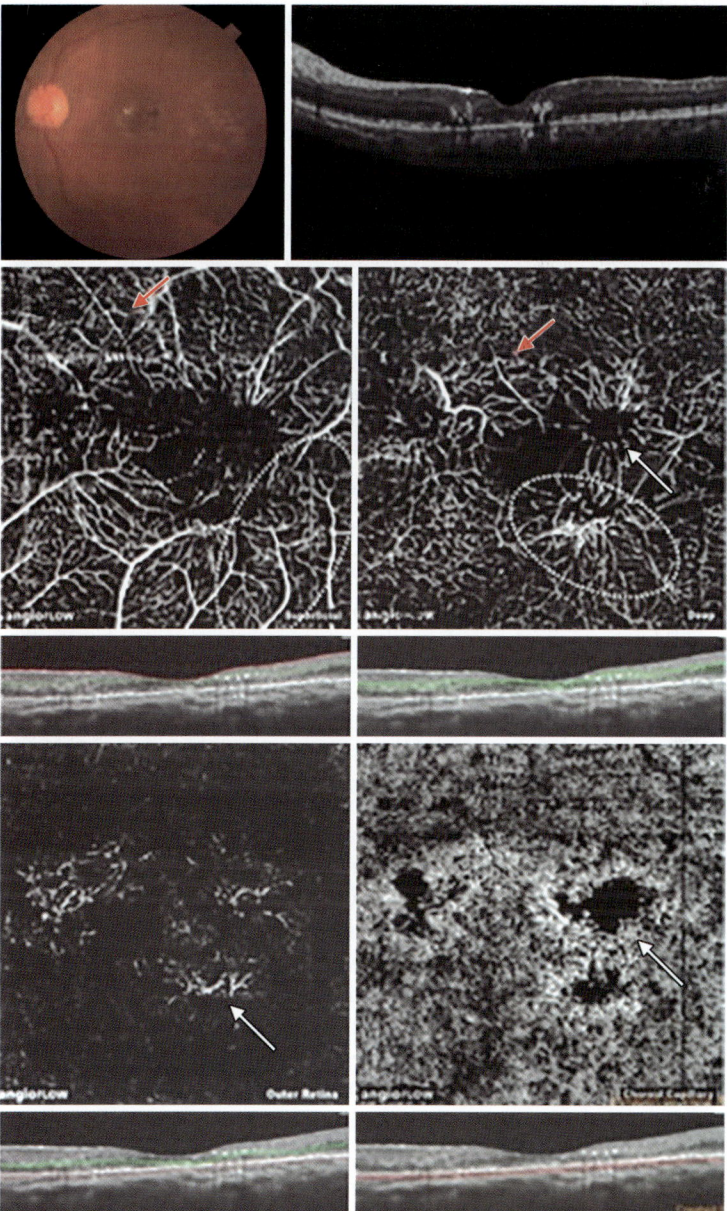

Fig. 12: MacTel Stage 4: Color fundus photo showing pigment clumps and retinal pigment epithelium (RPE) alteration at macula. Optical coherence tomography (OCT) shows intraretinal hyper-reflectivity with backscattering and disruption of photoreceptor layer with variable retinal thinning. OCTA shows increased foveal avascular zone diameter and intervascular spaces, more horizontally with complete loss of perifoveal regular capillary meshwork in the superficial and deep layers with prominent larger vessels. A brush-like localized branching of vessels (dotted circles) with right-angled dipping can be seen around darker areas (arrows) suggestive of RPE hyperplasia. Outer retina reveals blood vessels corresponding to areas around RPE hyperplasia (arrows). Choroid reveals dark areas surrounded by gross alteration of texture surrounding it. Red arrows depict the anastomosis between the superficial and deep layers.

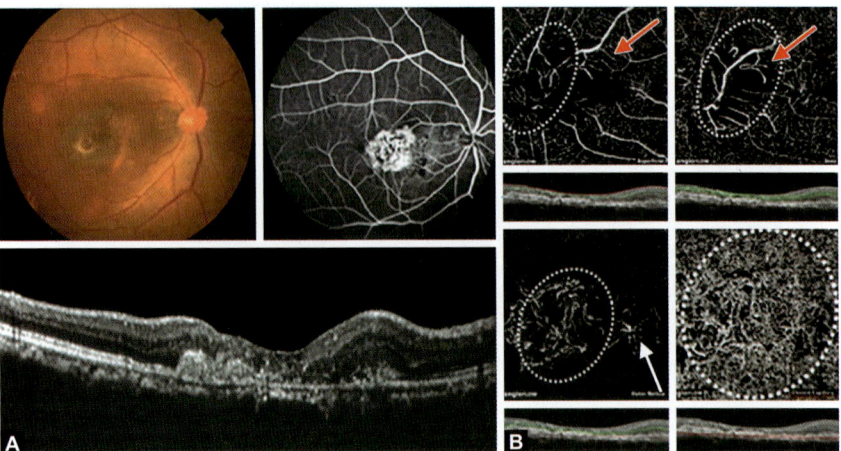

Figs. 13A and B: (A) MacTel Stage 5: A predominantly scarred neovascular membrane due to macular telangiectasia type 2 as seen on color fundus photo, mid-phase frame of fluorescein angiography and optical coherence tomography scan; (B) Superficial and deep layers show complete distortion of foveal avascular zone, gross capillary rarefaction and dilated vessels that can be traced through different layers with abnormal anastomosis (dotted circles). Outer retina shows dense vascular network corresponding to the area of the scar (dotted circles) with an additional area of network of vessels (white arrow) not corresponding to other layers suggestive of extensive areas of involvement. Choroid shows gross alterations in the texture with porous/spongy appearance, larger blood vessels with interspersed finer vessels in the area of the scar (larger dotted circle). Red arrows depict the anastomotic vessels between the superficial and deep network.

Outer retina: In the initial stages, it remains dark if the architecture is grossly maintained. A prominent vascular network with larger vessels that can be traced back to the superficial and deeper networks with a few bright and dark areas suggestive of scarring and RPE hyperplasia are seen in the later stages. The vascular network of the CNVM and the scarring stage with a dramatic and exemplary network of larger and smaller blood vessels across different quadrants can be seen. The vessels seen in these stages in the outer retina are not always well delineated as in the superficial and deeper networks, suggesting a wider area of involvement than expected

Choroid layer: The later stages with RPE hyperplasia and CNVM scarring show bright areas with altered choroidal architecture that are porous with a sponge-like or coral-like appearance with prominent larger vessels that seem embedded in the substance of choroid with a network of interspersed finer vessels corresponding to the area of the scar and the changes seen in the other layers

Dry Age-related Macular Degeneration

Dry age-related macular degeneration (AMD) is a disease affecting retina of elderly population characterized by drusen, pigmentary abnormalities, and photoreceptor/RPE damage leading to geographic atrophy (GA) and irreversible visual loss.[54]

Optical coherence tomography angiography shows a reduced vascular density in both retinal vascular plexuses among AMD patients. An altered blood flow in SVP, DCP, and CC is seen in early as well as later stages of AMD. In addition, the CC flow appears severely reduced in GA areas.[55,56]

Wet Age-related Macular Degeneration

Wet AMD is typically characterized by the presence of CNV, pigment epithelial detachment (PED), subretinal hemorrhages, and RPE tears; all leading to the irreversible visual loss from disciform scarring of the macula.[54]

Depending on the origin and anatomical relationship involved, CNV has been classified as type I, type II, and type III.

Type I or occult CNV is limited to sub-RPE space and is less distinct on FA. Type II CNV or classic CNV has proliferated through breaks in RPE into the subretinal space and grows in subretinal space. The third type, CNV III, also termed as retinal angiomatous proliferation (RAP) is the intraretinal type and characterized by intraretinal hemorrhages, exudation, and edema.

Type I Choroidal Neovascularization

Unlike FA and ICGA, type I CNV may take different distinctive appearances within CC slab on OCTA; as a highly organized complex of pruned vascular tree or tangled network or vascular loop. Often a central feeder vessel is seen with neovascular tree radiating centrifugally in a medusa pattern or branching in a sea-fan pattern. A hyporeflective halo surrounding the CNV has been also been described.[15,57] This halo might just be a shadow artifact from the RPE, or compression of CC or flow void area or a combination of all the above (Figs. 14A and B). Additionally type I CNV lesion tend to appear smaller on OCTA when compared to ICGA.[57] While OCTA can detect Type 1 CNV with similar sensitivity as ICG or OCT, combining imaging modalities may further improve sensitivity.[58]

Type II Choroidal Neovascularization

Type 2 lesions detected by OCTA present as a hyperflow lesion in the outer retina, with a glomerulus or medusa shape, surrounded by a dark halo. The superficial layer and the deep retina show no abnormal flow.[59] OCTA has also been used to document response of a mixed type I-II CNV to intravitreal vascular endothelial growth factor (VEGF) trap therapy. Although FA remains the gold standard for determining the presence of leakage and OCT easily shows fluid accumulation and its variations, OCTA offers noninvasive monitoring of the retinal and choriocapillaris microvasculature in patients with CNV, aiding in diagnosis and treatment decisions.

Type III Choroidal Neovascularization

Type III CNV, also known as RAP is considered as an AMD variant that may be sometimes difficult to distinguish from classic CNV. The sensitivity of OCTA in detecting type III CNV has been reported to range from 34% to 100%.[60] On OCTA, type III CNV appears as a neovascular complex in outer retinal segmentation as a tuft of bright, small, curvilinear vessels communicating

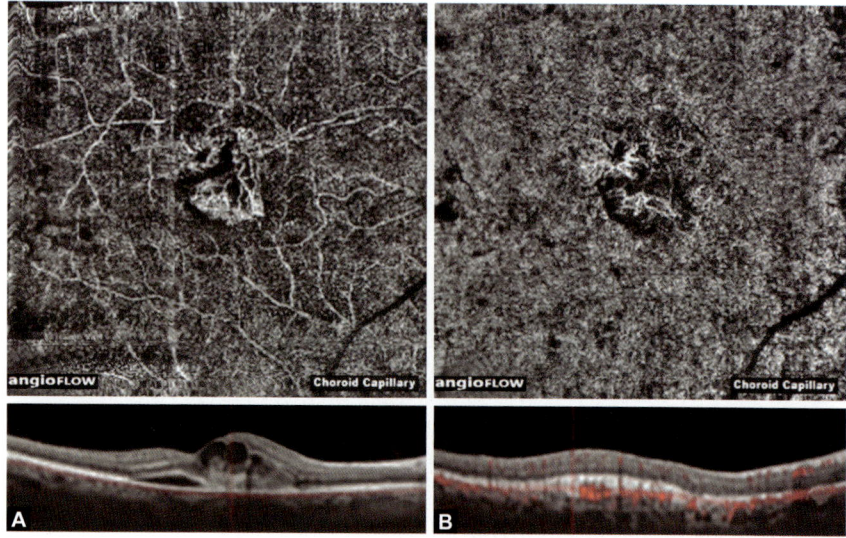

Figs. 14A and B: (A) OCTA images of the CC layer showing a well-defined network of fine vessels suggestive of CNVM complex. A hyporeflective halo surrounding the CNVM can also be made out; (B) OCTA image of the same eye 2 weeks postintravitreal anti-VEGF treatment showing decrease in the size of the CVVM complex.

(CC: choriocapillaris; CNVM: choroidal neovascular membrane; OCTA: optical coherence tomography angiography; VEGF: vascular endothelial growth factor)

with DCP through a feeder vessel. Often, a small clew-like lesion has been described in CC segmentation.[12]

Polypoidal Choroidal Vasculopathy

Polypoidal choroidal vasculopathy (PCV) is a disease entity characterized by multiple, bilateral, recurrent, serous, and serosanguineous RPE detachments in association with multiple polypoidal vascular abnormalities and branching vascular network (BVN) in the choroidal vasculature.

On OCTA, BVN is revealed as a hyperflow lesion in CC segmentation with better details, compared to ICGA (Fig. 15). Polyps have been described as hyperflow round lesions with surrounding dark halo in some cases and as hypoflow round structure in most of the cases. The BVN takes either a medusa or sea fan of tangled vascular pattern; while polypoidal lesions appear as nodular, ring or clustered configurations. In addition, the visibility/detection of polypoidal lesions can be improved by studying the outer retinal segmentation along with CC slab.[61] Though, OCTA can display BVN more clearly, it cannot detect polypoidal lesions with a sensitivity comparable to ICGA possibly due to low flood flow in some polyps.[61]

Central Serous Chorioretinopathy

Central serous chorioretinopathy (CSCR) is characterized by serous neurosensory macular separation and subretinal fluid (SRF) accumulation.

In acute stages of CSCR, SVP, deep capillary network, and outer retina show normal flow characteristics on OCTA. However, CC has been documented to

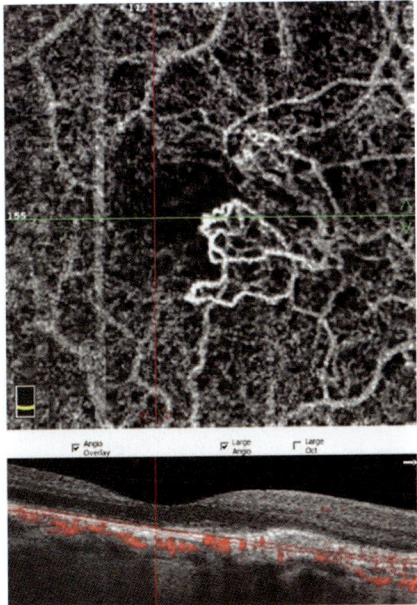

Fig. 15: OCTA demonstrating branched vascular network (BVN) as a hyperflow lesion in CC segmentation.
(CC: choriocapillaris; OCTA: optical coherence tomography angiography)

show altered texture and display dark areas and spots corresponding to flow reduction or shadowing from SRF or both.[62] CC slab may show dark areas, dark spots, and abnormal choroidal vessels. The dark areas correspond to diffuse or focal, foggy, ill-defined, and low-detectable flow areas. Abnormal choroidal vessels correspond to distinct, well-delineated, high-flow, tangled pattern areas in the choriocapillaries layer as well as an abnormal dilation of choroidal vessels (Fig. 16).

In chronic and long-standing course, CSRC may complicate by the development of CNV, persistent SRF and RPE alterations. SVP and DCP have been documented normal in all studies of CSCR. Conversely, abnormal flow signals in outer retinal slab, altered CC texture and higher flow signals may be seen in the chronic disease.[62-64] Signs consistent with CNV include abnormal flow in the avascular outer retinal slab, altered CC texture, and abnormal vasculature in CC. OCTA, in a number of studies, has demonstrated a great concordance to FA and ICGA in detecting CNV.[63] In all reported studies and cases, OCTA successfully detected CNV associated with CSCR in all cases.[18,62]

Optical coherence tomography angiography has been shown to be a useful imaging modality for the evaluation of several retinal diseases. In the future, newer algorithms are developed and as scanning speeds become faster, larger fields of view with higher resolution are bound to become available to the clinician. Thus, OCTA is poised to become an invaluable tool in imaging the retina.

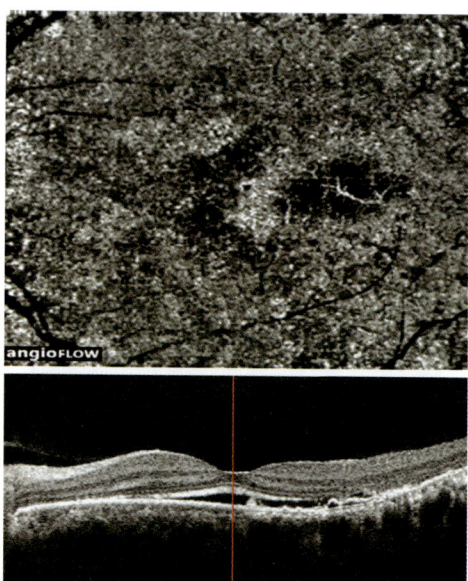

Fig. 16: A case of central serous chorioretinopathy showing a characteristic altered texture in the area involved. The PED seen as a dark well-circumscribed area on the choroidal level of the OCTA.

(PED: pigment epithelial detachment; OCTA: optical coherence tomography angiography)

REFERENCES

1. de Carlo TE, Romano A, Waheed NK, et al. A review of optical coherence tomography angiography (OCTA). Int J Retin Vitr. 2015;1(1):5.
2. Matsunaga D, Yi J, Puliafito CA, et al. OCT angiography in healthy human subjects. Ophthalmic Surg Lasers Imaging Retina. 2014;45(6):510-15.
3. Zhang A, Zhang Q, Chen C-L, et al. Methods and algorithms for optical coherence tomography-based angiography: a review and comparison. J Biomed Opt. 2015;20(10):100901.
4. Leitgeb R, Schmetterer L, Drexler W, et al. Real-time assessment of retinal blood flow with ultrafast acquisition by color Doppler Fourier domain optical coherence tomography. Opt Express. 2003;11(23):3116-21.
5. White B, Pierce M, Nassif N, et al. In vivo dynamic human retinal blood flow imaging using ultra-high-speed spectral domain optical coherence tomography. Opt Express. 2003;11(25):3490-7.
6. Fingler J, Zawadzki RJ, Werner JS, et al. Volumetric microvascular imaging of human retina using optical coherence tomography with a novel motion contrast technique. Opt Express. 2009;17(24):22190-200.
7. Schmitt JM, Xiang SH, Yung KM. Speckle in optical coherence tomography. J Biomed Opt. 1999;4(1):95.
8. Khan HA, Mehmood A, Khan QA, et al. A major review of optical coherence tomography angiography. Expert Rev Ophthalmol. 2017;12(5):373-85.
9. Jia Y, Tan O, Tokayer J, et al. Split-spectrum amplitude-decorrelation angiography with optical coherence tomography. Opt Express. 2012;20(4):4710.
10. Gao SS, Liu G, Huang D, et al. Optimization of the split-spectrum amplitude-decorrelation angiography algorithm on a spectral optical coherence tomography system. Opt Lett. 2015;40(10):2305.

11. Zhi Z, Qin W, Wang J, et al. 4D optical coherence tomography-based microangiography achieved by 16-MHz FDML swept source. Opt Lett. 2015;40(8):1779.
12. Miere A, Querques G, Semoun O, et al. Optical coherence tomography angiography in early type 3 neovascularization. Retina. 2015;35(11):2236-41.
13. Liu G, Jia Y, Pechauer AD, et al. Split-spectrum phase-gradient optical coherence tomography angiography. Biomed Opt Express. 2016;7(8):2943-54.
14. Wang X, Jia Y, Spain R, et al. Optical coherence tomography angiography of optic nerve head and parafovea in multiple sclerosis. Br J Ophthalmol. 2014;98(10):1368-73.
15. Jia Y, Bailey ST, Wilson DJ, et al. Quantitative optical coherence tomography angiography of choroidal neovascularization in age-related macular degeneration. Ophthalmology. 2014;121(7):1435-44.
16. Pechauer AD, Jia Y, Liu L, et al. Optical coherence tomography angiography of peripapillary retinal blood flow response to hyperoxia. Invest Ophthalmol Vis Sci. 2015;56(5):3287-91.
17. Jain N, Jia Y, Gao SS, et al. Optical coherence tomography angiography in choroideremia: Correlating choriocapillaris loss with overlying degeneration. JAMA Ophthalmol. 2016;134(6):697-702.
18. McClintic SM, Jia Y, Huang D, et al. Optical coherence tomographic angiography of choroidal neovascularization associated with central serous chorioretinopathy. JAMA Ophthalmol. 2015;133(10):1212-14.
19. Huang D, Jia Y, Rispoli M, et al. Optical coherence tomography angiography of time course of choroidal neovascularization in response to anti-angiogenic treatment. Retina. 2015;35(11):2260-4.
20. Agemy SA, Scripsema NK, Shah CM, et al. Retinal vascular perfusion density mapping using optical coherence tomography angiography in normals and diabetic retinopathy patients. Retina. 2015;35(11):2353-63.
21. Rosenfeld PJ, Durbin MK, Roisman L, et al. ZEISS Angioplex™ spectral domain optical coherence tomography angiography: Technical aspects. Dev Ophthalmol. 2016;56:18-29.
22. de Carlo TE, Salz DA, Waheed NK, et al. Visualization of the retinal vasculature using wide-field montage optical coherence tomography angiography. Ophthalmic Surg Lasers Imaging Retina. 2015;46(6):611-6.
23. Huang D, Jia Y, Gao SS, et al. Optical coherence tomography angiography using the optovue device. Dev Ophthalmol. 2016;56:6-12.
24. Gao SS, Jia Y, Zhang M, et al. Optical coherence tomography angiography. Invest Ophthalmol Vis Sci. 2016;57(9):27-36.
25. Choi WJ, Mohler KJ, Potsaid B, et al. Choriocapillaris and choroidal microvasculature imaging with ultrahigh speed OCT angiography. PLoS One. 2013;8(12):e81499.
26. Kraus MF, Potsaid B, Mayer MA, et al. Motion correction in optical coherence tomography volumes on a per A-scan basis using orthogonal scan patterns. Biomed Opt Express. 2012;3(6):1182.
27. Spaide RF, Fujimoto JG, Waheed NK. Image artifacts in optical coherence tomography angiography. Retina. 2015;35(11):2163-80.
28. Takusagawa HL, Liu L, Ma KN, et al. Projection-resolved optical coherence tomography angiography of macular retinal circulation in glaucoma. Ophthalmology. 2017;24:1589-99.
29. Bhavsar KV, Jia Y, Wang J, et al. Projection-resolved optical coherence tomography angiography exhibiting early flow prior to clinically observed retinal angiomatous proliferation. Am J Ophthalmol Case Rep. 2017;8:53-57.

30. Seknazi D, Coscas F, Sellam A, et al. Optical coherence tomography angiography in retinal vein occlusion: Correlations between macular vascular density, visual acuity, and peripheral nonperfusion area on fluorescein angiography. Retina. 2018:38:1562-70.
31. Matsunaga DR, Yi JJ, De Koo LO, et al. Optical coherence tomography angiography of diabetic retinopathy in human subjects. Ophthalmic Surg Lasers Imaging Retina. 2015;46(8):796-805.
32. Lee J, Rosen R. Optical coherence tomography angiography in diabetes. Curr Diab Rep. 2016;16(12):123.
33. Ishibazawa A, Nagaoka T, Takahashi A, et al. Optical coherence tomography angiography in diabetic retinopathy: A prospective pilot study. Am J Ophthalmol. 2015;160(1):35-44.
34. Lee H, Lee M, Chung H, et al. Quantification of retinal vessel tortuosity in diabetic retinopathy using optical coherence tomography angiography. Retina. 2018;38(5):976-85.
35. Hwang TS, Jia Y, Gao SS, et al. Optical coherence tomography angiography features of diabetic retinopathy. Retina. 2015;35(11):2371-6.
36. De Carlo TE, Chin AT, Bonini Filho MA, et al. Detection of microvascular changes in eyes of patients with diabetes but not clinical diabetic retinopathy using optical coherence tomography angiography. Retina. 2015;35(11):2364-70.
37. Bhanushali D, Anegondi N, Gadde SGK, et al. Linking retinal microvasculature features with severity of diabetic retinopathy using optical coherence tomography angiography. Invest Ophthalmol Vis Sci. 2016;57(9):519-25.
38. Choi W, Waheed NK, Moult EM, et al. Ultrahigh speed swept source optical coherence tomography angiography of retinal and choriocapillaris alterations in diabetic patients with and without retinopathy. Retina. 2017;37(1):11-21.
39. Ishibazawa A, Nagaoka T, Yokota H, et al. Characteristics of retinal neovascularization in proliferative diabetic retinopathy imaged by optical coherence tomography angiography. Invest Ophthalmol Vis Sci. 2016;57(14):6247.
40. Rispoli M, Savastano MC, Lumbroso B. Capillary network anomalies in branch retinal vein occlusion on optical coherence tomography angiography. Retina. 2015;35(11):2332-8.
41. Adhi M, Bonini Filho MA, Louzada RN, et al. Retinal capillary network and foveal avascular zone in eyes with vein occlusion and fellow eyes analyzed with optical coherence tomography angiography. Invest Ophthalmol Vis Sci. 2016;57(9):486-94.
42. Suzuki N, Hirano Y, Yoshida M, et al. Microvascular abnormalities on optical coherence tomography angiography in macular edema associated with branch retinal vein occlusion. Am J Ophthalmol. 2016;161:126-32e1.
43. Nobre Cardoso J, Keane PA, Sim DA, et al. Systematic evaluation of optical coherence tomography angiography in retinal vein occlusion. Am J Ophthalmol. 2016;163:93-107e6.
44. De Salles MC, Kvanta A, Amrén U, et al. Optical coherence tomography angiography in central retinal vein occlusion: Correlation between the foveal avascular zone and visual acuity. Invest Ophthalmol Vis Sci. 2016;57(9):242-6.
45. Coscas F, Glacet-Bernard A, Miere A, et al. Optical coherence tomography angiography in retinal vein occlusion: Evaluation of superficial and deep capillary plexa. Am J Ophthalmol. 2016;161:160-71e2.
46. De Castro-Abeger AH, De Carlo TE, Duker JS, et al. Optical coherence tomography angiography compared to fluorescein angiography in branch retinal artery occlusion. Ophthalmic Surg Lasers Imaging Retina. 2015;46(10):1052-4.

47. Bonini Filho MA, Adhi M, de Carlo TE, et al. Optical coherence tomography angiography in retinal artery occlusion. Retina. 2015;35(11):2339-46.
48. Lee AY, Zhang Q, Baughman DM, et al. Evaluation of bilateral central retinal artery occlusions with optical coherence tomography-based microangiography: A case report. J Med Case Rep. 2016;10(1):1-6.
49. Wolff B, Basdekidou C, Vasseur V, et al. "En face" optical coherence tomography imaging in type 2 idiopathic macular telangiectasia. Retina. 2014;34(10):2072-8.
50. Barthelmes D, Gillies MC, Sutter FKP. Quantitative OCT analysis of idiopathic perifoveal telangiectasia. Invest Ophthalmol Vis Sci. 2008;49(5):2156-62.
51. Thorell MR, Zhang Q, Huang Y, et al. Swept-source OCT angiography of macular telangiectasia type 2. Ophthalmic Surg Lasers Imaging Retina. 2014;45(5):369-80.
52. Spaide RF, Klancnik JM, Cooney MJ. Retinal vascular layers in macular telangiectasia type 2 imaged by optical coherence tomographic angiography. JAMA Ophthalmol. 2015;133(1):66-73.
53. Chidambara L, Gadde SGK, Yadav NK, et al. Characteristics and quantification of vascular changes in macular telangiectasia type 2 on optical coherence tomography angiography. Br J Ophthalmol. 2016;100(11):1482-8.
54. Ratnapriya R, Chew EY. Age-related macular degeneration-clinical review and genetics update. Clin Genet. 2013;84(2):160-6.
55. Toto L, Borrelli E, Di Antonio L, et al. Retinal vascular plexuses' changes in dry age-related macular degeneration, evaluated by means of optical coherence tomography angiography. Retina. 2016;36(8):1566-72.
56. Moult EM, Waheed NK, Novais EA, et al. Swept-source optical coherence tomography angiography reveals choriocapillaris alterations in eyes with nascent geographic atrophy and drusen-associated geographic atrophy. Retina. 36;2016:S2-S11.
57. Costanzo E, Miere A, Querques G, et al. Type 1 choroidal neovascularization lesion size: Indocyanine green angiography versus optical coherence tomography angiography. Invest Opthalmology Vis Sci. 2016;57(9):307.
58. Inoue M, Jung JJ, Balaratnasingam C, et al. A comparison between optical coherence tomography angiography and fluorescein angiography for the imaging of type 1 neovascularization. Invest Ophthalmol Vis Sci. 2016;57(9):314-23.
59. El Ameen A, Cohen SY, Semoun O, et al. Type 2 neovascularization secondary to age-related macular degeneration imaged by optical coherence tomography angiography. Retina. 2015;35(11):2212-8.
60. Kuehlewein L, Dansingani KK, de Carlo TE, et al. Optical coherence tomography angiography of type 3 neovascularization secondary to age-related macular degeneration. Retina. 2015;35(11):2229-35.
61. Kim JY, Kwon OW, Oh HS, et al. Optical coherence tomography angiography in patients with polypoidal choroidal vasculopathy. Graefe's Arch Clin Exp Ophthalmol. 2016;254(8):1505-10.
62. Costanzo E, Cohen SY, Miere A, et al. Optical coherence tomography angiography in central serous chorioretinopathy. J Ophthalmol. 2015;2015:134783.
63. Quaranta-El Maftouhi M, El Maftouhi A, Eandi CM. Chronic central serous chorioretinopathy imaged by optical coherence tomographic angiography. Am J Ophthalmol. 2015;160(3):581-7.e1.
64. de Carlo TE, Rosenblatt A, Goldstein M, et al. Vascularization of irregular retinal pigment epithelial detachments in chronic central serous chorioretinopathy evaluated with OCT angiography. Ophthalmic Surg Lasers Imaging Retina. 2016;47(2):128-33.

CHAPTER 17

Optical Coherence Tomography in Diabetic Retinopathy

Manila Khatri, Sandeep Saxena

■ INTRODUCTION

Diabetic retinopathy (DR) is an important cause of blindness, which is preventable.[1] Prevalence of diabetes mellitus (DM) has increased from 108 million to 422 million between 1980 and 2014.[2] As per WHO, diabetes mellitus will be the seventh important reason of death in 2030.[3]

Diabetic retinopathy is primarily a microvascular complication occurring in type 2 DM.[4] The changes in the structure of retina correlate with the severity of disease.[5] According to recent studies, DM is basically characterized by chronic subclinical inflammatory process. Increasing evidence suggests that chronic and subclinical inflammation plays an important part in the pathogenesis of retinopathy.[6]

Spectral domain-optical coherence tomography (SD-OCT) is an important diagnostic imaging modality that has made a significant impact in the evaluation DR.[7] It is (a) noninvasive, (b) noncontact, (c) transpupillary interferometric technique that provides in-vivo imaging of retinal microstructures in real time. SD-OCT has an important role in assessing the status of macula, as the retinopathy progresses. SD-OCT is now an essential and significant diagnostic modality for assessment of diabetic macular edema (DME). Present chapter summarizes the role of OCT in diagnosis, evaluation and management of DR.

■ SPECTRAL DOMAIN-OPTICAL COHERENCE TOMOGRAPHY ANALYSIS IN DIABETIC RETINOPATHY

Analysis in Cross Section

Vitreomacular Interface Analysis

Spectral domain-optical coherence tomography provides considerable analysis at vitreomacular interface (VMI) and offers an understanding into the strategic management approaches for DME.

Based on SD-OCT, the International Vitreomacular Traction Study Group has developed anatomic classification system for the diseases of the vitreomacular interface.[8] Vitreomacular adhesion (VMA) is defined as separation of perifoveal vitreous, characterized with remaining vitreomacular attachment and undisturbed morphologic features of fovea. Vitreomacular traction (VMT) is defined as abnormal detachment of posterior vitreous, which is accompanied by foveal distortion, anatomically (Figs. 1A and B). Various previous studies, in DME, have indicated the role of tangential traction applied by the posterior hyaloid on the retinal surface.[9,10] Hence, based on SD-OCT findings, in a clinical situation, it can be decided whether surgical intervention is required in DME. An indication for surgical intervention is the presence of vitreoretinal traction in DME, which is unresponsive to treatment. Vitrectomy is helpful in the following ways:

- Traction relief
- Removal of premacular hyaloid growth factor reservoir
- Improvement of retinal transvitreal oxygenation.[11,12]

Disorganization of Retinal Inner Layers

In eyes with center-involved DME, SD-OCT parameter, disorganization of the retinal inner layers (DRIL) has developed as a significant predictor of visual acuity (VA) (Figs. 2A and B).

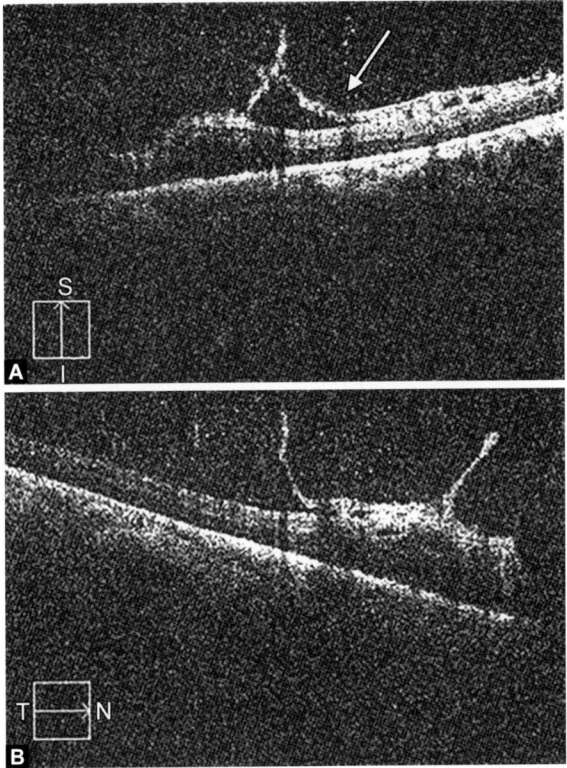

Figs. 1A and B: Spectral domain-optical coherence tomography (SD-OCT) shows vitreomacular traction (arrow).

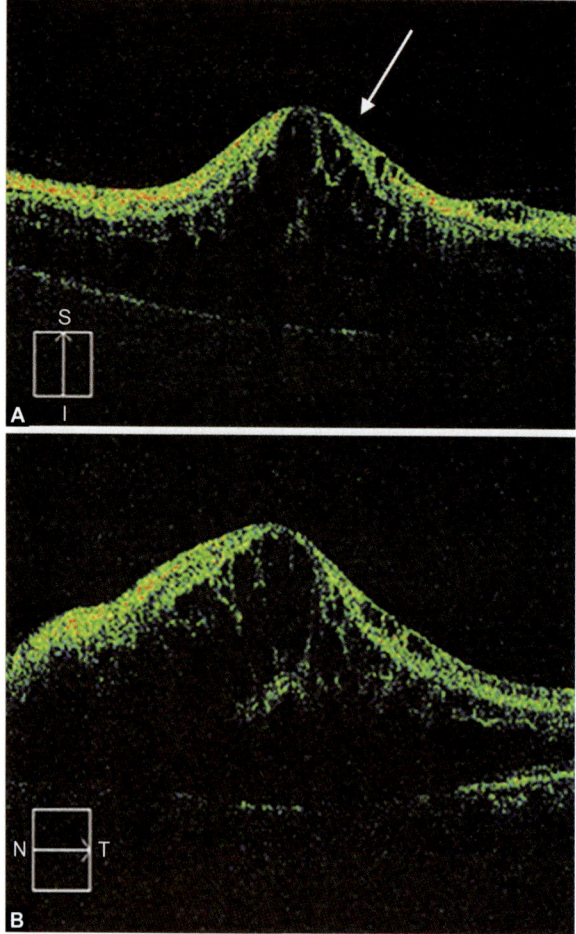

Figs. 2A and B: Spectral domain-optical coherence tomography (SD-OCT) showing disorganized retinal inner layers (arrow).

On the SD-OCT, the 1-mm-wide fovea-centered retinal area is assessed for the magnitude of DRIL. Sun et al. recognized that DRIL, in the 1-mm foveal area, is associated with decrease in VA. Occurrence of DRIL also predicts future change in VA. Early change in DRIL prospectively recognizes eyes with a high likelihood of resultant VA improvement or decline.[13]

Rodrigues et al. described early signs of neuroretinal changes in patients with early DR. They detected a significant thinning of different inner cell layers and central retina. Diabetic patients with no DR or mild DR were evaluated using four significant parameters: retinal nerve fiber layer (RNFL), ganglion cell layer (GCL) + inner plexiform layer (IPL), central subfoveal (CS) and retinal thickness (RT). Significant decline in RT was found in eyes with mild DR.[14]

Disruption of Outer Retinal Layers

On SD-OCT, the outer retina has been shown to have four discrete bands. The innermost, a linear convergence of junctional complexes between Müller cells and photoreceptors is the external limiting membrane (ELM).[15] The second hyper-reflective layer indicates the ellipsoid zone (EZ).[16,17] The third layer relates to the interdigitation zone between cone outer segment tips and apical processes of the retinal pigment epithelium (RPE). The outermost highly reflective zone signifies the RPE/Bruch's complex.[18] Clinical relevance to the subject can be attached with EZ and RPE.

A. *Ellipsoid zone*: Fernandez et al. used ultra-high resolution SD-OCT images of human foveal cone photoreceptors. They divided the inner segment of photoreceptors into ellipsoid and myoid segments.[19] Spaide and Curcio[18] established that the second band initially recognized as inner segment-outer segment junction (IS-OS) of photoreceptor was primarily the EZ of the photoreceptor. Statistically significant relationship between visual acuity and percentage of disruption of EZ was observed on multivariate analysis. This was based on cellular level resolution attained by OCT. Recently; significant correlation between macular thickness parameters and disruption of EZ has been acknowledged with increasing severity of diabetic retinopathy.[20]

Classification Systems for Ellipsoid Zone and External Limiting Membrane Disruption

Various classification systems have been developed to assess EZ and ELM disruption in DME. Significant impact on the visual prognosis has been observed with severity of disruption of these layers. An improved visual outcome can be predicted after anti-VEGF therapy or vitreoretinal surgery if the grade of disruption is improving. This observation is of clinical significance in prognosticating the visual outcome.

- Maheshwary et al. evaluated disruption of EZ of 500 microns in either direction of the fovea and graded EZ disruption from Grade 0–2:
  - *Grade 0:* Characterized with intact EZ.
  - *Grade 1:* Characterized with focal EZ disruption (200 microns or less in length).
  - *Grade 2:* Characterized with EZ disruption (greater than 200 microns in length).

  A statistically significant correlation between percentage disruption of the EZ and visual acuity was noted.[21]

- Sharma et al. put forward a simplified, all-inclusive and physician-friendly approach to grading EZ disruption (Figs. 3A to C):
  - *Grade 0:* Characterized with an intact EZ.
  - *Grade 1:* Characterized with focal disruption (localized, subfoveal EZ disruption).
  - *Grade 2:* Characterized with global disruption (generalized EZ disruption involving the whole of macular cube).

  Increase in the grade of subfoveal ELM and EZ disruption was found to be associated with increase in severity of diabetic retinopathy and a decrease in

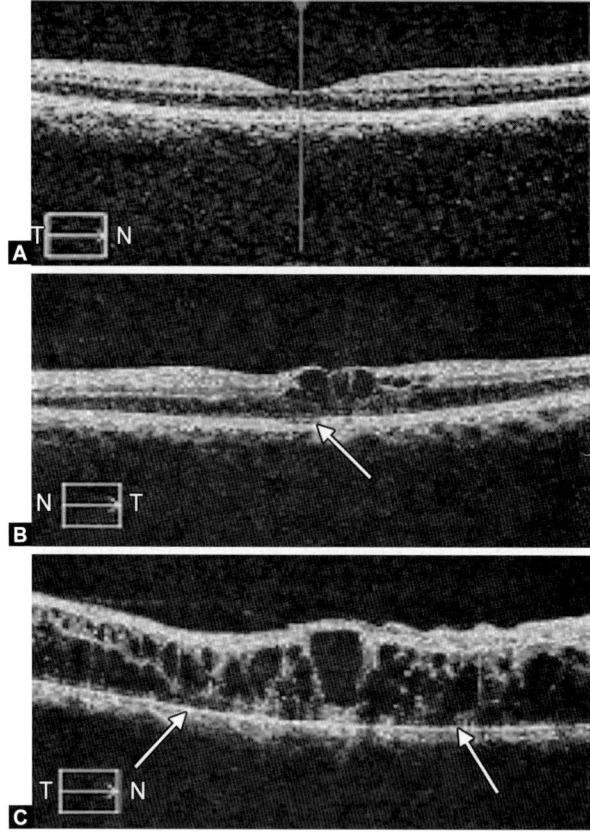

Figs. 3A to C: Spectral domain-optical coherence tomography (SD-OCT) macular cube shows ellipsoid zone (EZ). (A) Grade 0: intact EZ; (B) Grade 1: focal disruption (localized, subfoveal EZ disruption); (C) Grade 2: global disruption (generalized EZ disruption involving the whole of macular cube).

visual acuity. Also, "Global" EZ disruption was related with marked decrease in visual acuity as compared to "Focal" disruption.[22]

- Jain et al. graded disruption of ELM and EZ in patients with diabetic retinopathy and defined the mechanism of disruption of EZ too (Figs. 4A to C):
  - *Grade 0:* No disruption of ELM and EZ.
  - *Grade 1:* ELM disruption with an intact EZ.
  - *Grade 2:* Both ELM and EZ are disrupted.

  Decrease in VA and progression of diabetic retinopathy was found to be associated with increased grades of ELM and EZ disruption.[23]

- *Retinal pigment epithelium (RPE):* It plays a significant role in maintenance of a healthy retina. The RPE also constitutes the outer blood–retinal barrier (BRB). Vascular endothelial growth factor (VEGF) (an angiogenic factor) and PEDF (pigment epithelium derived factor; an antiangiogenic factor) are secreted by RPE. In diabetes mellitus, there is increase in advanced

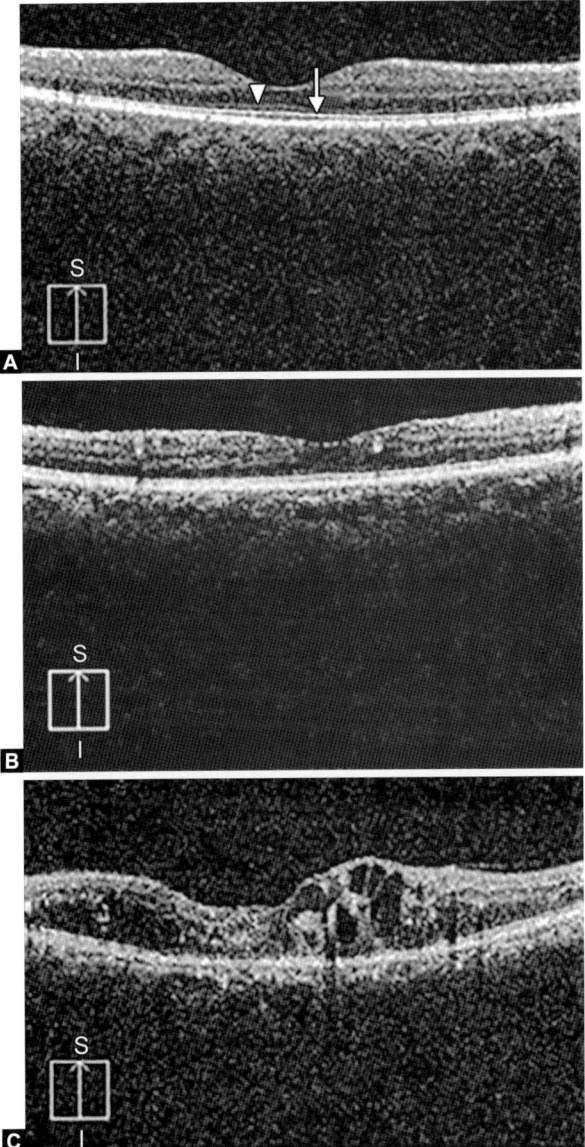

Figs. 4A to C: Spectral domain-optical coherence tomography (SD-OCT) macular cube showing grades of disruption of external limiting membrane (ELM) (arrow head) and ellipsoid zone (EZ) (arrow). (A) Grade 0: No disruption of ELM and EZ; (B) Grade 1: ELM disruption with an intact EZ; (C) Grade 2: Both ELM and EZ are disrupted.

glycation end-products (AGEs). These act on RPE and endothelial pericytes resulting in VEGF expression.[24,25] The consequential increased expression of VEGF leads to breakdown of outer BRB.[26] It has been found that there is decreased expression of PEDF due to elevated concentration of glucose. Thus, balance between VEGF and PEDF expression by RPE is crucial for the advancement of disease. VEGF secreted by RPE is important for the maintenance of the structural integrity of the outer retina as well as choriocapillaris.[27,28]

Topographic alterations in RPE can be evaluated by single layer retinal pigment epithelial (SL-RPE) map. Sharma et al. graded alteration of this layer[29] (Figs. 5A to C).

- *Grade 0:* Characterized by no RPE alteration.
- *Grade 1:* Characterized focal (alteration predominantly in up to two quadrants of the map).
- *Grade 2:* Characterized by global (alteration in more than two quadrants of the map).

Increase in the topographic alterations of RPE has been found to be correlated with increased severity of diabetic retinopathy and decrease in visual acuity.

SD-OCT-based Morphological Classification of Diabetic Macular Edema

Diabetic macular edema (DME) has been classified on the basis of following parameters: presence of retinal thickening, hard exudates, location with relation to the fovea, quantitative analysis of accumulation of fluid, morphological patterns of accumulation of fluid, changes in vitreomacular interface, and alterations in the microstructure of the retina.

In 1999, based on time domain OCT (TD-OCT), a classification for DME was proposed by Otani et al. This classification system was based on the retinal morphological changes (Table 1).[30]

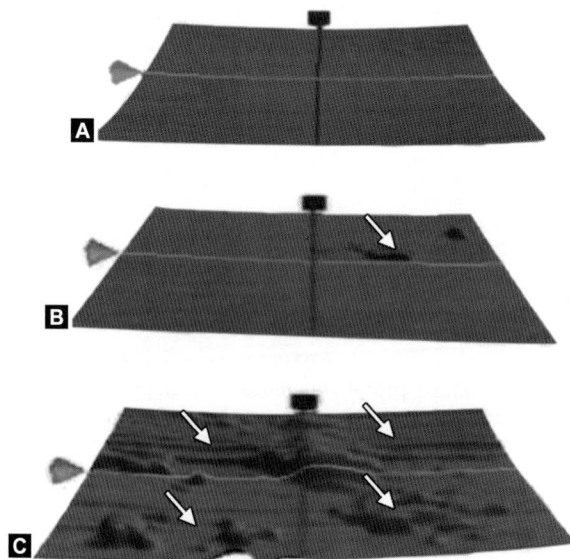

Figs. 5A to C: Spectral domain-optical coherence tomography (SD-OCT) macular cube shows grades of retinal pigment epithelium (RPE) alterations. (A) Grade 0: no RPE alteration; (B) Grade 1: focal (alterations predominantly in up to two quadrants of the map); (C) Grade 2: Global (alterations in more than two quadrants of the map).

Table 1: Optical coherence tomography (OCT)-based morphological classification of diabetic macular edema (DME) by Otani et al.

Type 1 (sponge-like swelling)	Thickening of the fovea, which is associated with homogeneous optical reflectivity
Type 2 (cystoid macular edema)	Thickening of the fovea, which is associated with markedly decreased optical reflectivity in outer layers
Type 3 (serous retinal detachment)	Thickening of the fovea, which is associated with subfoveal fluid accumulation and distinct outer border of detached neurosensory retina
Type 3A	Present without vitreofoveal traction
Type 3B	Present with apparent vitreofoveal traction

This simple classification helps in the assessment of the severity of DME and has prognostic implications.

Enface Optical Coherence Tomography

Spectral domain-optical coherence tomography imaging visualizes the retinal tissue in axial cross-sections. It also documents quantitative assessment of central submacular thickness, which correlates with visual acuity. This is useful in clinical management for DME.[31-39] However, these cross-sectional images do not allow for visualization of the full spatial extent of irregular or large pathologies at different retinal layers. Also, quantification of correlations between inner and outer retinal layer pathologies is also lacking. Recently developed image segmentation algorithms permit depth-resolved enface SD-OCT imaging. This imaging technique helps in viewing the retinal layers in the coronal plane. These enface SD-OCT "C-scans" have unique benefit of permitting quantifiable evaluation of individual retinal layers separated in depth. Several manual and semi-automated techniques have been evolved for evaluation of the retinal layers. This is aimed at improving the prognostic capability of SD-OCT imaging.[40-46]

Enface Thickness Maps and Reflectance Images

Segmentation of the retinal interfaces in the SD-OCT B-scans helps in the generation of enface thickness maps and reflectance images (Figs. 6A and B). Depth separation between the vitreous and internal limiting membrane (ILM) and retinal pigment epithelium (RPE) and choroid interfaces is contemplated as the total retinal (TR) thickness.

Advantages of Enface Optical Coherence Tomography
1. It allows uncovering of subtle retinal pathology that may be situated between standard OCT B-scans.
2. It allows visualization of the spatial extent of pathologies in different retinal layers. Thus, there is accurate monitoring of pathological changes over a period.
3. It allows study of change in choroidal thickness, which has been associated with severity of DR.

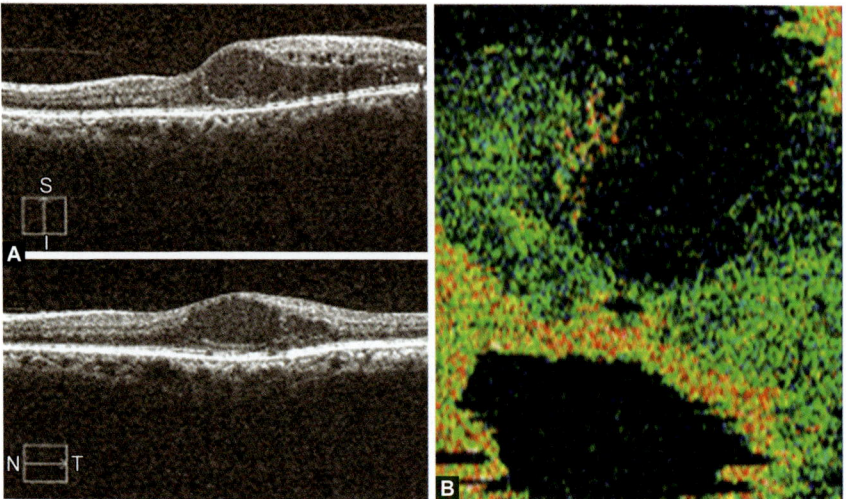

Figs. 6A and B: Enface optical coherence tomography (OCT): Cystic spaces observed on cross section (A) are visualized elegantly on enface view (B).

Three-dimensional SD-OCT

The 3D SD-OCT software provides a running B-scan and full-field 3D figures, and movies throughout the whole examined field in the macular cube (Figs. 7A to D). By "zooming out" the high-resolution minute vitreoretinal interface details, the full-field 3D figures and video clips enable viewing of the whole field under evaluation. These figures and movies provide an important guidance for DME management. 3D SD-OCT scans the field in a continuous fashion. It offers full-field 3D SD-OCT imaging as an important modality for decision-making in DME management.[47]

■ BIOIMAGING BIOMARKERS IN DIABETIC MACULAR EDEMA

WHO defines biomarkers as: "objective, quantifiable characteristics of a biological process, pathogenic process, or a pharmacologic response to a therapeutic intervention".[48]

Bioimaging biomarkers target the diseased organ or tissue and are hence specific indicators. Several bioimaging biomarkers have been recognized that have an important association with progression of diabetic retinopathy. These are macular central subfield thickness (CST) and cube average thickness (CAT).

Surrogate bioimaging biomarkers: SD-OCT based retinal structural alterations, that is, disruption of external limiting membrane (ELM) and ellipsoid zone (EZ), thinning of retinal nerve fiber layer (RNFL) and ganglion cell layer (GCL), choroidal surrogate endpoints and vitreoretinal interface endpoints are considered as surrogate markers.

Bioimaging Biomarkers

1. *Central subfield thickness and cube average thickness*: SD-OCT-based macular CST and CAT provide reliable, objective standard assessment for

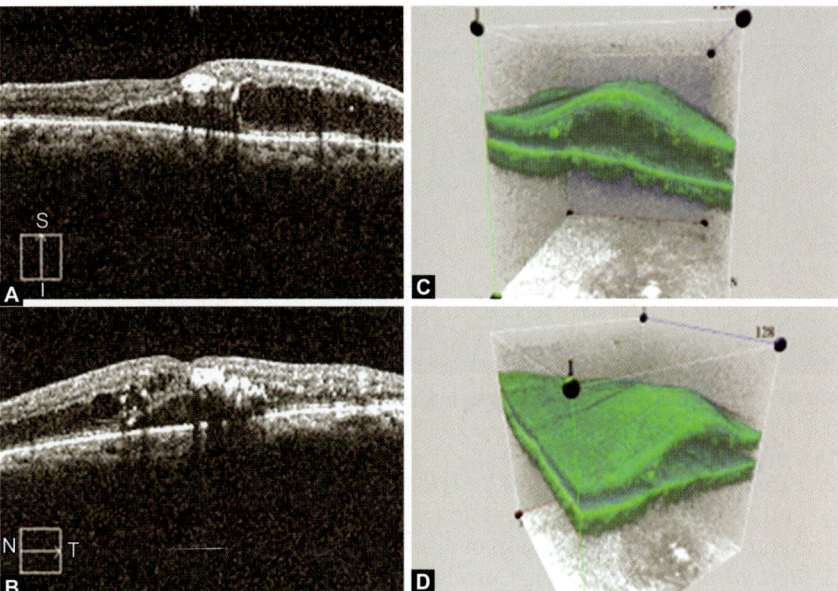

Figs. 7A to D: (A and B): Cross-sectional view shows diabetic macular edema; (C and D): 3D-optical coherence tomography (OCT) presents a global perspective of macular elevation in diabetic macular edema.

screening of diabetic macular edema.[49] Correlation between OCT-based retinal thickness and visual acuity in diabetic macular edema has been observed in several studies.[50-53] An increase in CST and CAT has been observed with increased severity of retinopathy. Targeted screening of diabetic macular edema, in a population, by these bioimaging biomarkers serve as a significant indicator for progression of disease process within the grade of retinopathy. This may not be evident clinically.

Bioimaging biomarkers have been assessed in anti-VEGF therapy. Anatomic outcomes in DRCR.net protocol T have been studied using central OCT thickness. At 1 year, it was observed that central OCT thickness decreased on an average by 169 µm (in aflibercept treated cases), 147 µm (ranibizumab treated cases) and 101 µm (bevacizumab treated cases).[54] Also, in eyes with center involving diabetic macular edema, disorganization of the foveal retinal inner layers and photoreceptor ELM disruption have been documented as significant SD-OCT-based bioimaging biomarkers for predicting visual outcome.

Cochrane database DME assessment: Recent Cochrane database study shows that central retinal thickness cut-off extracted in the documentation ranges between 230 µm and 300 µm, and has a median of 250 µm for the diagnosis of DME (Fig. 8).[55] This median value can be used for standard assessment of the macular thickness in DR and planning management strategies.

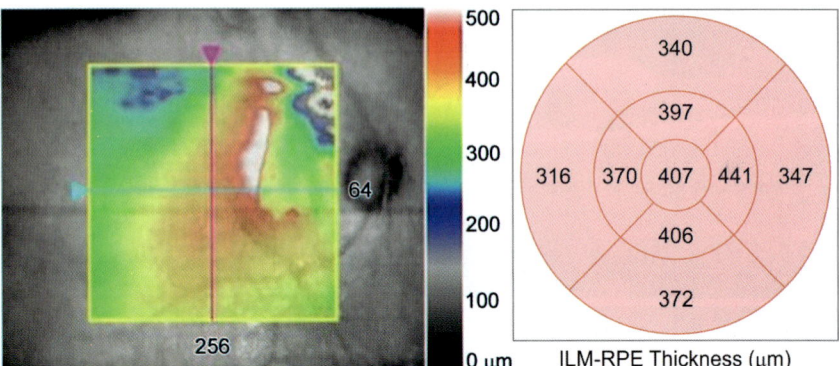

Fig. 8: Macular thickness map in diabetic macular edema.
(ILM-RPE: inner limiting layer–retinal pigment epithelium)

2. *External limiting membrane and ellipsoid zone*: Retinal photoreceptor ELM and EZ disruption grading systems may serve as surrogate biomarkers in determining the progression of disease.
3. *Retinal nerve fiber layer:* Correlation of RNFL thinning with severity of retinopathy on SD-OCT has been found in various studies.[56] A significant decrease in RNFL thickness with an increase in the severity of DR was observed. RNFL thinning has been found to be associated with progression of DR and poor glycemic control.[57]

Spectral domain-optical coherence tomography-based various parameters serve as significant indicators in prognosticating visual outcome in DME. SD-OCT imaging modality serves as an important diagnostic tool in deciding whether DME will benefit from anti-VEGF therapy, and laser or pars plana vitrectomy (PPV).

■ REFERENCES

1. Murakami T, Yoshimura N. Structural changes in individual retinal layers in diabetic macular edema. J Diab Res. 2013;920713:11
2. World Health Organization, Geneva 2016. (2016). Global report on diabetes. [online] Available from http://www.who.int/diabetes/global-report/en/. [Accessed November, 2018].
3. Mathers CD, Loncar D. Projections of global mortality and burden of disease from 2002 to 2030. PLoS Med. 2006;3:442.
4. Chowdhury TA, Hopkins D, Dodson PM, et al. The role of serum lipids in exudative diabetic maculopathy: is there a place for lipid lowering therapy? Eye (Lond). 2002;16:689-93.
5. King H, Aurbert RE, Herman WH. Global burden of diabetes: prevalence, numerical estimates and projections. Diabetes Care. 1998;21:1414-31.
6. Sinha S, Saxena S, Das S, et al. Antimyeloperoxidase antibody is a biomarker for progression of diabetic retinopathy. J Diabetes complications. 2016;30:700-4.
7. Ruia S, Saxena S, Cheung CM, et al. Spectral Domain Optical Coherence Tomography Features and Classification Systems for Diabetic Macular Edema: A Review. Asia-Pacific J Ophthalmol. 2016;5:360.

8. Duker JS, Kaiser PK, Binder S, et al. The International Vitreomacular Traction Study Group classification of vitreomacular adhesion, traction, and macular hole. Ophthalmology. 2013;120:2611-9.
9. Laidlaw DA. Vitrectomy for diabetic macular oedema. Eye (Lond). 2008;22: 1337-41.
10. Kaiser PK, Riemann CD, Sears JE, et al. Macular traction detachment and diabetic macular edema associated with posterior hyaloidal traction. Am J Ophthalmol. 2001;131:44-9.
11. Kishi S, Demaria C, Shimizu K. Vitreous cortex remnants at the fovea after spontaneous vitreous detachment. Int Ophthalmol. 1986;9:253-60.
12. Stefansson E. Ocular oxygenation and the treatment of diabetic retinopathy. Surv Ophthalmol. 2006;51:364-80.
13. Sun JK, Lin MM, Lammer J, et al. Disorganization of the retinal inner layers as a predictor of visual acuity in eyes with center-involved diabetic macular edema. JAMA Ophthalmol. 2014;132:1309-16.
14. Rodrigues EB, Urias MG, Penha FM, et al. Diabetes induces changes in neuroretina before retinal vessels: a spectral-domain optical coherence tomography study. Int J Retina Vitreous. 2015;1:4.
15. Drexler W, Sattmann H, Hermann B, et al. Enhanced visualization of macular pathology with the use of ultrahigh-resolution optical coherence tomography. Arch Ophthalmol. 2003;121:695-706.
16. Ko TH, Fujimoto JG, Duker JS, et al. Comparison of ultrahigh- and standard-resolution optical coherence tomography for imaging macular hole pathology and repair. Ophthalmology. 2004;111:2033-43.
17. Srinivasan VJ, Ko TH, Wojtkowski M, et al. Noninvasive volumetric imaging and morphometry of the rodent retina with high-speed, ultrahigh-resolution optical coherence tomography. Invest Ophthalmol Visual Sci. 2006;47:5522-8.
18. Spaide RF, Curcio CA. Anatomical correlates to the bands seen in the outer retina by optical coherence tomography: literature review and model. Retina. 2011;31:1609-19.
19. Fernandez EJ, Hermann B, Povazay B, et al. Ultrahigh resolution optical coherence tomography and pancorrection for cellular imaging of the living human retina. Opt Express. 2008;16:11083-94.
20. Meyer CH, Saxena S, Sadda SR. Spectral Domain Optical Coherence Tomography in Macular Diseases. Berlin, Germany: Springer; 2016.
21. Maheshwary AS, Oster SF, Yuson RM, et al. The association between percent disruption of the photoreceptor inner segment/outer segment and visual acuity in diabetic macular edema. Am J Ophthalmol. 2010;150:63-7.
22. Sharma SR, Saxena S, Mishra N, et al. The association of grades of photoreceptor inner segment-ellipsoid band disruption with severity of retinopathy in type 2 diabetes mellitus. J Case Rep Stud. 2014;2:205.
23. Jain A, Saxena S, Khanna VK, et al. Status of serum VEGF and ICAM-1 and its association with external limiting membrane and inner segment–outer segment junction disruption in type 2 diabetes mellitus. Mol Vis. 2013;19:1760-8.
24. Lu M, Kuroki M, Amano S, et al. Advanced glycation end products increase retinal vascular endothelial growth factor expression. J Clin Invest. 1998;101:1219-24.
25. Yamagishi S, Inagaki Y, Amano S, et al. Pigment epithelium-derived factor protects cultured retinal pericytes from advanced glycation end product induced injury through its antioxidative properties. Biochem Biophys Res Commun. 2002;296:877-82.

26. Hartnett ME, Lappas A, Darland D, et al. Retinal pigment epithelium and endothelial cell interaction causes retinal pigment epithelial barrier dysfunction via a soluble VEGF-dependent mechanism. Exp Eye Res. 2003;77:593-9.
27. Sebekova K, Schinzel R, Ling H, et al. Advanced glycated albumin impairs protein degradation in the kidney proximal tubules cell line LLC-PK1. Cell Mol Biol (Noisy-le-grand). 1998;44:1051-60.
28. Marneros AG, Fan J, Yokoyama Y, et al. Vascular endothelial growth factor expression in the retinal pigment epithelium is essential for choriocapillaris development and visual function. Am J Pathol. 2005;167:1451-9.
29. Sharma S, Saxena S, Srivastav K, et al. Nitric oxide and oxidative stress is associated with severity of diabetic retinopathy and retinal structural alterations. Clin Experiment Ophthalmol. 2015;43:429-36.
30. Otani T, Kishi S, Maruyama Y. Patterns of diabetic macular edema with optical coherence tomography. Am J Ophthalmol. 1999;127:688-93.
31. Mitchell P, Bandello F, Schmidt-Erfurth U, et al. The RESTORE study: ranibizumab monotherapy or combined with laser versus laser monotherapy for diabetic macular edema. Ophthalmology. 2011;118(4):615-25.
32. Massin P, Bandello F, Garweg JG, et al. Safety and efficacy of ranibizumab in diabetic macular edema (RESOLVE Study): a 12-month, randomized, controlled, double-masked, multicenter phase II study. Diabetes Care. 2010;33:2399-405.
33. Rajendram R, Fraser-Bell S, Kaines A, et al. A 2-year prospective randomized controlled trial of intravitreal bevacizumab or laser therapy (BOLT) in the management of diabetic macular edema: 24-month data: report 3. Arch Ophthalmol. 2012;130:972-9.
34. Brown DM, Nguyen QD, Marcus DM, et al. Long-term outcomes of ranibizumab therapy for diabetic macular edema: the 36-month results from two phase III trials: RISE and RIDE. Ophthalmology. 2013;120:2013-22.
35. Nguyen QD, Shah SM, Khwaja AA, et al. Two-year outcomes of the ranibizumab for edema of the macula in diabetes (READ-2) study. Ophthalmology. 2010;117:2146-51.
36. Elman MJ, Ayala A, Bressler NM, et al. Intravitreal Ranibizumab for diabetic macular edema with prompt versus deferred laser treatment: 5-year randomized trial results. Ophthalmology. 2015;122:375-81.
37. Jampol LM, Glassman AR, Bressler NM. Comparative Effectiveness Trial for Diabetic Macular Edema: Three Comparisons for the Price of 1 Study from the Diabetic Retinopathy Clinical Research Network. JAMA Ophthalmol. 2015;133(9):983-4.
38. Lim LT, Chia SN, Ah-Kee EY, et al. Advances in the management of diabetic macular edema based on evidence from the Diabetic Retinopathy Clinical Research Network. Singapore Med J. 2015;56:237-47.
39. Wells JA, Glassman AR, Ayala AR, et al. Aflibercept, bevacizumab, or ranibizumab for diabetic macular edema. N Engl J Med. 2015;372:1193-203.
40. Wanek J, Zelkha R, Lim JI, et al. Feasibility of a method for en face imaging of photoreceptor cell integrity. Am J Ophthalmol. 2011;152:807-14.
41. Lim JI, Zelkha R, Niec M, et al. Inner and outer retinal thickness mapping of nonproliferative diabetic retinopathy by spectral-domain optical coherence tomography. Ophthalmic Surg Lasers Imaging Retina. 2015;46:316-20.
42. Huang Y, Danis RP, Pak JW, et al. Development of a semi-automatic segmentation method for retinal OCT images tested in patients with diabetic macular edema. PLoS One. 2013;8:e82922.

43. Chiu SJ, Allingham MJ, Mettu PS, et al. Kernel regression based segmentation of optical coherence tomography images with diabetic macular edema. Biomed Opt Express. 2015;6:1172-94.
44. Chiu SJ, Li XT, Nicholas P, et al. Automatic segmentation of seven retinal layers in SDOCT images congruent with expert manual segmentation. Opt Express. 2010;18:19413-28.
45. Garvin MK, Abràmoff MD, Wu X, et al. Automated 3-D intraretinal layer segmentation of macular spectral-domain optical coherence tomography images. IEEE Trans Med Imaging. 2009;28:1436-47.
46. Vermeer KA, van der Schoot J, Lemij HG, et al. Automated segmentation by pixel classification of retinal layers in ophthalmic OCT images. Biomed Opt Express. 2011;2:1743-56.
47. Ophir A. Full-Field 3-D Optical Coherence Tomography Imaging and Treatment Decision in Diffuse Diabetic Macular Edema. Invest Ophthalmol Visual Sci. 2014;55:3052-3.
48. Ruia S, Saxena S. Targeted screening of macular edema by spectral domain optical coherence tomography for progression of diabetic retinopathy. Indian J Ocular Biol. 2016;1:102-7.
49. Diabetic Retinopathy Clinical Research Network; Browning DJ, Glassman AR, et al. Relationship between optical coherence tomography-measured central retinal thickness and visual acuity in diabetic macular edema. Ophthalmology. 2007;114:525-36.
50. Pelosini L, Hull CC, Boyce JF, et al. Optical coherence tomography may be used to predict visual acuity in patients with macular edema. Invest Ophthalmol Vis Sci. 2011;52:2741-8.
51. Alkuraya H, Kangave D, El-Asrar AM. The correlation between optical coherence tomographic features and severity of retinopathy, macular thickness and visual acuity in diabetic macular edema. Int Ophthalmol. 2005;26:93-9.
52. Ruia S, Saxena S, Prasad S, et al. Correlation of biomarkers thiobarbituric acid reactive substance, nitric oxide and central subfield and cube average thickness in diabetic retinopathy: a cross-sectional study. Int J Retina Vitreous. 2016;2:1.
53. The Diabetic Retinopathy Clinical Research Network; Wells JA, Glassman AR, et al. Aflibercept, bevacizumab, or ranibizumab for diabetic macular edema. N Engl J Med. 2015;372(13):1193-203.
54. Virgili G, Menchini F, Casazza G, et al. Optical coherence tomography (OCT) for detection of macular oedema in patients with diabetic retinopathy. Cochrane Database Syst Rev. 2015;1:CD008081.
55. Oshitari T, Hanawa K, Adachi-Usami E. Changes of macular and RNFL thicknesses measured by Stratus OCT in patients with early stage diabetes. Eye. 2009;23:884-9.
56. Srivastav K, Saxena S, Mahdi AA, et al. Increased serum urea and creatinine levels correlate with decreased retinal nerve fibre layer thickness in diabetic retinopathy. Biomarkers. 2015;20:470-3.
57. Srivastav K, Saxena S, Ruia S, et al. Correlation of retinal Nerve fibre layer thinning and central subfield thickness with type 2 diabetic retinopathy on spectral domain optical coherence tomography. Open Sci J Clin Med. 2015;3:194-8.

CHAPTER
18

Necrotizing Retinopathies

Rajesh Babu B, Saurabh Mistry, Sudharshan S

■ INTRODUCTION

Retinitis/retinopathies are most commonly caused due to herpetic viruses and uncommonly due to nonherpetic viruses like chikungunya, dengue and West Nile virus.

■ HERPETIC RETINITIS

Herpetic viruses are deoxyribonucleic acid (DNA) viruses belonging to herpesviridae. They consist of herpes simplex viruses (HSV) types 1 and 2, varicella zoster virus (VZV), cytomegalovirus (CMV), and Epstein–Barr virus (EBV). These herpetic viral agents are important causes of ocular inflammatory disorders worldwide. A wide range of posterior segment manifestations are caused by them, from the aggressive acute retinal necrosis (ARN) to the slow progressing necrotizing and non-necrotizing types of inflammation.[1]
Broadly, necrotizing herpetic retinopathies group (Flowchart 1) consists of:
- Acute retinal necrosis (ARN)
- Progressive outer retinal necrosis (PORN)
- Cytomegalovirus retinitis (CMVR).[2]

■ HISTORICAL BACKGROUND

Cytomegalovirus was first isolated in the year 1957. Earliest descriptions of CMVR were in 1970s much before these lesions were described in patients with HIV/AIDS.[3]

Akira Urayama and colleagues of Tohoku University of Japan were the first to report six cases of ARN in 1971. Their patients had acute unilateral panuveitis, retinal periarteritis progressing to diffuse necrotizing retinitis and retinal detachment. They named it Kirisawa–Urayama uveitis in honor of their teacher Professor Naganori Kirisawa, the Professor of Ophthalmology at Tohoku University.[4] In 1978, Young and Bird described patients with bilateral ARN and called them "BARN".[5] In 1982, the findings by Culbertson et al. led to initiation of specific antiviral therapy for the disease.[6] In 1990, Forster et al. were the first to observe similar findings in two patients with human immunodeficiency virus (HIV). The unique feature in their patients was that it involved only the outer retina initially with minimal to no intraocular

Flowchart 1: Herpetic retinopathies.

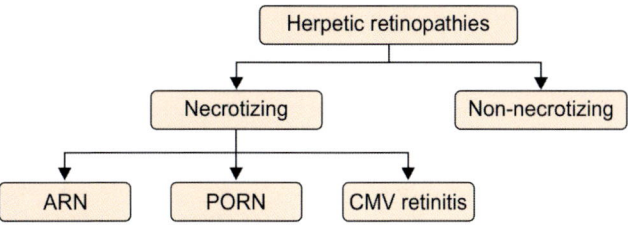

(ARN: acute retinal necrosis; CMV: cytomegalovirus; PORN: progressive outer retinal necrosis)

inflammation. The inner retinal layers and retinal vessels were affected only late in the disease[7] and they termed it as "PORN".

The standard diagnostic criteria for ARN were in 1994 by the Executive Committee of the American Uveitis Society.[8]

Acute retinal necrosis was defined based on characteristics and disease course:
- One or more foci of retinal necrosis in the peripheral retina with discrete borders
- Rapid progression in the absence of antiviral therapy
- Circumferential spread
- Occlusive vasculopathy with both arterial and venous involvement
- Prominent anterior and vitreous inflammatory reaction.

Currently though considering the multiple presentations of the same, they have been named as necrotizing herpetic retinopathies and graded according to the site and size of presentation.

The term ARN (Fig. 1) is used only when there is characteristic triad of moderate-to-severe vitritis, peripheral coalescing necrotizing retinitis, and periarteritis and periphlebitis.

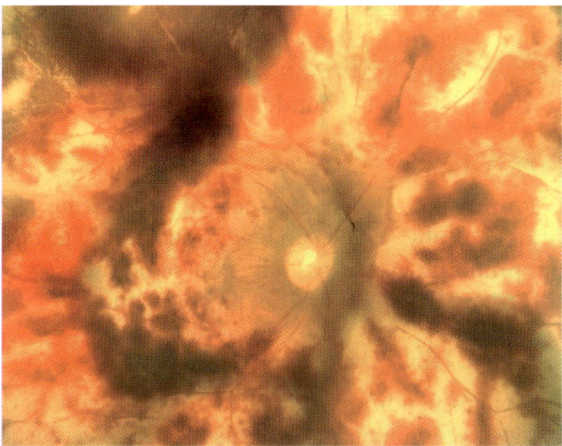

Fig. 1: Active herpetic phase of acute retinal necrosis characterized by full thickness retinal whitening that tend to enlarge over time and associated with large areas of retinal hemorrhage with severe overlying vitritis.

Flowchart 2: Clinical presentation of herpetic retinopathies.

```
                    Herpetic retinopathies
                    /                    \
        Normal immune              Immunodepressed
           status                      status
          /      \                    /        \
        ARN    Non-                 CMV        PORN
             necrotizing          retinitis
```

(ARN: acute retinal necrosis; CMV: cytomegalovirus; PORN: progressive outer retinal necrosis)

ETIOLOGY

Clinical presentation may vary based on the patient's immune status (Flowchart 2). PORN and CMVR are seen in immunocompromised patients such as those with HIV/AIDS, systemic diseases (e.g. lymphoma) or those on immunosuppressives for other systemic diseases such as nephrotic syndrome, rheumatoid arthritis, and graft-versus-host disease after bone marrow transplantation, etc. After CMVR, PORN is the second most common infectious retinitis, in immunosuppressed HIV patients. It presents more aggressively than CMV retinitis and can have even more severe consequences.[9,10] PORN is usually caused by the VZV, although other rare causes are reported.[10,11]

In contrast, ARN usually is seen in immunocompetent individuals, more commonly in males as reported in some studies.[12] The disease affects typically young adults and is uncommon in the pediatric population. A bimodal age distribution has been described with peaks between 20 years and 50 years of age.[13,14]

Varicella zoster virus is the most common cause followed by HSV-1 or -2, and less commonly, CMV and EBV infections.[15]

A study by Ganatra et al. from intraocular specimens (aqueous and vitreous) by polymerase chain reaction (PCR) showed that in middle and older aged patients, VZV and HSV-1 are more common while in children and young adults HSV-2 is more likely to be found.[14]

CLINICAL FEATURES

Characteristic fundus picture usually seen in necrotizing retinopathies is progressive retinal atrophy, which can lead to secondary retinal detachment (RD) leading to profound visual loss. The course of disease varies based on the causative virus and immune status of the individual.

ACUTE RETINAL NECROSIS

Acute retinal necrosis syndrome typically presents with periorbital pain, redness in the eye, photophobia, and diminished vision. It is usually unilateral and in up to one-third of patients, other eye may be affected, even as early as 1–6 weeks. Second eye involvement as late as 20 years after the first eye has also been reported.[16]

There are two phases:
1. *Acute herpetic phase*: It is caused by the viral particles infiltrating the retina and vitreous causing an inflammatory reaction. Anterior-segment findings at this stage include episcleritis, scleritis, keratitis, and/or a nongranulomatous or granulomatous type of anterior chamber inflammation.[16] Patients typically complain of floaters and decreased vision due to vitritis, which worsens as disease progresses. Early retinal lesions are well demarcated with small full thickness patchy, white-yellow areas. These increase with size and number and coalesce over a period of time. They usually start in the mid-periphery although uncommonly occur in the posterior pole, and most importantly do not follow the retinal vessels architecture. Retinal vasculitis characterized by vascular sheathing and small intraretinal hemorrhages are also seen. Characteristically, arteries are more affected than veins. Periphlebitis, capillary nonperfusion as demonstrated by fundus fluorescein angiography (FFA) and venous occlusions are less commonly described. Optic neuropathy is a frequent and important component of ARN syndrome. Disk edema is an early finding and presence of an afferent pupillary defect and/or severe loss despite minimal fundus findings should lead to a suspicion of optic nerve involvement.
2. *Late cicatricial phase*: Acute inflammatory phase resolves over several months with or without therapy. With treatment, resolution of ARN starts in about 3 weeks while, in untreated patients it may take up to 2–3 months. The course of the disease has a definite correlation with the number of clock hours of necrotizing retinitis. This phase depends upon the changes in the way the vitreous is organized in the acute phase. Formation of contractile membranes can occur in the vitreous and on the thinned and necrotic retinal surface. Retinal thinning and atrophy starts in the periphery moving gradually toward the center. Retinal pigment epithelium perturbation develops with areas of clearing forming the characteristic "swiss cheese appearance".

Atrophy of the retina leads to retinal holes or tears, usually at the junction of normal and necrotic retina. Multiple sieve-like retinal holes are quite typical. The pathomechanism of development of retinal complications are explained in Flowchart 3. Subsequent proliferative vitreoretinopathy changes with fibrosis and traction also leads to retinal detachment in up to 75% cases.[17,18]

PROGRESSIVE OUTER RETINAL NECROSIS

Progressive outer retinal necrosis is commonly caused by VZV and is predominantly seen in people with AIDS, usually in the late stages when patient is severely immunodeficient. In their study of 38 patients with AIDS and PORN, the median CD4 lymphocyte count at presentation of the disease was 21 cells/mm^3 (0–130 cells/mm).[3,10] In their study, 61% of the patients who had unilateral presentation initially eventually had bilateral involvement.[10] Affected patients tend to complain of blurred vision or constricted visual

Flowchart 3: Mechanism of retinal detachment in acute retinal necrosis (ARN).

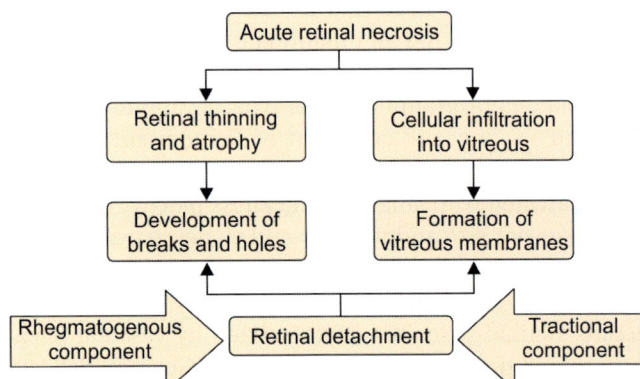

field. In some patients, the disease is asymptomatic at presentation. Pain and photophobia that are typically present in ARN are notably absent in PORN, since the anterior segment is not involved commonly.

A characteristic hallmark of PORN is lack of inflammation. Examination usually reveals a quiet anterior segment with minimal or no vitritis. Scleritis is typically absent, which is a possible reflection of the severely immunocompromised state. The hallmark sign is multifocal, opaque yellow-white necrotic lesions usually starting off initially in either the posterior pole in about one-third cases and/or in the periphery in the rest.[19] The lesions involve outer retinal layers in the early stages, which can involve the full thickness progressively over the next few days to weeks. These lesions coalesce, rapidly progressing toward the macula, with accompanying loss in vision. Perivenular sparing gives the characteristic "cracked mud appearance".[20] Early removal of necrotic debris or edema from the perivascular retina is thought to be the cause of perivascular sparing.[20]

The natural course of the disease is rapid progression leading to blindness. Without therapy, the necrosis rapidly progresses circumferentially to involve the entire retina. Similar to ARN, the development of optic atrophy and retinal detachments is the rule, occurring in greater than 70% of cases. The final outcome is a blind eye with atrophic retina and a pale optic nerve. Even with prompt antiherpetic therapy, the prognosis is guarded.

The differentiating features of the varieties of herpetic retinopathies are summarized in Table 1.

Diagnosis

The diagnosis of necrotizing retinitis is mostly based on characteristic ocular features (Table 1). PCR analysis of the intraocular specimen for identification of specific virus has helped to confirm etiology and initiate early and appropriate therapy.

Table 1: Differentiating features of herpetic retinopathies.[11]

	ARN	PORN	CMV retinitis
Immune status	Healthy	Immunosuppressed state	Immunosuppressed state
Laterality	Bilateral 30–80%	Bilateral 71%	Bilateral 30–50%
Visual loss	Severe	Early loss of vision	Only if it involves macula
Symptoms	Periorbital pain	No pain	Often asymptomatic
Anterior uveitis	Mild to moderate	Mild	Mild
Vitreous reaction	Significant vitritis	Minimal/No vitritis	Minimal/No vitritis
Retinal involvement	Full thickness	Deep outer retinal involvement	Full thickness involvement with granular border
Classic appearance	Swiss cheese	Cracked mud	Pizza pie
Vasculitis	Common	Uncommon	Seen but not common
Retinal hemorrhages	Common	Uncommon	Seen in active lesions
Retinal detachment	Common	Common	Less common
Progression	Rapid	Rapid	Slow

(ARN: acute retinal necrosis; CMV: cytomegalovirus; PORN: progressive outer retinal necrosis)

Treatment[21]

Systemic Therapy

Goals:

- To inhibit replication of the virus
- To stop progression of the disease
- To prevent other eye involvement

Intravenous acyclovir (1,500 mg/m^2/day) for 2–3 weeks, followed by oral acyclovir (800 mg five times/day) for 4–6 weeks. Systemic acyclovir therapy has been shown to fulfill the goals.

Oral acyclovir has poor bioavailability in plasma when compared to valacyclovir (pro-drug). Valacyclovir is capable of achieving plasma levels comparable to intravenous acyclovir.

It is an excellent oral alternative avoiding the need for hospitalization as is required for intravenous acyclovir. Oral valacyclovir (1 gram TID) can reach adequate concentrations in the vitreous and achieve inhibitory ranges of HSV-1, HSV-2 and VZV.[22]

Oral famciclovir (pro-drug for penciclovir) has also been found to be effective in successful management of ARN.[23]

Foscarnet, being a DNA polymerase inhibitor, is not dependent viral thymidine kinase for activation. Intravenous foscarnet[24] is reserved for patients who have failed traditional antiviral therapy and is more effective in treating resistant strains.

Adjunctive Therapies

The mainstay is aggressive, adequate, and appropriate antiviral therapy. Systemic corticosteroids, aspirin, warfarin, prophylactic laser, and vitrectomy are adjuvant therapies and are required for various reasons at various stages of the disease.

Steroids are the mainstay for inflammation control but have to be used under great caution. It can be administered in topical and oral form as per the requirement. Too early initiation with inadequate antiviral therapy can aggravate and accelerate the progress of the retinal necrosis as it carries the risk of potentiating viral replication and causing rapid progression of retinitis. Periocular and intravitreal forms are best avoided. Timing is crucial and oral corticosteroids can only be added 48–72 hours after initiation of antivirals.

The pathogenesis of ARN involves vascular occlusion manifesting as retinal ischemia. Hyperaggregation of platelets is hypothesized to be one of the causative factors and thus anticoagulants have also been considered as adjuvant drugs.[24,25] Since there is no conclusive evidence "for" the same, it has to be weighed with the risks associated with its use vis-à-vis the systemic condition of the patient.[21]

SURGICAL MANAGEMENT OF ACUTE RETINAL NECROSIS

Atrophic retinal holes and rhegmatogenous retinal detachments (RRD) that develop secondary to retinal necrosis are among the most dreaded complications. This can lead to retinal atrophy and vitreoretinal traction changes. Multiple options to prevent such complications are considered with variable benefits.[21]

Prophylactic laser photocoagulation has been used to create strong chorioretinal adhesions posterior to the area of the involved retina. The limiting factors for adequate laser photocoagulation are the presence of severe vitritis preventing the view fundus. Better outcomes are in patients with less inflammation and limited spread of retinal necrosis.

Prophylactic pars plana vitrectomy has also been suggested with varied results by some authors. This helps by removing inflammatory material and risk factors for retinal detachment.[26,27]

Combination Systemic and Intravitreal Antiviral Therapy

Combined systemic and intravitreal antiviral therapy has increasingly been adopted for quicker control of infection for patients with ARN. A long-term follow-up study showed that patients receiving combination therapy showed a higher incidence of two line or greater visual acuity and decreased incidence of retinal detachment and severe visual acuity loss to 20/200 or poorer when compared to patients who received systemic antiviral alone.[28]

CYTOMEGALOVIRUS RETINITIS

Cytomegalovirus (CMV) retinitis (Fig. 2) is the most common opportunistic ocular infection. It is an AIDS-defining illness. The Longitudinal Study of Ocular Complications of AIDS (LSOCA) found that CD4+ T-cell count below

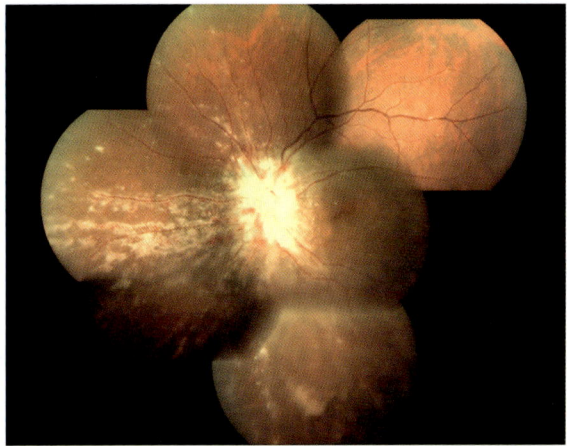

Fig. 2: Montage fundus photo of cytomegalovirus retinitis involving the optic disc and peripapillary retina, also note the vascular sheathing in the blood vessels in the nasal side of the retina.

50 cells/mL was the most important risk factor for the development of CMV retinitis.[29] It occurs due to systemic reactivation of latent infection. It can be often asymptomatic or patients can present with decreased vision, floaters, and scotomata.

Typically CMV retinitis is described as a necrotizing retinitis, which may or may not be hemorrhagic and tends to follow retinal vasculature. Histologically, CMV retinitis appears as areas of full-thickness retinal necrosis and edema or exudative detachment. Ophthalmoscopically, there are several recognized patterns:

- Brush-fire pattern—Wedge-shaped areas of whitening with retinal hemorrhages (Pizza-pie appearance)
- Granular type—Small dot-like lesions (granular type) with minimal hemorrhages
- Frosted branch angiitis—uncommon presenting with retinal vasculitis with perivascular sheathing.

It usually begins in the peripheral retina and progresses centrifugally toward the posterior pole at an average rate of 24 mm per day.[30] Activity of the retinitis and disease progression or relapse occurs at the border of the lesion and if left untreated, expands in size and leaves behind necrotic, atrophic, and nonfunctional retina. There can be presence of a subtle retinal edema and therefore regular fundus examination is necessary.

Angiographically frosted branch angiitis variant demonstrates findings of normal vascular filling pattern in early stages, followed by leakage of fluorescein from the affected vessels in later stages. Kyriele's plaques (segmental retinal periarteritis), which is usually seen in patients with toxoplasmic retinochoroiditis may also be seen uncommonly in patients with CMV retinitis. This can be differentiated from retinal vasculitis on FA by the absence of leakage.[31-34]

Significant visual impairment is caused when macula or optic nerve is involved (zone 1 disease). Vision loss or blindness may also occur as a result of RD, cataract formation or epiretinal membrane.

Treatment
Intravenous ganciclovir and valganciclovir[31] (pro-drug of ganciclovir) are the first-line therapy in CMV retinitis. IV ganciclovir 5 mg/kg/day in two divided doses for 1–2 weeks followed by systemic valganciclovir is the standard protocol currently.

Valganciclovir has excellent bioavailability and has been shown to be as efficacious as intravenous ganciclovir for the treatment of CMV retinitis. The induction dose is tablet valganciclovir 900 mg BD, followed by maintenance dose of 900 mg OD.

Intravitreal Therapy
Intravitreal ganciclovir 2,000 IU can be used as complimentary therapy in addition to systemic therapy. Intravitreal therapy has an advantage of providing direct and immediate therapy to the area of active infection, which may be necessary given the aggressive nature of the disease and is also helpful in resource constraint settings.[21]

OTHER RETINITIS/RETINOPATHIES

Chikungunya Retinitis
Ocular lesions of chikungunya retinitis mimic herpetic or CMV retinitis. It is diagnosed based on a history of a previous episode of systemic illness with chikungunya disease. With such a history and clinical features, detection of specific antibodies to the virus from serum or intraocular fluid is confirmatory. Various authors have described the occurrence of retinitis, choroiditis, panuveitis, and neuroretinitis following systemic history of chikungunya disease.[35-39]

The intraocular inflammation is often self-limiting and supportive anti-inflammatory therapy is the mainstay. No vaccines or antiviral agents specific to chikungunya are available as yet. Currently, treatment is mainly only symptomatic such as analgesics, antipyretics and/or anti-inflammatory agents although sometimes empirical antiviral therapy is also advised. Clinical role of antivirals like ribavarin and interferons in chikungunya retinitis is not known.[31,40]

West Nile Virus Retinopathy
The causative agent West Nile virus (WNV) is a single-stranded RNA flavivirus, which belongs to the Japanese encephalitis serogroup. It is a zoonotic disease most commonly transmitted by the bite of the *Culex* genus of mosquitoes (especially *Culex pipiens*).[41-46] The most common ocular manifestations of WNV infection is asymptomatic multifocal chorioretinitis seen in up to 80% of patients (80%).[41-46] Other ocular complications of WNV infection include anterior uveitis, subconjunctival hemorrhage, retinal vasculitis,

neurophthalmic manifestations such as optic neuritis, cranial nerve palsies especially 6th nerve, nystagmus, and congenital chorioretinal scarring.[41-46]

Chorioretinal lesions seen in WNV are typically linearly arranged or scattered lesions. Active lesions are deep in location, creamy and circular whereas the inactive ones are atrophic, pigmented partially and have a targetoid appearance.[46]

Patients with macular involvement come with complaints of redness in the eyes, decreased vision, floaters, and visual field defects or diplopia. Irreversible vision loss can occur due to complications such as foveal scarring, choroidal neovascularization, vitreous hemorrhage, tractional retinal detachment, ischemic maculopathy, optic atrophy, and retrogeniculate damage.[41-46]

Rathinam et al. described discrete, superficial, white retinitis; arteritis; phlebitis; and retinal hemorrhages with or without macular star. In their patients, optical coherence tomography (OCT) revealed inner retinal layer edema in active inflammation and retinal atrophy in late stage.[47]

There is no proven treatment for WNV infection. Systemic disease management consists of supportive anti-inflammatory treatment and fluid management systemically. In case of retinal complications like choroidal neovascular membrane, anti-VEGF treatment is advised.

Dengue Virus Retinopathy

The pathological process of dengue ophthalmic complications is complex and clinical manifestations varied. Ophthalmic complications are usually seen in young adults who often present at the nadir of thrombocytopenia. Hemorrhages associated with dengue-related maculopathy are mostly intraretinal and can take the form of dot, blot, or flame-shaped hemorrhages.[48,49]

Vascular sheathing[48,50-52] and vasculitis[48,53,54] were often found in association with macular hemorrhage. Dengue-related foveolitis refers to the yellow-orange lesion at the fovea of patients with dengue maculopathy. OCT reveals disruption of the outer neurosensory retina in these patients.[51] Dengue-related maculopathy commonly presents with macular edema.[49,52,53]

OTHER RARE CAUSES

Retinitis has been reported rarely in associated with other febrile illnesses like malaria,[55,56] typhoid[57,58] among others and they mainly cause retinopathy rather than typical necrotizing type of retinitis. The treatment is of the primary disease with anti-infective agents and supportive anti-inflammatory therapy for the ocular and systemic condition.

REFERENCES

1. Wensing B, de Groot-Mijnes JDF, Rothova A. Necrotizing and nonnecrotizing variants of herpetic uveitis with posterior segment involvement. Arch Ophthalmol Chic Ill 1960. 2011;129(4):403-8.
2. Ittner EA, Bhakhri R, Newman T. Necrotising herpetic retinopathies: a review and progressive outer retinal necrosis case report: A review of necrotising herpetic retinopathies Ittner, Bhakhri and Newman. Clin Exp Optom. 2016;99(1):24-9.

3. Ho M. The history of cytomegalovirus and its diseases. Med Microbiol Immunol (Berl). 2008;197(2):65-73.
4. Urayama A, Yamada N, Sasaki T. Unilateral acute uveitis with retinal periarteritis and detachment. Jpn J Clin Ophthalmol. 1971;25:607-19.
5. Young NJ, Bird AC. Bilateral acute retinal necrosis. Br J Ophthalmol. 1978;62(9):581-90.
6. Culbertson WW, Blumenkranz MS, Haines H, et al. The acute retinal necrosis syndrome. Part 2: Histopathology and etiology. Ophthalmology. 1982;89(12):1317-25.
7. Forster DJ, Dugel PU, Frangieh GT, et al. Rapidly progressive outer retinal necrosis in the acquired immunodeficiency syndrome. Am J Ophthalmol. 1990;110(4):341-8.
8. Holland GN. Standard diagnostic criteria for the acute retinal necrosis syndrome. Executive Committee of the American Uveitis Society. Am J Ophthalmol. 1994;117(5):663-7.
9. Weinberg DV, Lyon AT. Repair of retinal detachments due to herpes varicella-zoster virus retinitis in patients with acquired immune deficiency syndrome. Ophthalmology. 1997;104(2):279-82.
10. Engstrom RE, Holland GN, Margolis TP, et al. The progressive outer retinal necrosis syndrome. A variant of necrotizing herpetic retinopathy in patients with AIDS. Ophthalmology. 1994;101(9):1488-502.
11. Austin RB. Progressive outer retinal necrosis syndrome: a comprehensive review of its clinical presentation, relationship to immune system status, and management. Clin Eye Vis Care. 2000;12(3-4):119-29.
12. Fisher JP, Lewis ML, Blumenkranz M, et al. The acute retinal necrosis syndrome. Part 1: Clinical manifestations. Ophthalmology. 1982;89(12):1309-16.
13. Ganatra JB, Chandler D, Santos C, et al. Viral causes of the acute retinal necrosis syndrome. Am J Ophthalmol. 2000;129(2):166-72.
14. Wong RW, Jumper JM, McDonald HR, et al. Emerging concepts in the management of acute retinal necrosis. Br J Ophthalmol. 2013;97(5):545-52.
15. Van Gelder RN, Willig JL, Holland GN, et al. Herpes simplex virus type 2 as a cause of acute retinal necrosis syndrome in young patients. Ophthalmology. 2001;108(5):869-76.
16. Schlingemann RO, Bruinenberg M, Wertheim-van Dillen P, et al. Twenty years' delay of fellow eye involvement in herpes simplex virus type 2-associated bilateral acute retinal necrosis syndrome. Am J Ophthalmol. 1996;122(6):891-2.
17. Clarkson JG, Blumenkranz MS, Culbertson WW, et al. Retinal detachment following the acute retinal necrosis syndrome. Ophthalmology. 1984;91(12):1665-8.
18. Lau CH, Missotten T, Salzmann J, et al. Acute retinal necrosis features, management, and outcomes. Ophthalmology. 2007;114(4):756-62.
19. Moorthy RS, Weinberg DV, Teich SA, et al. Management of varicella zoster virus retinitis in AIDS. Br J Ophthalmol. 1997;81(3):189-94.
20. Margolis TP, Lowder CY, Holland GN, et al. Varicella-zoster virus retinitis in patients with the acquired immunodeficiency syndrome. Am J Ophthalmol. 1991;112(2):119-31.
21. Shantha JG, Weissman HM, Debiec MR, et al. Advances in the management of acute retinal necrosis. Int Ophthalmol Clin. 2015;55:1-13.
22. Aizman A, Johnson MW, Elner SG. Treatment of acute retinal necrosis syndrome with oral antiviral medications. Ophthalmology. 2007;114(2):307-12.

23. Figueroa MS, Garabito I, Gutierrez C, et al. Famciclovir for the treatment of acute retinal necrosis (ARN) syndrome. Am J Ophthalmol. 1997;123(2):255-7.
24. Kawaguchi T, Spencer DB, Mochizuki M. Therapy for acute retinal necrosis. Semin Ophthalmol. 2008;23(4):285-90.
25. Ando F, Kato M, Goto S, et al. Platelet function in bilateral acute retinal necrosis. Am J Ophthalmol. 1983;96(1):27-32.
26. Ishida T, Sugamoto Y, Sugita S, et al. Prophylactic vitrectomy for acute retinal necrosis. Jpn J Ophthalmol. 2009;53(5):486-9.
27. Iwahashi-Shima C, Azumi A, Ohguro N, et al. Acute retinal necrosis: factors associated with anatomic and visual outcomes. Jpn J Ophthalmol. 2013;57(1):98-103.
28. Yeh S, Suhler EB, Smith JR, et al. Combination systemic and intravitreal antiviral therapy in the management of acute retinal necrosis syndrome. Ophthalmic Surg Lasers Imaging Retina. 2014;45(5):399-407.
29. Sugar EA, Jabs DA, Ahuja A, et al. Incidence of cytomegalovirus retinitis in the era of highly active antiretroviral therapy. Am J Ophthalmol. 2012;153(6):1016-24.e5.
30. Holland GN, Shuler JD. Progression rates of cytomegalovirus retinopathy in ganciclovir-treated and untreated patients. Arch Ophthalmol Chic Ill 1960. 1992;110(10):1435-42.
31. Patil AJ, Sharma A, Kenney MC, et al. Valganciclovir in the treatment of cytomegalovirus retinitis in HIV-infected patients. Clin Ophthalmol. 2010;4:111-9.
32. Walker S, Iguchi A, Jones NP. Frosted branch angiitis: a review. Eye Lond Engl. 2004;18(5):527-33.
33. Patel A, Pomykala M, Mukkamala K, et al. Kyrieleis plaques in cytomegalovirus retinitis. J Ophthalmic Inflamm Infect. 2011;1(4):189-91.
34. Banker AS. Posterior segment manifestations of human immunodeficiency virus/acquired immune deficiency syndrome. Indian J Ophthalmol. 2008;56(5):377-83.
35. Mahendradas P, Ranganna SK, Shetty R, et al. Ocular manifestations associated with chikungunya. Ophthalmology. 2008;115:287-91.
36. Murthy KR, Venkataraman N, Satish V, et al. Bilateral retinitis following chikungunya fever. Indian J Ophthalmol. 2008;56:329-31.
37. Lalitha P, Rathinam S, Banushree K, et al. Ocular involvement associated with an epidemic outbreak of Chikungunya virus infection. Am J Ophthalmol. 2008;144(4):552-6.
38. Mahesh G, Giridhar A, Shedbele A, et al. A case of bilateral presumed chikungunya neuroretinitis. Indian J Ophthalmol. 2009;57:148-50.
39. Chanana B, Azad RV, Nair S. Bilateral macular choroiditis following chikungunya virus infection. Eye (Lond). 2007;21(7):1020-1.
40. Abdelnabi R, Neyts J, Delang L. Antiviral Strategies against Chikungunya Virus. In: Chu J, Ang S (Eds). Chikungunya Virus. Methods in Molecular Biology, vol 1426. New York, NY: Humana Press; 2016.
41. Bakri SJ, Kaiser PK. Ocular manifestations of West Nile virus. Curr Opin Ophthalmol. 2004;15:537-40.
42. Garg S, Jampol LM. Systemic and intraocular manifestations of West Nile virus infection. Surv Ophthalmol. 2005;50:3-13.
43. Khairallah M, Ben Yahia S, Ladjimi A, et al. Chorioretinal involvement in patients with West Nile virus infection. Ophthalmology. 2004;111:2065-70.
44. Khairallah M, Yahia SB, Letaief M, et al. A prospective evaluation of factors associated with chorioretinitis in patients with West Nile virus infection. Ocul Immunol Inflamm. 2007;15:435-9.

45. Yahia SB, Khairallah M. Ocular manifestations of West Nile virus infection. Int J Med Sci. 2009;6:114-5.
46. Bains HS, Jampol LM, Caughron MC, et al. Vitritis and chorioretinitis in a patient with West Nile virus infection. Arch Ophthalmol. 2003;121(2):205-7.
47. Sivakumar RR, Prajna L, Arya LK, et al. Molecular Diagnosis and Ocular Imaging of West Nile Virus retinitis and neuroretinitis. Ophthalmology. 2013;120(9): 1820-6.
48. Bacsal KE, Chee SP, Cheng CL, et al. Dengue-associated maculopathy. Arch Ophthalmol. 2007;125:501-10.
49. Su DH, Bacsal K, Chee SP, et al. Prevalence of dengue maculopathy in patients hospitalized for dengue fever. Ophthalmology. 2007;114:1743-7.
50. Lim WK, Mathur R, Koh A, et al. Ocular manifestations of dengue fever. Ophthalmology. 2004;111:2057-64.
51. Loh BK, Bacsal K, Chee SP, et al. Foveolitis associated with dengue fever: a case series. Ophthalmologica. 2008;222:317-20.
52. Quek DT, Barkham T, Teoh SC. Recurrent bilateral dengue maculopathy following sequential infections with two serotypes of dengue virus. Eye (Lond). 2009;23:1471-2.
53. Teoh SC, Chan DP, Nah GK, et al. Eye institute dengue-related ophthalmic complications workgroup. A re-look at ocular complications in dengue fever and dengue haemorrhagic fever. Dengue Bull. 2006;30:184-93.
54. Tan CS, Teoh SC, Chan DP, et al. Dengue retinopathy manifesting with bilateral vasculitis and macular oedema. Eye (Lond). 2007;21:875-7.
55. Beare NA, Taylor TE, Harding SP, et al. Malarial retinopathy: a newly established diagnostic sign in severe malaria. Am J Trop Med Hyg. 2006;75:790-7.
56. Beare NA, Harding SP, Taylor TE, et al. Perfusion abnormalities in children with cerebral malaria and malarial retinopathy. J Infect Dis. 2009;199(2):263-71.
57. Relhan N, Pathengay A, Albini T, et al. A case of vasculitis, retinitis and macular neurosensory detachment presenting post typhoid fever. J Ophthalmic Inflamm Infect. 2014;4:23.
58. Prabhushanker M, Topiwala TT, Ganesan G, et al. Bilateral retinitis following typhoid fever. Int J Retina Vitreous. 2017;3:11.

CHAPTER 19

Nyctalopia

Avinash Pathengay, Sharat Hegde, Shreyansh Doshi

■ INTRODUCTION

Nyctalopia (night blindness), derived from Greek "nyct" (night) + "aloas" (blind) + "opsis" (vision), is impaired vision in dark environment as a result of inability to adapt to low illumination. This occurs because of absence or subnormal activity of rod photoreceptors. Night blindness should be differentiated with blurred vision made worse by low light (pseudonight blindness), which occurs in patients with cataract, high myopia, and glaucoma where patient experiences decreased vision in dark environment.

■ ETIOLOGY

Nyctalopia may be true or pseudo. It may be congenital or acquired. Main causes of true nyctalopia are presented in Flowchart 1.

The classification and causes of pseudonyctalopia are shown in Flowchart 2.

Flowchart 1: Classification and causes of nyctalopia.

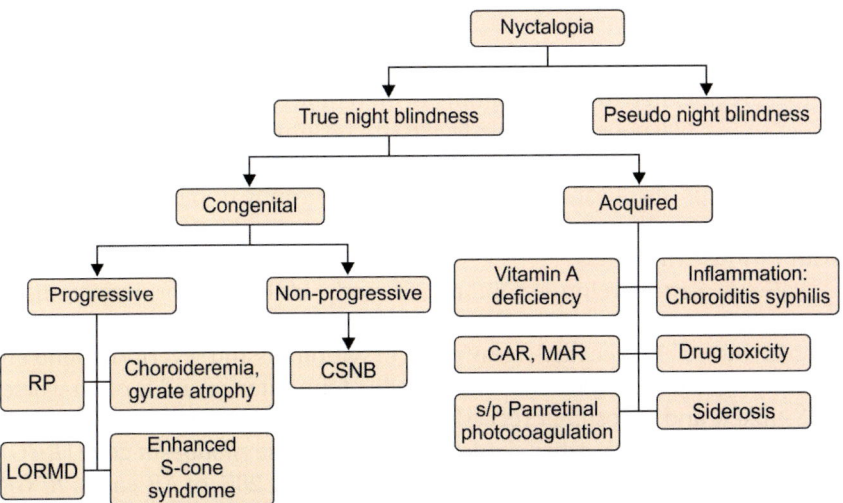

(RP: retinitis pigmentosa; LORMD: late onset retinal macular degeneration; CSNB: congenital stationary night blindness; CAR: carcinoma-associated retinopathy; MAR: melanoma-associated retinopathy; s/p: status post)

Flowchart 2: Classification and causes of pseudonyctalopia.

```
                    Pseudo night
                      blindness
          ┌──────────────┼──────────────┐
        Ocular     Psychological:    Malingering
                     Hysteresis
    ┌─────────┐
 Glaucoma ─── Optic atrophy
 Cataract ─── Miotic pupil
 Multifocal IOL
```

(IOL: intraocular lens)

Symptom of night blindness can be seen in various etiologies, which affects retinal pigment epithelium (RPE) and rod photoreceptors either directly or indirectly. In certain conditions like congenital stationary night blindness (CSNB), it can be stationary and in condition like retinitis pigmentosa (RP) and choroideremia, symptom of night blindness progresses with age. Symptoms of night blindness can develop in early childhood, while some may remain asymptomatic until adulthood.

Majority of the conditions causing night blindness are hereditary like RP, choroidal dystrophies choroideremia and CSNB, RP being most common. Acquired conditions include vitamin A deficiency, cancer-associated retinopathy, inflammatory choroiditis, and siderosis.[1]

CLINICAL FEATURES OF SPECIFIC DISORDERS CAUSING NYCTALOPIA

Retinitis Pigmentosa

These are the heterogenous group of hereditary retinal dystrophies that affect ~1 in 4,000 people worldwide.[2,3] It can be inherited either as autosomal dominant (AD), autosomal recessive (AR), X-linked or rarely mitochondrial inherited. It is also termed as tapetoretinal dystrophy or pigmentary retinal dystrophy. Some patients can have an atypical presentation and be associated with various syndromes.

Patients can develop symptoms in early childhood or may remain asymptomatic until adulthood with progression to legal blindness usually seen in the 3rd–6th decade.[4] Age of onset of symptoms and severity depend on underlying genetic abnormality and mode of inheritance and is often worse in X-linked and autosomal recessive RP. Many genes have been identified, which lead to RP with other syndromes. Out of these *rhodopsin* gene (*RHO*) account for 25% of AD cases, *USH2A* gene around 20% of AR cases, *RPGR* gene around 70% of X-linked cases and *RPE65* gene.[5,6]

Typical Retinitis Pigmentosa

Typical RP is characterized by night blindness in childhood or young adulthood with profound visual loss or blindness in middle or late life. It presents progressive contraction of peripheral visual field with relative preservation of central vision leading to tunnel-like vision.[2,7] It is also associated with high myopia. Fundus in early stage shows progressive narrowing of peripheral retinal blood vessels and bony spicules—like pigmentary migration in mid-peripheral retina. This later leads to extensive pigmentation of retina with waxy pallor optic disk atrophy (Figs. 1A to D). The patient can develop posterior polar cataract and multiple vitreous opacities.[8] Electroretinogram (ERG) shows a reduced or extinguished amplitude of photoreceptors in scotopic vision with normal or reduced amplitudes in photopic vision (Fig. 2).[2,9] Early central visual loss can be due to cystoid macular edema, epiretinal membrane, and atrophic changes in RPE at the macula.[10]

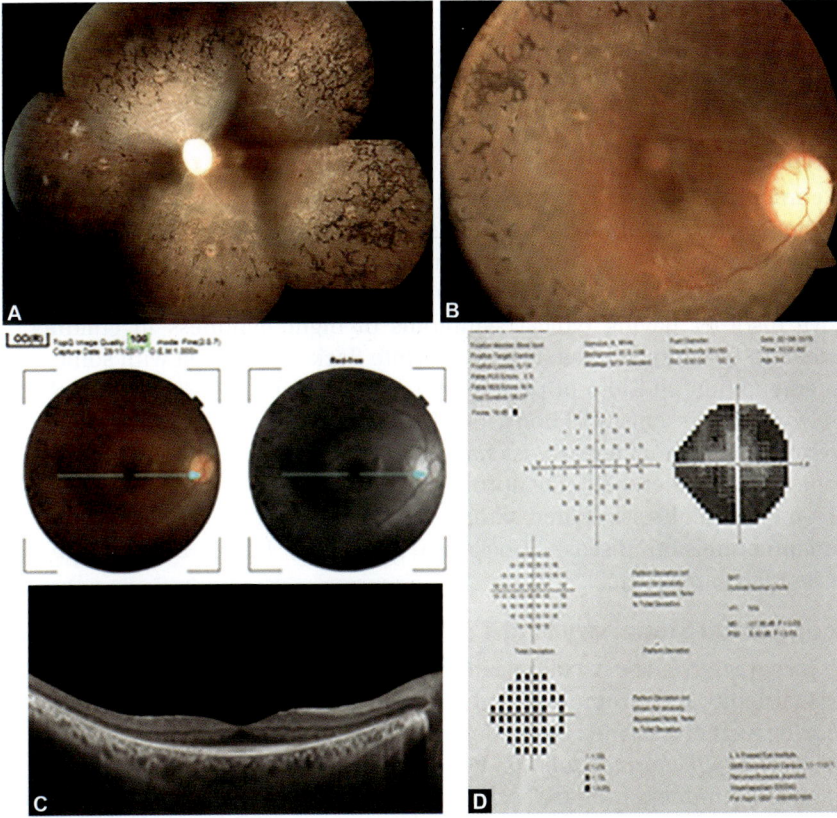

Figs. 1A to D: (A and B) Fundus picture of typical retinitis pigmentosa (RP) showing waxy disk pallor with bony spicule pigmentation and severe arteriolar attenuation; (C) Optical coherence tomography (OCT) showing loss of photoreceptors sparing fovea; (D) Visual field 242 shows tunnel vision with loss of midperipheral field.

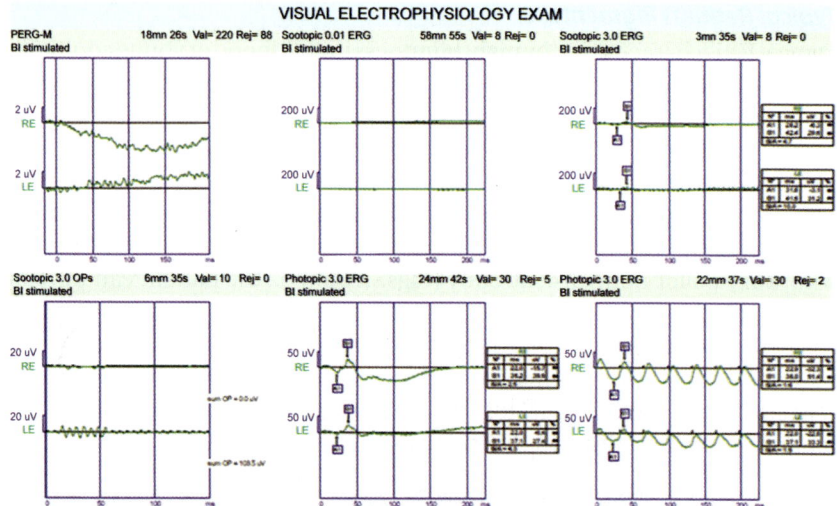

Fig. 2: Electroretinogram (ERG) changes in typical retinitis pigmentosa (RP) showing extinguished "a" and "b" waves in scotopic response and decrease amplitudes of "a" and "b" waves in photopic response.

Atypical Retinitis Pigmentosa

Retinitis pigmentosa can present with various atypical presentations. The patients with *RP sine pigmento* have symptoms of night blindness and visual field constriction, but there is absence of bony spicule pigmentation with arteriolar attenuation. *Retinitis punctate albescens* is an autosomal recessive disorder having typical symptoms of night blindness in childhood, wherein fundus shows small gray or white flecks over retina with some RPE pigmentation and loss of peripheral field of vision (Figs. 3A to D).[11-13] The *sectoral RP* presents with bony spicule pigmentation only in one quadrant of retina,[14] while unilateral RP is characterized by typical features of RP only in one eye and other eye being normal including ERG and visual fields.[15,16]

The RP can be associated with various syndromes like Usher's syndrome, infantile Refsum disease, Cockayne syndrome, Bardet–Biedl syndrome, Friedrich's ataxia, etc.[17-20]

Congenital Stationary Night Blindness

It is characterized by nyctalopia in childhood. Patients usually maintain good visual acuity and symptom of night blindness do not progress with age. CSNB can be further classified based on retinal changes as:

- *CSNB with normal fundus*: Patients have symptoms of nonprogressive night blindness from early childhood. On examination, fundus shows no abnormality. ERG, AD variant (Riggs type) shows a reduced but normal appearing photoreceptor response under photopic condition, and poor or absent b-wave amplitude under scotopic condition.[21] AR variant (Schubert–Bornschein type) shows progressive increase in a wave and not in b-wave in scotopic response called as negative ERG.[22]

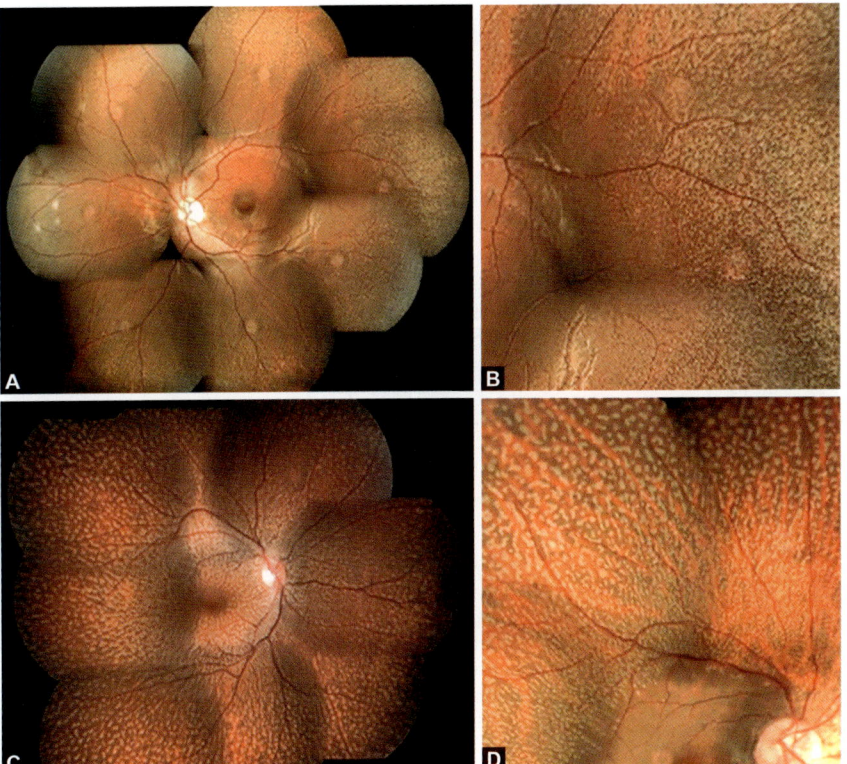

Figs. 3A to D: (A and B) Atypical form of retinitis pigmentosa (RP), retinitis punctate albescens with tiny yellow flecks with arteriolar attenuation; (C and D) Fundus albipunctatus with yellow flecks, which is coarse and large more toward periphery sparing macula.

- **CSNB with abnormal fundus:**
  - *Oguchi's disease*: Oguchi's disease is characterized by night blindness with normal visual acuity, visual fields, and color vision. Fundus reveals golden yellow sheen in light adapted state and which returns to normal after dark adaptation of 30 minutes to few hours (Figs. 4A to D). This characteristic feature is called as Mizuo phenomenon.[23,24] Retinal vessels stand out in bold and arteries and veins may look similar. ERG shows subnormal rod responses that usually normalize after prolonged dark adaptation. It is caused by abnormality in photoreceptor transduction due to abnormality in the rhodopsin kinase or arrestin gene.[25-27]
  - *Fundus albipunctatus*: Patient can have history of night blindness from early childhood or may be identified on regular checkup as his/her visual acuity is usually good. The disease is characterized by a number of discrete, small, punctate yellowish white spots deep in the retina, extending from posterior pole to periphery (Figs. 3C and D). Maximum density of flecks is noted in the posterior pole but the center of macula is spared.[28-30] Optical coherence tomography (OCT) shows flecks are confined at the photoreceptor outer segment continuous with RPE.[31] ERG shows marked delay in regeneration of both the rod

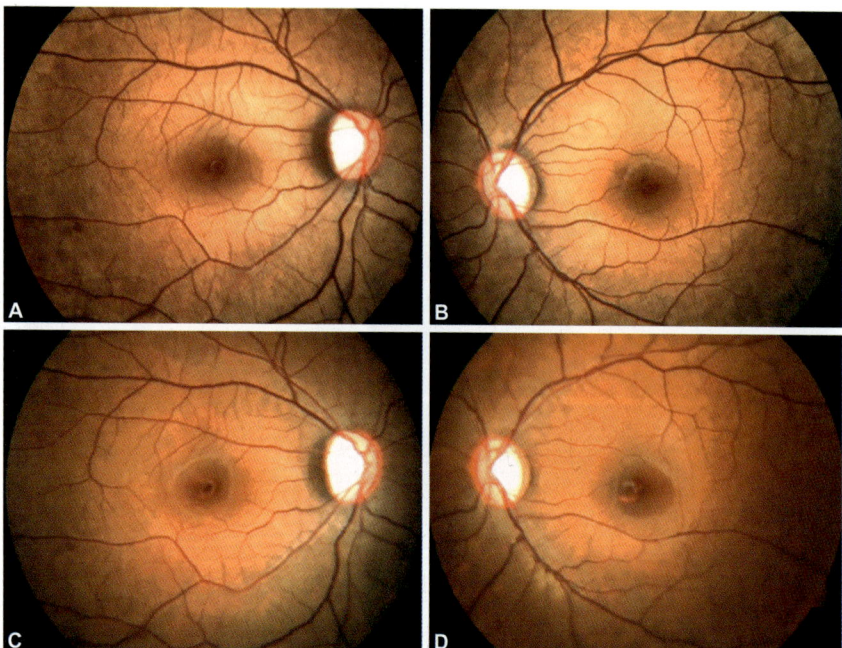

Figs. 4A to D: (A and B) Mizuo phenomenon in Oguchi disease characterized by golden yellow sheen reflex; (C and D) It becomes normal on dark adaptation.

and cone visual pigments, which is because of defect in 11 cis retinol dehydrogenase (*RDS65*) gene.[32,33]

Cone-rod Dystrophy

Cone-rod dystrophy is characterized by early loss of visual acuity, night blindness, and impaired color vision with progressive peripheral visual field loss.[34] Fundus shows variable degree of peripheral pigmentary changes with macular atrophy and pigmentation. ERG shows marked reduction or absence of cone response in photopic response with relatively less reduction in rod response.[35] It can be due to AD, AR, or X-linked with mutation in gene *GUCY2D*.[36]

Vitamin A Deficiency

Patients with vitamin A deficiency can present with typical symptoms such as progressive night blindness, delayed dark adaptation, and dryness in the eyes. On evaluation, there can be presence of Bitot's spots, corneal xerosis, which can complicate to corneal ulcer and peculiar multiple yellow white granular spots in the fundus xerophthalmicus/Uyemura's syndrome).[37-39] There is marked constriction of visual fields and delayed dark adaptation. ERG shows disappearance of "a" wave followed by loss of "b" wave with greater reduction of scotopic than photopic response (Figs. 5A to C). A decrease in serum vitamin A levels (less than 0.7 μmol/L) may be found. It may be due to inadequate dietary intake, malabsorption status due to various etiology, chronic liver

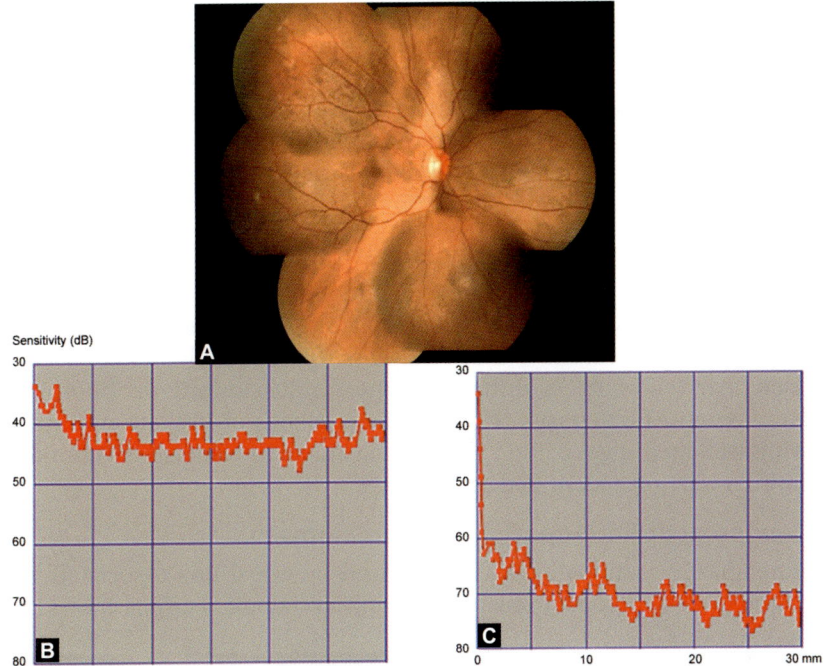

Figs. 5A to C: Vitamin A deficiency: (A) Fundus shows very small discrete white flecks; (B) Dark adaptation test showing delayed dark adaptation curve; (C) Dark adaptation becoming normal after vitamin A treatment.

disease, postbariatric surgery, etc.[39,40] Vitamin A (retinol) is needed in phototransduction cycle to produce essential protein by photoreceptor. The deficiency thus leads to disruption of phototransduction cycle, which in turn leads to night blindness. Following administration of vitamin A, there may be complete or partial reversal of fundus and ERG changes.

Choroideremia

Choroideremia is a X-linked recessive chorioretinal dystrophy[41,42] caused by mutation in *CHM* gene localized to long arm of chromosome Xq21.2.[43,44] Affected males usually note the onset of night blindness between 10 years and 30 years of age. Early disease characterized by mottled depigmentation of RPE and in later stages, severe RPE and choroidal atrophy develops in mid-periphery of fundus and spreads gradually in anterior and posterior directions, eventually sparing stellate area of relatively normal choroid and RPE in macular area (Fig. 6A). ERG shows reduced amplitude with delay in "b" wave implicit time.[41,45]

Gyrate Atrophy

Gyrate atrophy is characterized by nyctalopia, high myopia, and progressive constriction of visual fields. Early changes include well-circumscribed scalloped region of chorioretinal dystrophy with hyperpigmented margins in midperiphery of fundus. These regions enlarge and coalesce in scalloped pattern, spread anteriorly and posteriorly (Fig. 6B). ERG shows early impaired scotopic and photopic response which extinguish as disease progresses.[46] Etiology is attributed to high levels of ornithine due to autosomal recessive deficiency in ornithine delta aminotransferase enzyme linked to chromosome 10q26.[47,48] The treatment is aimed toward reducing plasma ornithine levels. Giving pyridoxine supplements and diet restricted in arginine may help to decrease the plasma ornithine levels.[48]

Late-onset Retinal Macular Degeneration

In late-onset retinal macular degeneration (LORMD), patients develop symptoms of delayed dark adaptation at 5th–6th decade, which slowly progress to night blindness over few years. Early retinal changes include drusen like yellow spots throughout the fundus toward periphery that represent sub-RPE deposits (Fig. 6C). Soon islands of RPE atrophy ensue, leaving scalloped edges of RPE.[49] It has been linked with autosomal dominant condition with gene identified as *CTRD5*.[50,51]

Paraneoplastic Retinopathy with Carcinoma

Paraneoplastic retinopathy is characterized by visual loss associated with bizarre visual symptoms (phosphenes) and nyctalopia. Fundus shows pro-

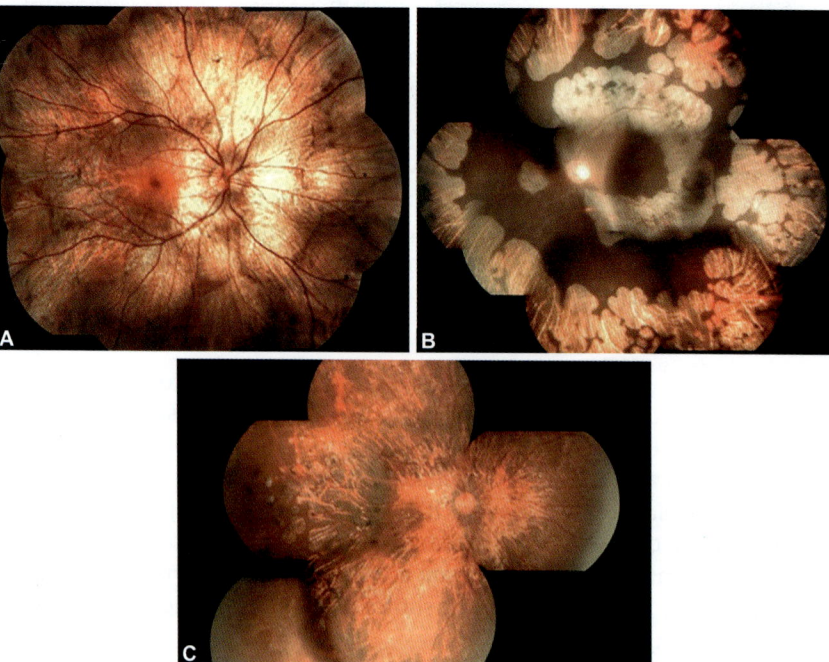

Figs. 6A to C: (A) Choroideremia with stellate macula and surrounding retinal pigment epithelium (RPE) atrophy; (B) Gyrate atrophy: characteristic scalloped margin RPE atrophy in midperiphery; (C) Late-onset retinal macular degeneration (LORMD): RPE atrophy with scalloped edges in periphery with scalloped edges.

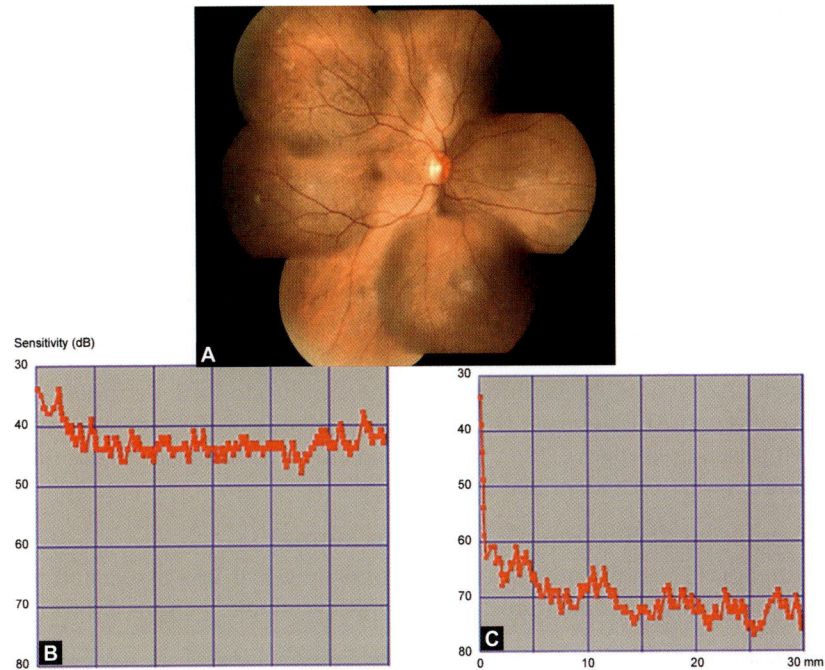

Figs. 5A to C: Vitamin A deficiency: (A) Fundus shows very small discrete white flecks; (B) Dark adaptation test showing delayed dark adaptation curve; (C) Dark adaptation becoming normal after vitamin A treatment.

disease, postbariatric surgery, etc.[39,40] Vitamin A (retinol) is needed in phototransduction cycle to produce essential protein by photoreceptor. The deficiency thus leads to disruption of phototransduction cycle, which in turn leads to night blindness. Following administration of vitamin A, there may be complete or partial reversal of fundus and ERG changes.

Choroideremia

Choroideremia is a X-linked recessive chorioretinal dystrophy[41,42] caused by mutation in *CHM* gene localized to long arm of chromosome Xq21.2.[43,44] Affected males usually note the onset of night blindness between 10 years and 30 years of age. Early disease characterized by mottled depigmentation of RPE and in later stages, severe RPE and choroidal atrophy develops in mid-periphery of fundus and spreads gradually in anterior and posterior directions, eventually sparing stellate area of relatively normal choroid and RPE in macular area (Fig. 6A). ERG shows reduced amplitude with delay in "b" wave implicit time.[41,45]

Gyrate Atrophy

Gyrate atrophy is characterized by nyctalopia, high myopia, and progressive constriction of visual fields. Early changes include well-circumscribed scalloped region of chorioretinal dystrophy with hyperpigmented margins in midperiphery of fundus. These regions enlarge and coalesce in scalloped pattern, spread anteriorly and posteriorly (Fig. 6B). ERG shows early impaired scotopic and photopic response which extinguish as disease progresses.[46] Etiology is attributed to high levels of ornithine due to autosomal recessive deficiency in ornithine delta aminotransferase enzyme linked to chromosome 10q26.[47,48] The treatment is aimed toward reducing plasma ornithine levels. Giving pyridoxine supplements and diet restricted in arginine may help to decrease the plasma ornithine levels.[48]

Late-onset Retinal Macular Degeneration

In late-onset retinal macular degeneration (LORMD), patients develop symptoms of delayed dark adaptation at 5th–6th decade, which slowly progress to night blindness over few years. Early retinal changes include drusen like yellow spots throughout the fundus toward periphery that represent sub-RPE deposits (Fig. 6C). Soon islands of RPE atrophy ensue, leaving scalloped edges of RPE.[49] It has been linked with autosomal dominant condition with gene identified as *CTRD5*.[50,51]

Paraneoplastic Retinopathy with Carcinoma

Paraneoplastic retinopathy is characterized by visual loss associated with bizarre visual symptoms (phosphenes) and nyctalopia. Fundus shows pro-

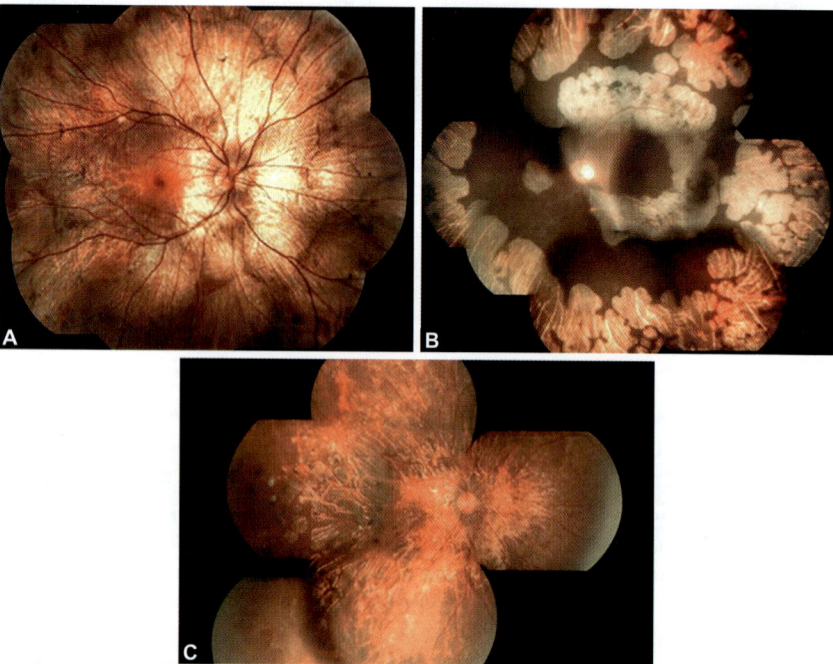

Figs. 6A to C: (A) Choroideremia with stellate macula and surrounding retinal pigment epithelium (RPE) atrophy; (B) Gyrate atrophy: characteristic scalloped margin RPE atrophy in midperiphery; (C) Late-onset retinal macular degeneration (LORMD): RPE atrophy with scalloped edges in periphery with scalloped edges.

gressive retinal vessels narrowing and no or minimal changes in RPE and optic disk. ERG shows markedly decreased "b" wave with normal "a" wave. The retinopathy is most frequently noted with small cell carcinoma of lung. It has been proposed that this is due to an autoimmune mechanism where antibodies are formed against bipolar cells of retina.[52-54] Night blindness has also been associated with metastatic cutaneous melanoma.[54-58] It is characterized with features of acute anterior and posterior uveitis, patchy depigmentation of choroid, vitiligo, dysacousia, and severe visual loss.

Siderosis

Siderosis is caused secondary to retained intraocular iron foreign body characterized by iris heterochromia, atonic pupil, and brown deposits over anterior capsular region of the lens.[59,60] Fundus in early stage may present optic disk hyperemia with no other change. While in the late stage, it simulates degeneration of retina with RPE pigmentation, arteriolar narrowing, and loss of peripheral visual field. ERG in the early phase has transient increase in both "a" and "b" waves. With time, "b" wave decreases and may be extinguished.[60,61] Retinal changes occur due to oxidative cell death because of free radicals resulting from ferrous oxidation, which gets deposited in intraocular epithelial structures.

Drug Toxicity

Patients on more than 800 mg/day of thioridazine can develop thioridazine toxicity characterized by night blindness and blurring of central vision.[62,63] Early toxicity shows few areas of pigmentation, which become coarser as condition progresses. In the advanced stage, it simulates fundus picture of choroideremia with diffuse atrophy of choriocapillaris and RPE. ERG shows decreased amplitude of both rod and cone responses where both "a" and "b" waves are decreased. Similar features can be seen in chlorpromazine and chloroquine toxicity.

■ PATHOPHYSIOLOGY

The pathophysiology of night blindness is complex and depends on the underlying disease process. Inherited gene mutations produce abnormal or absent versions of proteins essential for photoreceptor function. Many gene mutations have been identified in RP, choroideremia, and CSNB.[64] Vitamin A (retinol) is required for photoreceptors to produce essential proteins involved in the phototransduction cycle, deficiency of which causes photoreceptor dysfunction, which can result in the symptom of night blindness. In gyrate atrophy, high levels of ornithine due to deficiency in ornithine delta aminotransferase enzyme lead to night blindness. Antibodies against retinal cells in paraneoplastic retinopathy can lead to night blindness, while degeneration of photoreceptors occurs due to oxidative damage in patient with a retained intraocular iron foreign body.

APPROACH TO THE PATIENT OF NYCTALOPIA
History
A history of the onset, duration, and progression of night blindness should be noted. The patient should be asked about reduced vision during the daytime or problems in distinguishing color. A past ophthalmic history is important to exclude conditions that may cause blurred vision at low light levels (rather than true night blindness), like history of previous refractive surgery.[65] The patient's past medical history including any previous history of gastric or abdominal surgery, alcohol intake, and symptoms of intestinal malabsorption; identify possible cause of vitamin A deficiency. Any history of previous treatment for cancer should also be excluded, specifically malignant melanoma.[55] A detailed family history should be taken as many conditions are inherited and mode of inheritance should be identified.[1]

Examination
Ocular examination, including the patient's visual acuity, pupillary responses, lens opacity, visual fields, and detailed fundus evaluation should be done. ERG and dark adaptation tests help to confirm the diagnosis of night blindness and also the extent of rod and cone involvement. Visual field is recorded for determination of peripheral field loss and OCT helps to check for macular changes.

A general medical examination should be carried out to exclude a systemic cause for the night blindness, or to document associated systemic findings in an inherited retinal condition or if syndromic association is suspected. Measurement of serum vitamin A (retinol) may be indicated, if the patient has a known risk factor for its deficiency. Genetic testing to confirm the gene involved is available for inherited diseases such as CSNB, RP, choroideremia, and gyrate atrophy.

TREATMENT
Treatment varies according to the underlying etiology. Various treatment modalities have been tried in RP like vitamin A, oral supplementation of docosahexaenoic acid, and lutein supplements.[66,67] But till date, there is no definite therapy for RP and other genetic disorders. Recently, new gene therapy has been approved by Food and Drug Administration (FDA) (*RPE65* gene defect using AAV2 viral vector).[68,69] Children above the age of 1 year with vitamin A deficiency receive 2,00,000 IU of vitamin A orally on day 1, 2, and 8, and 1,00,000 IU if age is below 1 year.[37,70] In gyrate atrophy, arginine-restricted diet with pyridoxine supplements may help. For paraneoplastic retinopathy, treatment for primary condition along with steroids, immunosuppression and immunoglobulins has been tried.[71,72] Stopping the drugs in early stage may reverse the condition in drug toxicity.

Emerging Treatment

Gene Therapy: Adeno-associated Viral Vectors

Adeno-associated viral (AAV) vectors can be used to transfer genes to the photoreceptors and RPE cells. This treatment has been used in rats with different types of retinal degeneration. Clinical trials have also started in patients with X-linked choroideremia.[73] Voretigene neparvovec (Luxturna) has been FDA approved for gene therapy of *RPE65* gene defect in RP using AAV2 viral vector.

Stem-cell Therapy, Transplantation, and Artificial Vision

Stem cell transplantation have been tried from bone marrow,[74] adult brain derived neural progenitor cells, mesenchymal stem cells, and pluripotent stem cells but with limited success.[75,76] Neuroprotective agent, ciliary neurotrophic factor (CNTF) has been experimented in animals with minimal success and also been tried in human with encapsulated cell technology.[77,78]

Retinal Implants

Patients with extreme loss of vision, retinal implants like ARGUS II, and subretinal implants like Boston retinal implant demonstrated significant improvement in recognizing letters, spatial motor tasks but with limited visual field.[79,80]

SUMMARY

- Nyctalopia (night blindness) is impaired vision in dark environment as a result of inability to adapt to low illumination.
- Various acquired and inherited conditions cause night blindness, RP being most common.
- Mizuo phenomenon characteristically seen in Oguchi disease and also seen in cone dystrophy, enhanced S-cone syndrome, and juvenile retinoschisis.
- Appropriate history including family history and drug history has to be documented.
- Electroretinogram helps to confirm the diagnosis of night blindness and extent of cone and rod involvement.
- Hopefully, intractable conditions like, RP, choroideremia, gyrate atrophy, etc. may be managed by gene therapy and stem transplantation.

REFERENCES

1. Petzold A, Plant GT. Clinical disorders affecting mesopic vision. Ophthalmic Physiol Opt. 2006;26(3):326-41.
2. Hartong DT, Berson EL, Dryja TP. Retinitis pigmentosa. Lancet. 2006;368 (9549):1795-809.
3. Gartner S, Henkind P. Pathology of Retinitis Pigmentosa. Ophthalmology. 1982; 89(12):1425-32.

4. Berson EL. Retinitis pigmentosa: unfolding its mystery. Proc Natl Acad Sci USA. 1996;93(10):4526-8.
5. Bunker CH, Berson EL, Bromley WC, et al. Prevalence of Retinitis Pigmentosa in Maine. Am J Ophthalmol. 1984;97(3):357-65.
6. GRøNDAHL J. Estimation of prognosis and prevalence of retinitis pigmentosa and Usher syndrome in Norway. Clin Genet. 2008;31(4):255-64.
7. Jacobson SG, Kemp CM, Sung C-H, et al. Retinal Function and Rhodopsin Levels in Autosomal Dominant Retinitis Pigmentosa with Rhodopsin Mutations. Am J Ophthalmol. 1991;112(3):256-71.
8. Spalton DJ, Rahi AH, Bird AC. Immunological studies in retinitis pigmentosa associated with retinal vascular leakage. Br J Ophthalmol. 1978;62(3):183-7.
9. Birch DG, Fish GE. Rod ERGs in retinitis pigmentosa and cone-rod degeneration. Invest Ophthalmol Vis Sci. 1987;28(1):140-50.
10. Fishman GA, Gilbert LD, Fiscella RG, et al. Acetazolamide for Treatment of Chronic Macular Edema in Retinitis Pigmentosa. Arch Ophthalmol. 1989;107(10):1445.
11. Hamel C, Dessalces E, Meunier I. Retinitis Punctata Albescens. In: Peuch B, De Laey JJ, Holder GE (Eds). Inherited Chorioretinal Dystrophies. Berlin, Heidelberg: Springer Berlin Heidelberg; 2014. pp. 135-41.
12. Standish M. Retinitis Punctata Albescens. Trans Am Ophthalmol Soc. 1893;6:534-7.
13. Souied E, Soubrane G, Benlian P, et al. Retinitis punctata albescens associated with the Arg135Trp mutation in the rhodopsin gene. Am J Ophthalmol. 1996;121(1):19-25.
14. Heckenlively JR, Rodriguez JA, Daiger SP. Autosomal Dominant Sectoral Retinitis Pigmentosa. Arch Ophthalmol. 1991;109(1):84.
15. Fishman GA, Alexander KR, Milam AH, et al. Acquired unilateral night blindness associated with a negative electroretinogram waveform. Ophthalmology. 1996;103(1):96-104.
16. Mukhopadhyay R, Holder GE, Moore AT, et al. Unilateral retinitis pigmentosa occurring in an individual with a germline mutation in the RP1 gene. Arch Ophthalmol. 2011;129(7):954-6.
17. Boughman JA, Vernon M, Shaver KA. Usher syndrome: Definition and estimate of prevalence from two high-risk populations. J Chronic Dis. 1983;36(8):595-603.
18. Koenig R. Bardet-Biedl Syndrome and Usher Syndrome. In: Wissinger S, Kohl S, Langenbeck U (Eds). Genetics in Ophthalmology. Basel: KARGER; 2003. pp. 126-40.
19. Weleber RG, Gupta N, Trzupek KM, et al. Electroretinographic and clinicopathologic correlations of retinal dysfunction in infantile neuronal ceroid lipofuscinosis (infantile Batten disease). Mol Genet Metab. 2004;83(1-2):128-37.
20. Aleman TS, Cideciyan AV, Volpe NJ, et al. Spinocerebellar Ataxia Type 7 (SCA7) Shows a Cone–Rod Dystrophy Phenotype. Exp Eye Res. 2002;74(6):737-45.
21. Noble KG, Carr RE, Siegel IM. Autosomal dominant congenital stationary night blindness and normal fundus with an electronegative electroretinogram. Am J Ophthalmol. 1990;109(1):44-8.
22. Miyake Y, Yagasaki K, Horiguchi M, et al. Congenital Stationary Night Blindness with Negative Electroretinogram. Arch Ophthalmol. 1986;104(7):1013.
23. Wilder H. Oguchi's disease. Am J Ophthalmol. 1953;36(5):718-9.
24. Yamanaka M. Histologic Study of Oguchi's Disease: Its Relationship to Pigmentary Degeneration of the Retina. Am J Ophthalmol. 1969;68(1):19-26.

25. Dryja TP. Molecular genetics of Oguchi disease, fundus albipunctatus, and other forms of stationary night blindness: LVII Edward Jackson Memorial Lecture. Am J Ophthalmol. 2000;130(5):547-63.
26. Miyake Y, Horiguchi M, Suzuki S, et al. Electrophysiological findings in patients with Oguchi's disease. Jpn J Ophthalmol. 1996;40(4):511-9.
27. Nakamura M, Yamamoto S, Okada M, et al. Novel mutations in the arrestin gene and associated clinical features in Japanese patients with Oguchi's disease. Ophthalmology. 2004;111(7):1410-4.
28. Marmor MF. Long-term follow-up of the physiologic abnormalities and fundus changes in fundus albipunctatus. Ophthalmology. 1990;97(3):380-4.
29. Levy NS, Toskes PP. Fundus albipunctatus and vitamin A deficiency. Am J Ophthalmol. 1974;78(6):926-9.
30. Nakamura M, Miyake Y. Macular dystrophy in a 9-year-old boy with fundus albipunctatus. Am J Ophthalmol. 2002;133(2):278-80.
31. Pachydaki SI, Klaver CC, Barbazetto IA, et al. Phenotypic Features of Patients With NR2E3 Mutations. Arch Ophthalmol. 2009;127(1):71.
32. Dryja TP. Molecular genetics of Oguchi disease, fundus albipunctatus, and other forms of stationary night blindness: LVII Edward Jackson Memorial Lecture. Am J Ophthalmol. 2000;130(5):547-63.
33. Yamamoto H, Yakushijin K, Kusuhara S, et al. A novel *RDH5* gene mutation in a patient with fundus albipunctatus presenting with macular atrophy and fading white dots. Am J Ophthalmol. 2003;136(3):572-4.
34. Krill AE, Deutman AF, Fishman M. The cone degenerations. Doc Ophthalmol. 1973;35(1):1-80.
35. Berson EL, Gouras P, Gunkel RD. Progressive Cone-Rod Degeneration. Arch Ophthalmol. 1968;80(1):68-76.
36. Moore AT. Cone and cone-rod dystrophies. J Med Genet. 1992;29(5):289-90.
37. Sommer A. Vitamin a deficiency and clinical disease: an historical overview. J Nutr. 2008;138(10):1835-9.
38. Law WC, Rando RR. The molecular basis of retinoic acid induced night blindness. Biochem Biophys Res Commun. 1989;161(2):825-9.
39. Lee WB, Hamilton SM, Harris JP, et al. Ocular Complications of Hypovitaminosis A after Bariatric Surgery. Ophthalmology. 2005;112(6):1031-4.
40. Mele L, West KP, Kusdiono, et al. Nutritional and household risk factors for xerophthalmia in Aceh, Indonesia: a case-control study. The Aceh Study Group. Am J Clin Nutr. 1991;53(6):1460-5.
41. Harris GS, Miller JR. Choroideremia. Arch Ophthalmol. 1968;80(4):423.
42. Ghosh M, McCulloch JC. Pathological findings from two cases of choroideremia. Can J Ophthalmol. 1980;15(3):147-53.
43. Ponjavic V, Abrahamson M, Andréasson S, et al. Phenotype variations within a choroideremia family lacking the entire CHM gene. Ophthalmic Genet. 1995;16(4):143-50.
44. Seabra MC, Ho YK, Anant JS. Deficient geranylgeranylation of Ram/Rab27 in choroideremia. J Biol Chem. 1995;270(41):24420-7.
45. Renner AB, Kellner U, Cropp E, et al. Choroideremia: Variability of Clinical and Electrophysiological Characteristics and First Report of a Negative Electroretinogram. Ophthalmology. 2006;113(11):2066-2073.e2.
46. Berson EL, Schmidt SY, Shih VE. Ocular and Biochemical Abnormalities in Gyrate Atrophy of the Choroid and Retina. Ophthalmology. 1978;85(10):1018-27.

47. Takki K, Simell O. Genetic aspects in gyrate atrophy of the choroid and retina with hyperornithinaemia. Br J Ophthalmol. 1974;58(11):907-16.
48. Javadzadeh A, Gharabaghi D. Gyrate atrophy of the choroid and retina with hyper-ornithinemia responsive to vitamin B6: a case report. J Med Case Rep. 2007;1(1):27.
49. Milam AH, Curcio CA, Cideciyan AV, et al. Dominant late-onset retinal degeneration with regional variation of sub-retinal pigment epithelium deposits, retinal function, and photoreceptor degeneration. Ophthalmology. 2000;107(12): 2256-66.
50. Borooah S, Collins C, Wright A, et al. Late-onset retinal macular degeneration: clinical insights into an inherited retinal degeneration. Br J Ophthalmol. 2009;93(3):284-9.
51. Soumplis V, Sergouniotis PI, Robson AG, et al. Phenotypic findings in *C1QTNF5* retinopathy (late-onset retinal degeneration). Acta Ophthalmol. 2013;91(3):e191-5.
52. Kornguth SE, Kalinke T, Grunwald GB, et al. Anti-neurofilament antibodies in the sera of patients with small cell carcinoma of the lung and with visual paraneoplastic syndrome. Cancer Res. 1986;46(5):2588-95.
53. Grunwald GB, Kornguth SE, Towfighi J, et al. Autoimmune basis for visual paraneoplastic syndrome in patients with small cell lung carcinoma. Retinal immune deposits and ablation of retinal ganglion cells. Cancer. 1987;60(4): 780-6.
54. Rush JA. Paraneoplastic retinopathy in malignant melanoma. Am J Ophthalmol. 1993;115(3):390-1.
55. Klopfer M, Schmidt T, Leipert KP, et al. Melanoma-associated retinopathy with night blindness. Case report. Ophthalmologe. 1997;94(8):563-7.
56. Keltner JL, Thirkill CE, Yip PT. Clinical and Immunologic Characteristics of Melanoma-associated Retinopathy Syndrome: Eleven New Cases and a Review of 51 Previously Published Cases. J Neuroophthalmol. 2001;21(3):173-87.
57. Singh AD, Milam AH, Shields CL, et al. Melanoma-associated retinopathy. Am J Ophthalmol. 1995;119(3):369-70.
58. Borkowski LM, Grover S, Fishman GA, et al. Retinal findings in melanoma-associated retinopathy. Am J Ophthalmol. 2001;132(2):273-5.
59. Sandhu HS, Young LH. Ocular Siderosis. Int Ophthalmol Clin. 2013;53(4): 177-84.
60. Hope-Ross M, Mahon GJ, Johnston PB. Ocular siderosis. Eye. 1993;7(3):419-25.
61. Weiss MJ, Hofeldt AJ, Behrens M, et al. Ocular siderosis. Diagnosis and management. Retina. 1997;17(2):105-8.
62. Tekell JL, Silva JA, Maas JA, et al. Thioridazine-induced retinopathy. Am J Psychiatry. 1996;153(9):1234-5.
63. Hamilton JD. Thioridazine retinopathy within the upper dosage limit. Psychosomatics. 1985;26(10):823-4.
64. Goodwin P. Hereditary retinal disease. Curr Opin Ophthalmol. 2008;19(3): 255-62.
65. Alió JL, Piñero D, Muftuoglu O. Corneal Wavefront-guided Retreatments for Significant Night Vision Symptoms after Myopic Laser Refractive Surgery. Am J Ophthalmol. 2008;145(1):65-74.e1.
66. Hoffman DR, Locke KG, Wheaton DH, et al. A randomized, placebo-controlled clinical trial of docosahexaenoic acid supplementation for X-linked retinitis pigmentosa. Am J Ophthalmol. 2004;137(4):704-18.

67. Berson EL, Rosner B, Sandberg MA, et al. Clinical trial of docosahexaenoic acid in patients with retinitis pigmentosa receiving vitamin A treatment. Arch Ophthalmol. 2004;122(9):1297-305.
68. Russell S, Bennett J, Wellman JA, et al. Efficacy and safety of voretigene neparvovec (AAV2-hRPE65v2) in patients with RPE65-mediated inherited retinal dystrophy: a randomised, controlled, open-label, phase 3 trial. Lancet. 2017;390(10097):849-60.
69. Dias MF, Joo K, Kemp JA, et al. Molecular genetics and emerging therapies for retinitis pigmentosa: Basic research and clinical perspectives. Prog Retina Eye Res. 2017;63:107-31.
70. Apushkin MA, Fishman GA. Improvement in visual function and fundus findings for a patient with vitamin A-deficient retinopathy. Retina. 2005;25(5):650-2.
71. Guy J, Aptsiauri N. Treatment of Paraneoplastic Visual Loss with Intravenous Immunoglobulin. Arch Ophthalmol. 1999;117(4):471.
72. Keltner JL, Thirkill CE, Tyler NK, et al. Management and Monitoring of Cancer-associated Retinopathy. Arch Ophthalmol. 1992;110(1):48-53.
73. MacLaren RE, Groppe M, Barnard AR, et al. Retinal gene therapy in patients with choroideremia: initial findings from a phase 1/2 clinical trial. Lancet. 2014;383(9923):1129-37.
74. Kicic A, Shen W-Y, Wilson AS, et al. Differentiation of marrow stromal cells into photoreceptors in the rat eye. J Neurosci. 2003;23(21):7742-9.
75. Lu B, Wang S, Girman S, et al. Human adult bone marrow-derived somatic cells rescue vision in a rodent model of retinal degeneration. Exp Eye Res. 2010;91(3):449-55.
76. Joe AW, Gregory-Evans K. Mesenchymal Stem Cells and Potential Applications in Treating Ocular Disease. Curr Eye Res. 2010;35(11):941-52.
77. Sieving PA, Caruso RC, Tao W, et al. Ciliary neurotrophic factor (CNTF) for human retinal degeneration: phase I trial of CNTF delivered by encapsulated cell intraocular implants. Proc Natl Acad Sci U S A. 2006;103(10):3896-901.
78. Peterson WM, Wang Q, Tzekova R, et al. Ciliary neurotrophic factor and stress stimuli activate the Jak-STAT pathway in retinal neurons and glia. J Neurosci. 2000;20(11):4081-90.
79. Ahuja AK, Dorn JD, Caspi A, et al. Blind subjects implanted with the Argus II retinal prosthesis are able to improve performance in a spatial-motor task. Br J Ophthalmol. 2011;95(4):539-43.
80. Rizzo JF, Wyatt J, Loewenstein J, et al. Perceptual efficacy of electrical stimulation of human retina with a microelectrode array during short-term surgical trials. Invest Opthalmol Vis Sci. 2003;44(12):5362.

CHAPTER

20

Management of Ocular Burns: A Practical Approach

Jayesh Vazirani

■ INTRODUCTION

Ocular chemical and thermal injuries (collectively called ocular burns) constitute a grave hazard to the eye and form a significant proportion of overall ocular trauma. Children and young adults tend to be the demographic most likely to suffer from ocular burns. A hospital-based study from north India on pediatric ocular burns concluded that preschool age children are the likeliest to be affected, and severe visual loss is a common consequence.[1]

Ocular burns affect the entire ocular surface unit, including the periocular skin, lids and lid margins, conjunctiva, limbus and the cornea. The most profound long-term impact on the eye is limbal stem cell deficiency (LSCD). A large cohort study from India found ocular burns to be the leading cause of both unilateral and bilateral LSCD. The most common causative agent was found to be *"chuna"* (lime).[2]

■ EMERGENCY AND ACUTE PHASE MANAGEMENT

With a genuine ophthalmic emergency like burns, the immediate management is of critical importance. This makes it vital to have clear, sensible, and practical guidelines for management in the prehospital setting. The first and the most important thing to do is to limit exposure to the offending agent, and to irrigate the ocular surface with copious amounts of fluid. In most circumstances, water is the only fluid available. It is acceptable to rinse the eyes with copious amounts of water immediately following ocular burns. Provided that there are no other life-threatening injuries or severe skin burns, the patient should be subsequently shifted as soon as possible to an eye care facility.

In the clinic, following a cursory examination to rule out open globe injury, it is advisable to copiously irrigate the ocular surface with available fluids, even if it has been done earlier. Although various fluids have been concocted for this purpose, the average eye clinic is likely to have saline, Ringer lactate, or balanced salt solution readily available. Any of these may be used to irrigate the eyes for at least 20–30 minutes. Simultaneously, residual chemical particles ought to be removed from the surface and fornices after double eversion of the eyelids. Children may not allow this in the clinic, and an examination under anesthesia is imperative in such cases. Once ocular surface irrigation is complete, a detailed eye examination should be carried out, with emphasis on detecting incomplete lid closure due to eyelid burns and surface staining using fluorescein. Ocular surface staining helps to assess and classify the severity of ocular burns, according to the amount of corneal, limbal, and conjunctival surface involved[3] (Table 1).

The analog scale records accurately the limbal involvement in clock hours of affected limbus/percentage of conjunctival involvement. While calculating percentage of conjunctival involvement, only involvement of bulbar conjunctiva, up to and including the conjunctival fornices is considered.

The aims of therapy in the acute phase of ocular burns are to control inflammation, promote epithelial healing, and prevent stromal lysis. The list of agents that are believed to be useful in acute ocular burns is long, and includes artificial tears, antibiotics, topical and systemic ascorbate, acetylcysteine, cycloplegic agents, autologous serum, other biological fluids, etc. We believe the most important component in the medical therapy of acute ocular burns is the use of steroids. For severe burns, 1 hourly application of prednisolone eye drops is recommended. This may be tapered by the clinician based on evaluation of the ocular surface inflammation over time. Recent researches suggest that inflammatory cytokines released during the acute phase of ocular burns play an important role in damaging retinal ganglion cells. Administration of tissue necrosis factor (TNF)-alpha inhibition in acute burns as well as lowering of intraocular pressure provides retinal protection.[4]

It is important to serially evaluate the eye with ocular burns using fluorescein staining. Milder degrees of burns may do well with just medical therapy—

Table 1: Classification of ocular surface burns.

Grade	Prognosis	Clinical findings	Conjunctival involvement	Analog scale
I	Very good	0 clock hours of limbal involvement	0%	0/0%
II	Good	≤3 clock hours of limbal involvement	≤30%	0.1–3/1–29.9%
III	Good	>3–6 clock hours of limbal involvement	>30–50%	3.1–6/31–50%
IV	Good to guarded	>6–9 clock hours of limbal involvement	>50–75%	6.1–9/51–75%
V	Guarded to poor	>9 to <12 clock hours of limbal involvement	>75 to <100%	9.1–11.9/75.1–99.9%
VI	Very poor	Total limbus (12 clock hours) involved	Total conjunctiva (100%) involved	12/100%

Source: Dua HS, King AJ, Joseph A. A new classification of ocular surface burns. Br J Ophthalmol. 2001;85(11):1379-83.

mainly control of surface inflammation using topical steroid. Severe burns involving half or more of the limbus with adjacent corneal and conjunctival epithelial damage usually need adjunctive measures to aid epithelial healing (Fig. 1). These may include use of a bandage contact lens or application of amniotic membrane over the ocular surface. This may be combined with a lateral, or in very severe cases, a central permanent tarsorrhaphy (Fig. 2). Even after application of amniotic membrane, serial assessment of the surface is mandatory, as the procedure may have to be repeated in case of persistent epithelial defects. Perforations may necessitate the use of corneal or scleral grafts, and loss of eyelid tissue may require reconstruction using a pedicle skin flap, a free flap, or a mucous membrane graft.

The endpoint of therapy in acute ocular burns is when the ocular surface is completely covered by epithelium, there is no recurrent epithelial breakdown

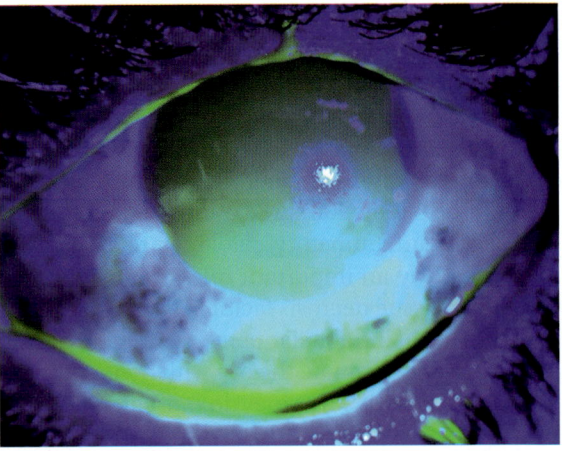

Fig. 1: Fluorescein staining of the ocular surface in acute ocular burns showing extent of corneal, limbal, and conjunctival involvement.

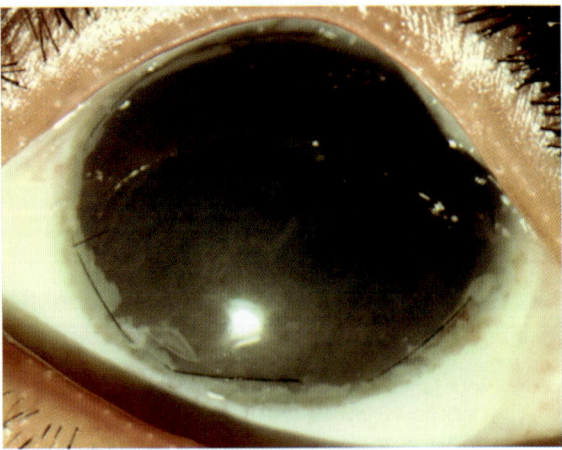

Fig. 2: Amniotic membrane application over the cornea for severe ocular burns.

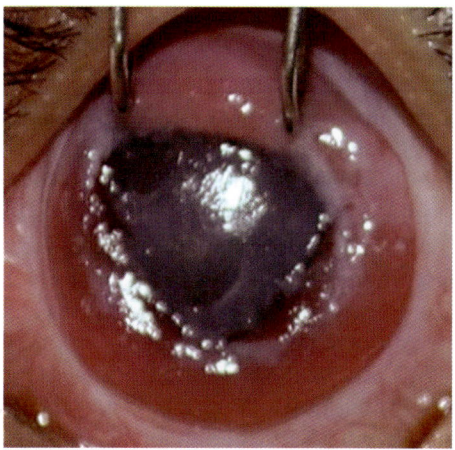

Fig. 3: Limbal stem cell deficiency after ocular burns.

and ocular surface inflammation has subsided. In the best case scenario, the limbal stem cells would repopulate the corneal surface with epithelium of a corneal epithelial phenotype. In cases with severe limbal damage, the cornea would be covered by conjunctiva, fibrovascular pannus or skin—hallmarks of LSCD (Fig. 3). These outcomes are also acceptable, as stromal lysis and perforation are prevented.

■ OCULAR SURFACE RECONSTRUCTION AND VISION RESTORATION AFTER SEVERE OCULAR BURNS

Severe degrees of ocular burns may result in damage to the periocular skin, eyelids, conjunctiva, limbus, and the cornea. Eyelid and adnexal issues should be addressed before attempting ocular surface reconstruction. Eyelid malpositions, entropion, ectropion, and lagophthalmos may need surgical correction. Once this is done, surgery for vision restoration may be contemplated. It is prudent to wait for the surface inflammation to settle down and the final extent of damage to emerge prior to reconstructive surgery—a process that usually takes a few months.

The major cause of poor vision following ocular burns is LSCD, which manifests as persistent epithelial defects, corneal vascularization, fibrovascular pannus formation over the cornea, and conjunctivalization. It is important to assess the extent of LSCD and whether it is unilateral or bilateral. Partial LSCD, in which a few clock hours of the limbus are affected, results in pannus covering some part of the cornea. Such cases may simply be observed, if the vision is good. In cases with partial LSCD with pannus encroaching on the visual axis, excision of the pannus with autologous limbal transplantation using donor limbus from the healthy part of the same eye or the fellow eye gives good results.[5]

Unilateral total LSCD secondary to ocular burns is best managed using autologous limbal tissue from the fellow eye to restore the corneal surface after pannus excision. A keratoplasty, if required for stromal scarring, is best performed later after stabilization of the ocular surface. The standard of care technique for limbal transplantation is simple limbal epithelial transplantation (SLET), which combines the benefits of earlier techniques such as conjunctival limbal autografting (CLAU) and cultivated limbal epithelial transplantation (CLET), while obviating the disadvantages of each. Using just 2 × 2 mm of donor limbal tissue, the recipient corneal surface is restored by *in vivo* expansion of limbal tissue, which is cut into multiple pieces and placed on the ocular surface after pannus excision, using amniotic membrane as a scaffold[6] (Fig. 4). The technique is highly successful in stabilizing the ocular surface as well as in improving visual acuity.[7,8]

For cases with significant bilateral LSCD, the choices for vision restoration are either allogeneic limbal transplantation or a type-1 Boston keratoprosthesis (Kpro) surgery. Donor tissue for allogeneic limbal transplantation can be from a cadaveric source or a live donor, preferably related. Results are comparable to autologous limbal transplantation, with the caveat that the recipient needs long-term systemic immunosuppressive therapy.[9] The type-1 Kpro is essentially an optically clear poly(methyl methacrylate) (PMMA) cylinder that is supported by a back plate (PMMA or titanium). The entire assembly is held in place and secured to the recipient eye using a rim of donor corneal tissue (Fig. 5). Prerequisites for implanting a type-1 Kpro are a wet ocular surface, healthy fornices, and the ability of the patient to follow-up frequently. The surgery is similar to a penetrating keratoplasty, and vision restoration is almost instantaneous. Major concerns are retrokeratoprosthetic membrane formation, glaucoma, endophthalmitis, tissue melts around the Kpro cylinder, and device extrusion.[10]

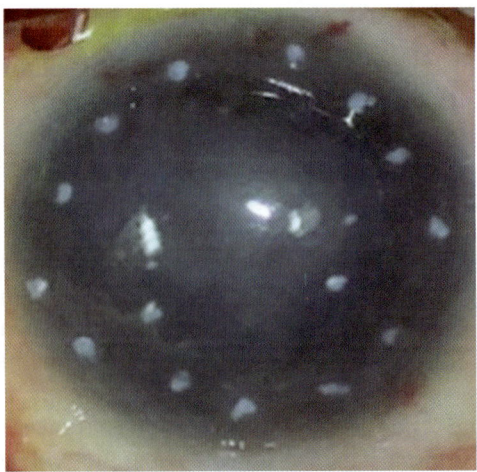

Fig. 4: Limbal transplants visible on ocular surface after simple limbal epithelial transplantation.

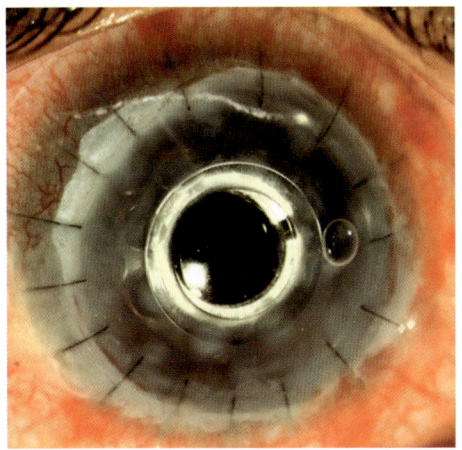

Fig. 5: Type-1 keratoprosthesis.

SUMMARY

To summarize, ocular burns constitute a genuine ophthalmic emergency. Prompt and appropriate management in the emergency and acute phases of burns can help salvage the eye. The major long-term consequence of ocular burns is LSCD. Cell-based therapy and keratoprosthesis surgery provide options for vision restoration in such cases.

REFERENCES

1. Vajpayee RB, Shekhar H, Sharma N, et al. Demographic and clinical profile of ocular chemical injuries in the pediatric age group. Ophthalmology. 2014;121(1):377-80.
2. Vazirani J, Nair D, Shanbhag S, et al. Limbal Stem Cell Deficiency-Demography and Underlying Causes. Am J Ophthalmol. 2018;188:99-103.
3. Dua HS, King AJ, Joseph A. A new classification of ocular surface burns. Br J Ophthalmol. 2001;85(11):1379-83.
4. Dohlman CH, Cade F, Regatieri CV, et al. Chemical Burns of the Eye: The Role of Retinal Injury and New Therapeutic Possibilities. Cornea. 2018;37(2):248-51.
5. Vazirani J, Basu S, Kenia H, et al. Unilateral partial limbal stem cell deficiency: contralateral versus ipsilateral autologous cultivated limbal epithelial transplantation. Am J Ophthalmol. 2014;157(3):584-90.
6. Sangwan VS, Basu S, MacNeil S, et al. Simple limbal epithelial transplantation (SLET): a novel surgical technique for the treatment of unilateral limbal stem cell deficiency. Br J Ophthalmol. 2012;96(7):931-4.
7. Vazirani J, Ali MH, Sharma N, et al. Autologous simple limbal epithelial transplantation for unilateral limbal stem cell deficiency: multicentre results. Br J Ophthalmol. 2016;100(10):1416-20.
8. Basu S, Sureka SP, Shanbhag SS, et al. Simple Limbal Epithelial Transplantation: Long-Term Clinical Outcomes in 125 Cases of Unilateral Chronic Ocular Surface Burns. Ophthalmology. 2016;123(5):1000-10.

9. Basu S, Fernandez MM, Das S, et al. Clinical outcomes of xeno-free allogeneic cultivated limbal epithelial transplantation for bilateral limbal stem cell deficiency. Br J Ophthalmol. 2012;96(12):1504-9.
10. Shanbhag SS, Saeed HN, Paschalis EI, et al. Boston keratoprosthesis type 1 for limbal stem cell deficiency after severe chemical corneal injury: A systematic review. Ocul Surf. 2018;16(3):272-81.

CHAPTER 21

Cerebral Angiography in Neuro-ophthalmology

Hima Pendharkar

■ INTRODUCTION

Wilhelm Conrad Röntgen's discovery of X-rays in 1895 revolutionized the world of medicine. The history of angiography which is the fluoroscopic visualization of the vascular system—arterial or venous—by the introduction of contrast medium dates back to 1927 when Egaz Moniz pioneered cerebral angiography. By the early 1950s crude fluoroscopy was available for clinical use and two simultaneous developments gave added impetus to the refinement of diagnostic angiography. In 1952, the first synthetic vascular bypass graft was placed and, in 1953, Seldinger described the use of a hollow-bore needle and guidewire system for accessing the femoral artery. Dotter percutaneously dilated a tight localized stenosis of the superficial femoral artery and thus on 16th January 1964 a new specialty was born which was formally named as "Interventional Radiology" by Alexander Margulis.

A thorough clinical evaluation of a patient presenting with symptoms referable to the ophthalmic system is indispensable to arrive at differential diagnoses. Cross-sectional imaging with either computed tomography (CT) and/or magnetic resonance imaging (MRI) with dedicated protocols is then performed to localize the lesion. Contrast administration is essential for complete evaluation of the lesion. Vascular lesions form a significant part of the spectrum of lesions identified on cross-sectional imaging. CT angiogram or MR angiogram are noninvasive modalities that help characterize the lesions well. However, the role of cerebral angiography (CA) remains indispensable in certain cases. With the advent of endovascular techniques many lesions of this spectrum can be treated completely. CA is an invasive procedure and needs careful patient selection though the risk is significantly reduced in experienced hands. A biplane catheter laboratory is the standard of operation presently; the importance of an equally competent radiologist to perform the procedures cannot be overlooked. The after care of patients plays an equally important role in obtaining good results.

INDICATIONS FOR CEREBRAL ANGIOGRAPHY

In the present time with state of art CT machines for noninvasive angiograms, the indications for a diagnostic CA are limited and include:
- To assess the hemodynamics of a given lesion
- To study the angioarchitecture of various fistulous lesions such as carotid-cavernous fistula (CCF), pial arteriovenous fistula or dural arteriovenous fistula (DAVF) and lesion such as arteriovenous malformation (AVM)
- Evaluate a vascular lesion (aneurysm) if high-end CT machine is not available.
- Evaluation of spinal vascular malformations
- Plan therapeutic endovascular procedure for complex vascular lesions.

Review of cross-sectional imaging that the patient might have with him/her is mandatory before proceeding with the angiogram.

CONTRAINDICATIONS

Absolute: Uncorrectable coagulation disorders.
Relative:
- Severe atherosclerotic disease of the access vessel
- Local infection
- Access site aneurysm.

PREPROCEDURAL WORKUP

- Complete hemogram
- Coagulation profile [prothrombin time (PT), partial thromboplastin time (PTT), and international normalized ratio (INR), platelets]
- Renal function tests
- Electrolyte status
- Human immunodeficiency virus (HIV)/hepatitis B surface antigen (HBsAg) status
- Further tests can be tailored according to the patient's condition
- The patient's drug history is required with special reference to any known drug allergies.

Consent

An informed consent from the immediate relatives after detailing the requirement of procedure, the technique, expected outcome and associated complications is absolutely essential before proceeding with the CA.

Angiography Machine

Digital subtraction angiography (DSA) is a technique for showing contrast-filled vessels without any interfering background mainly the bones. Present day DSA systems are based on digital fluoroscopy systems, which are equipped with high-end software and display facilities. The latest machines are biplane machines with flat panel detectors.[1]

Anesthesia

Most diagnostic procedures are done under local anesthesia, however at times depending on the condition of the patient, sedation or general anesthesia may be required.

Patient Position

The patient should be positioned on the table comfortably with the head secured in a special head rest. A strap should be applied if necessary to immobilize the head. The patient must be informed preprocedure about the possible sensation of the contrast including metallic taste in the mouth, warm sensation on the side of the head and face where the vessels will be injected. The patient's eyes should be covered with a blindfold to avoid apprehension that comes with seeing unfamiliar environment of the catheter laboratory.

Arterial Access

Vascular access is gained from one of the arteries—mostly the femoral artery in the groin. The brachial artery route might be used rarely as in a patient with occlusion of aortic bifurcation. However, accessing the cerebral vessels via brachial route is challenging, hence alternate imaging such as CT angiography should be considered in these patients.

■ PROCEDURE

Once the femoral artery is punctured, a sheath is placed *in situ* for continued arterial access. Heparin is administered as per standard protocol. The cerebral diagnostic catheter is then passed through this sheath and navigated under fluoroscopic guidance to the area of interest. Using a nonionic contrast medium angiography is carried out (Figs. 1A to C).

The CA begins with acquiring the anteroposterior (AP) and lateral views of the right carotid bifurcation. If there are no plaques at the bifurcation, selective right external carotid artery (ECA) and internal carotid artery (ICA) are then carried out in AP and lateral views. This is followed by the injection of the left carotid system (Figs. 2A and B) followed by the dominant-usually left vertebral artery (VA) (Figs. 2C to H). The angiogram has four phases—(1) arterial, (2) capillary, (3) early venous and (4) late venous phase and is analyzed in both AP (Figs. 3A to D) and lateral views (Figs. 4A to D) for all arteries. The amount of contrast used is approximately 8 mL for ICA and VA and about 4 mL for ECA injections. At times additional projections, three-dimensional (3D) acquisitions, selective arterial injections (may include microcatheter injection) and magnified views are also taken. Adequate knowledge of the catheters and wires to be used are absolutely essential especially when accessing tortuous arteries. After the angiogram, the sheath is removed and hemostasis achieved by manual compression of puncture site or at times by use of closure devices. Adequate measures are taken to minimize radiation exposure to all present in the catheter laboratory.

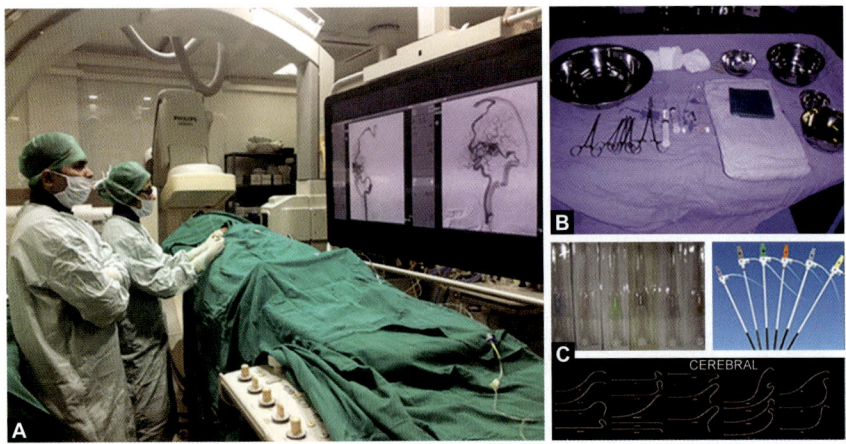

Figs. 1A to C: (A) A cerebral angiogram is in progress. The two tubes of the machine are toward the head end of the patient. A large screen with multiformatting capabilities displays angiographic images; (B) The preparation for proceeding with an angiogram; (C) Clockwise: the needles, sheaths, and catheters that are used for a cerebral angiogram. These are color coded for easy identification.

Pediatric Patient

The angiographic protocol *per se* remains the same. However, the choice of puncture needle, access sheath, diagnostic catheter, heparin dosage, and contrast used are all tailored as per the weight of the child.

COMPLICATIONS

The CA is an invasive procedure. The stated risk of complications associated with a CA is 1.3%.[2] General complications of any angiographic procedure include:
- Puncture site hematoma
- Arterial thrombosis
- Pseudoaneurysm
- Arteriovenous fistula
- Contrast reaction
- Contrast-induced renal failure

A Word of Caution

Clinical examination should identify markers such as abnormal facies in a given patient to identify those with a connective tissue disorder such as Ehlers-Danlos syndrome. Given the vascular fragility in these patients causing arterial dissections[3] and attendant complications, diagnostic CA should never be considered as first investigation for vascular evaluation. CT angiogram provides similar necessary information.

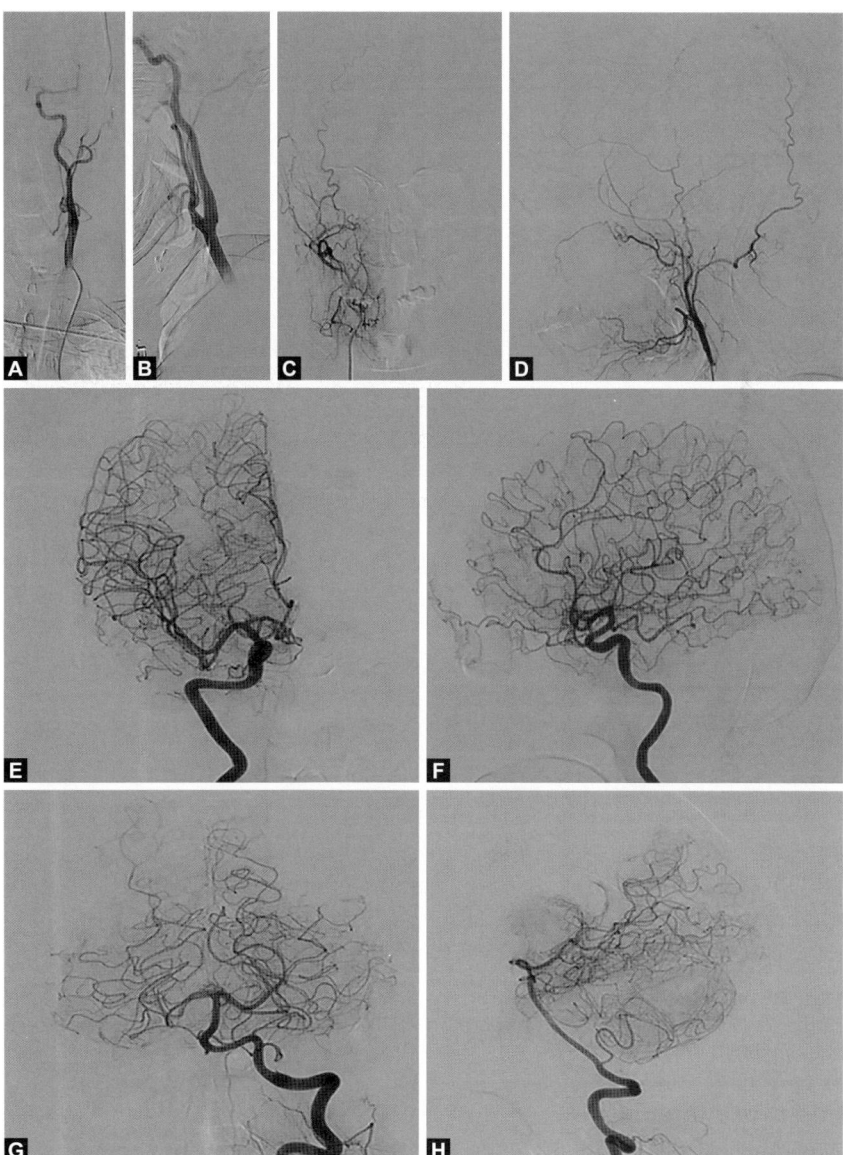

Figs. 2A to H: (A) Anteroposterior; (B) Lateral view of the left carotid bifurcation show a normal luminal contour; (C and D) Right external carotid artery (RECA) anteroposterior and lateral view: normal filling of branches of the external carotid artery (ECA); (E and F) Right internal carotid artery (RICA) anteroposterior and lateral view: normal filling of the intracranial branches in anterior cerebral artery (ACA) and middle cerebral artery (MCA) territory. *Note:* Fetal posterior cerebral artery (PCA) supplying the corresponding right territory; (G and H) Left vertebral artery (VA) anteroposterior and lateral view: normal filling of the posterior fossa parenchyma.

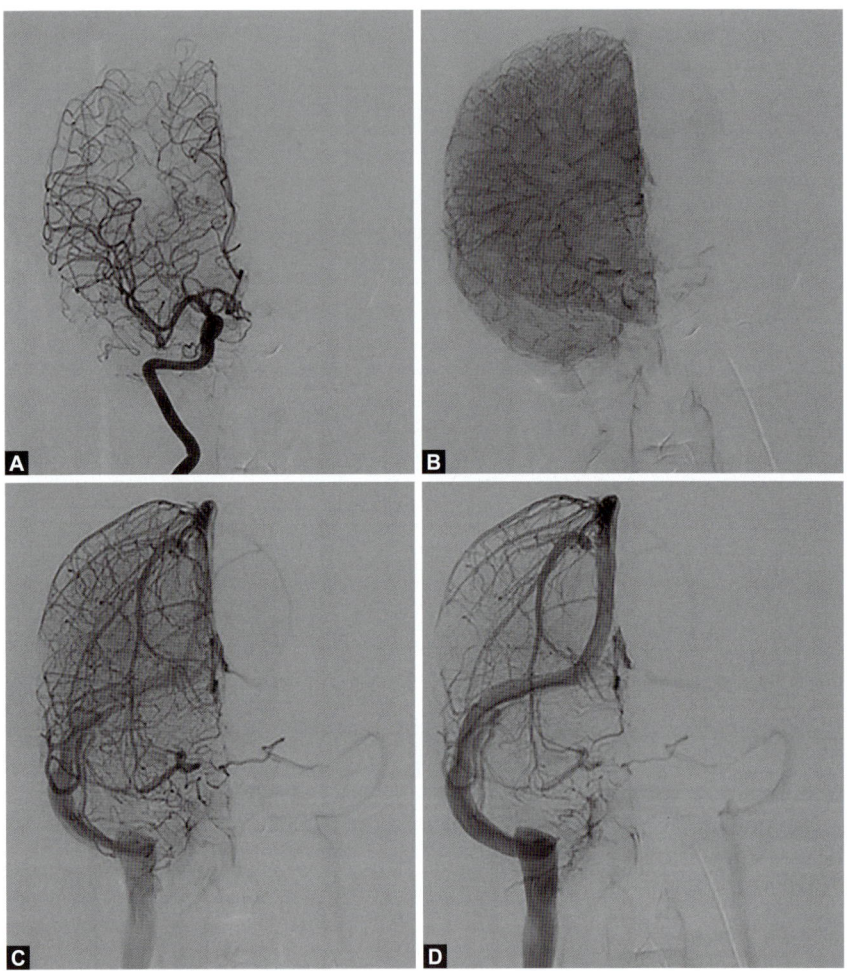

Figs. 3A to D: Right internal carotid artery (RICA) anteroposterior (AP) view: (A) Arterial phase; (B) Capillary phase; (C) Early venous phase; (D) Late venous phase of a normal cerebral angiogram.

Postprocedure Care

A patient who has undergone an uncomplicated CA can be monitored in the ward. The leg in which the artery was accessed should be immobilized for 8 hours. Any bleeding from puncture site, change in neurological status or absence of a peripheral pulse that was palpable preprocedure need to be informed to the radiologist immediately. Antibiotics are not routinely administered after a diagnostic CA.

Report

A report detailing the findings should be provided to the patient. Relevant images depicting the lesions should also be given to the patient for reference and records.

Cerebral Angiography in Neuro-ophthalmology

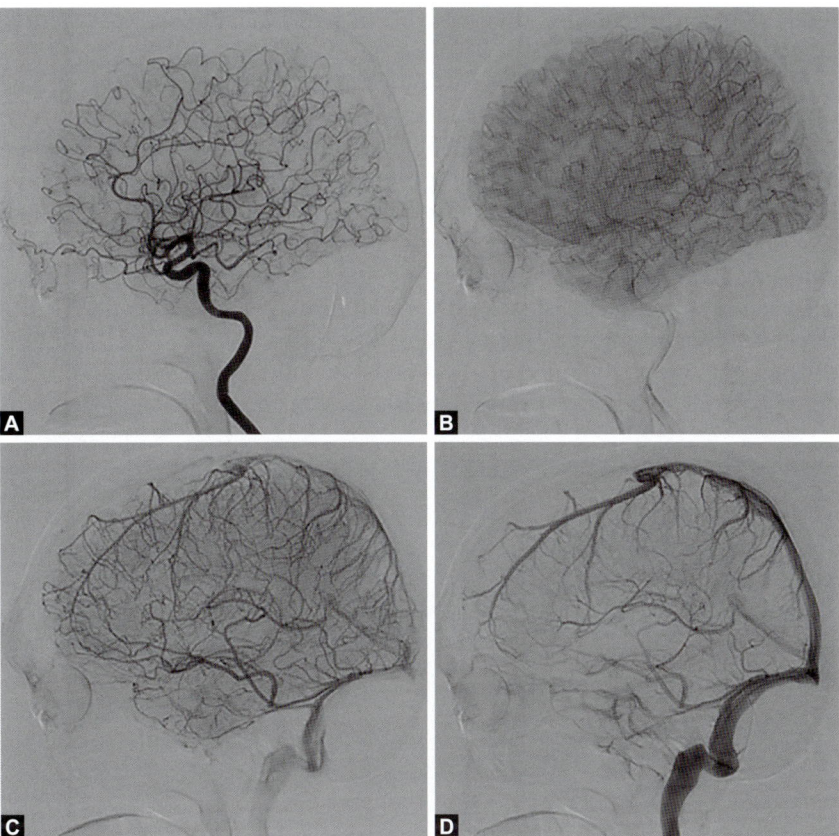

Figs. 4A to D: Right internal carotid artery (RICA) lateral view: (A) Arterial phase; (B) Capillary phase; (C) Early venous; (D) Late venous phase of a normal cerebral angiogram. *Note:* The hypoplastic anterior-third of the superior sagittal sinus; the frontal lobe is drained by a prominent parietal vein, which joins the sagittal sinus at its mid segment, variant anatomy.

ADVANCES IN CEREBRAL ANGIOGRAPHY: 3D-DIGITAL SUBTRACTION ANGIOGRAPHY

With the patient supine on the table, the right femoral artery is accessed with a 6F sheath. A 5F standard angiographic catheter is navigated to the artery of interest and connected to a pressure injector. For 3D-DSA, an initial rotational acquisition (a 200° rotation of the AP X-ray tube around the patient's head (angular velocity, 40° per second) is obtained before administration of the contrast agent and serves as a mask sequence for the subsequent subtraction process. A second identical rotational acquisition is performed as the contrast agent selectively flows through the arterial tree of interest. Volumes of contrast agent and rates for rotational acquisitions are as per standard institutional protocols. Subtracting the mask images from the contrast-enhanced images with matching angles then creates rotational DSA images. A detailed 3D representation of the vascular tree is finally generated from the rotational DSA dataset by using a 3D reconstruction algorithm. This mode of reconstruction produces the 3D images available on most modern angiographic units.[4]

Three-dimensional-DSA has now become an established tool in routine cerebral angiography. It provides more-detailed vascular information than standard two-dimensional (2D) angiography. It allows the possibility of free rotation of images, exquisite anatomic information, the lack of over projecting bony structures and extensive postprocessing capabilities all of which help in choosing the most appropriate working projection for subsequent endovascular therapy.[4-8] Postprocessing tools provide images in formats such as shaded surface display (SSD), maximum intensity projection (MIP), translucent rendering, etc. (Figs. 5A to E).

However, the limitation of 3D-DSA is the inability to provide information about osseous structures surrounding the aneurysm. 3D digital angiograms

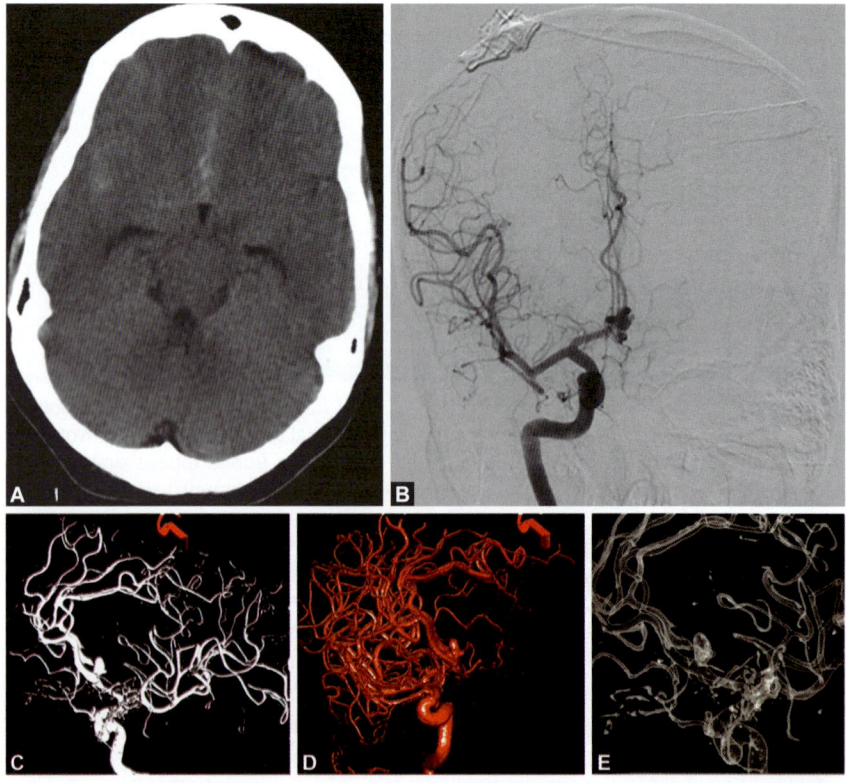

Figs. 5A to E: (A) Noncontrast computed tomography (CT) shows diffuse subarachnoid hemorrhage (SAH) in the anterior interhemispheric fissure and the right sylvian fissure; (B) Right internal carotid artery (RICA) anteroposterior (AP) view: the aneurysm was elongated, measured 6 mm × 4 mm and was directed cranially; (C) Right internal carotid artery (RICA) shaded surface display (SSD): the two daughter blebs along its posterior surface are best depicted in this figure; (D) Right internal carotid artery (RICA) injection: a different colored image of the shaded surface display (SSD) in a different projection also shows relevant details of the aneurysm; (E) Right internal carotid artery (RICA) injection: a transparent rendering of the 3D images can also be obtained.

(3D-DA) overcome this limitation. 3D-DA is a new reconstruction algorithm that allows simultaneous 3D display of the osseous and vascular information acquired through a rotational CA. Because 3D-DA uses a part of the dataset necessary to generate 3D-DSA images, both 3D-DA and 3D-DSA images can be reconstructed from a single rotational angiogram. The concomitant representation of vascular structures and their osseous surroundings allows 3D-DA to combine the spatial resolution of 3D-DSA with the topographic information previously offered by only CT angiography.[4]

A biplane DSA machine with features of 3D-DSA and 3D-DA eventually leads to a decrease in total number of DSA exposures in every procedure—diagnostic and during endovascular procedures which eventually reduces the number of exposures thus limiting the side effects of radiation.[8]

■ CASE STUDIES

Case 1

A 50-year-old male presented with sudden severe headache and transient loss of consciousness on the prior evening. He then underwent a DSA which revealed an aneurysm of the anterior communicating artery. Various reconstruction algorithms were used to demonstrate different aspects of aneurysm morphology in this patient (Figs. 5A to E). He subsequently underwent surgical clipping of the aneurysm.

Case 2

A 25-year-old female presented with right-sided headache on and off for 1 year. MRI brain revealed a large AVM in the region of the right basal ganglia, hypothalamus and thalamus. She was subjected to a CA (Figs. 6A to J) which revealed multiple AVMs.

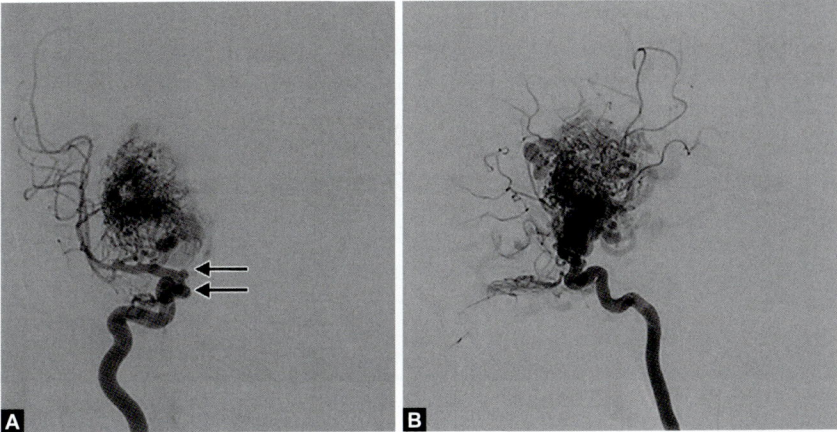

Figs. 6A and B: (A) Right internal carotid artery (RICA) anteroposterior (AP) view: revealed the feeders from hypertrophied lenticulostriate arteries. Aneurysms (arrows) were noted at the communicating segment of the right internal carotid artery (ICA) and at right ICA bifurcation [because of increased hemodynamic flow to the arteriovenous malformation (AVM)]; (B) Right internal carotid artery (RICA) lateral view: in addition to the arterial feeders it also demonstrates abnormal vessels from the right ophthalmic artery (OA) to the right orbital region.

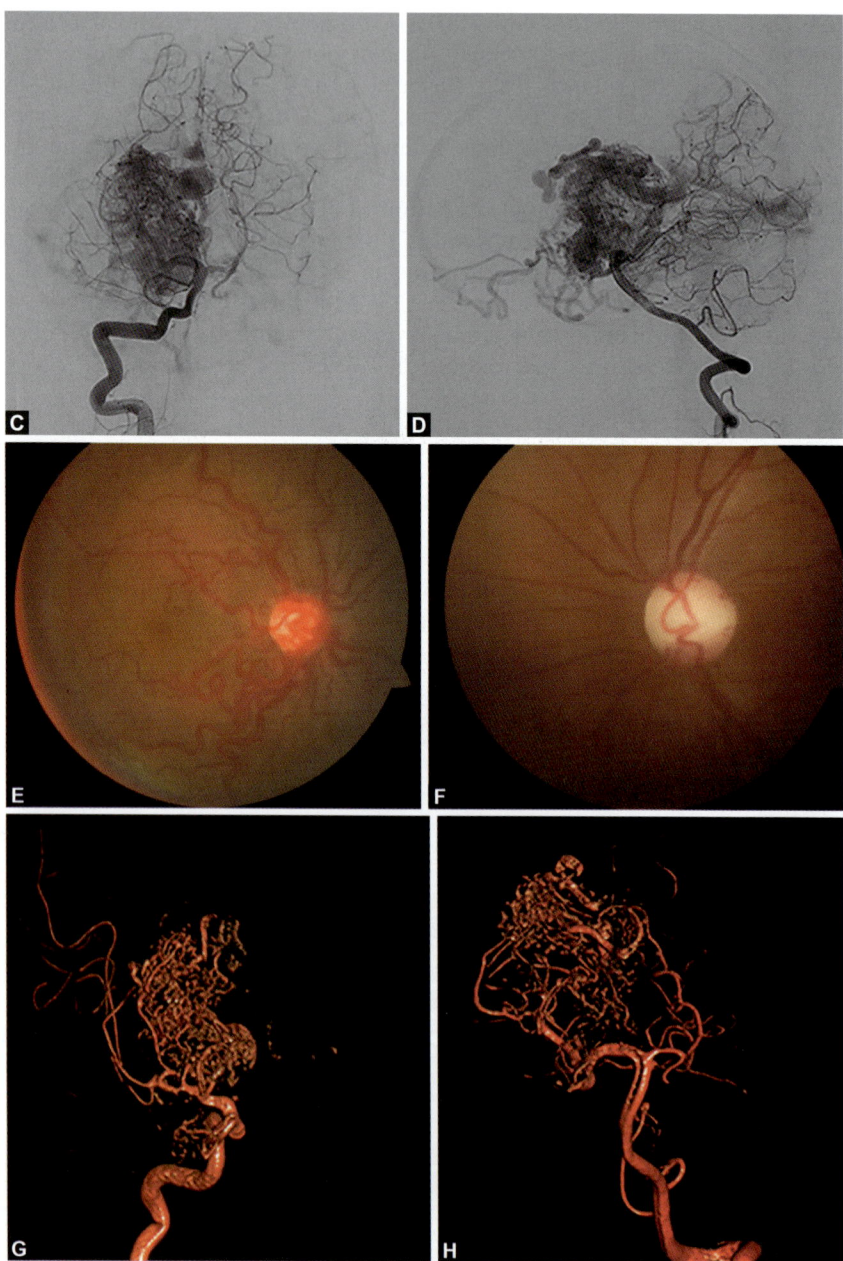

Figs. 6C to H: (C) Right vertebral artery (RVA) anteroposterior (AP) view: shows the contribution from the thalamoperforators; (D) Right vertebral artery (RVA) lateral view: shows the arterial feeders, the arteriovenous malformation (AVM) nidus and the venous drainage of the AVM to the vein of Galen as also to the anterior-third of the superior sagittal sinus; (E) The fundus revealed a retinal arteriovenous malformation (AVM) on the right. (F) Note the normal vessels of the left fundus; (G) 3D reconstructed images of the angiogram of this patient demonstrate the internal carotid artery (ICA) aneurysms well in addition to the details of the arterial feeders; (H) Vertebral artery (VA) anteroposterior view.

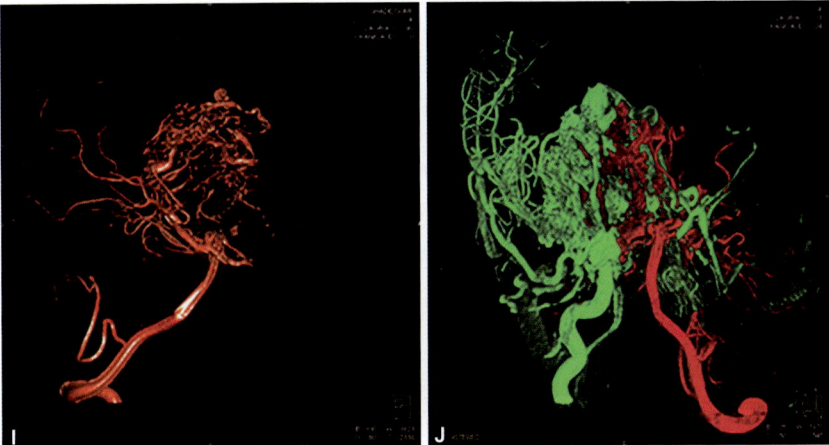

Figs. 6I and J: (I) VA lateral view demonstrates in exquisite detail the anatomy of the feeding artery and the nidus. Rotation and manipulation of these images on work station provide additional information that is required for endovascular management; (J) Fused 3D image: internal carotid artery (ICA) (green color) and the vertebral artery (VA) (red color) acquisitions are fused on the work station using vendor-specific software to assess the differential contribution of various arteries to arteriovenous malformation (AVM) that involve larger anatomic regions.

This was a case of a type 2 cerebral arterial metameric syndrome (CAMS). This is a condition where AVM is noted involving the lateral prosencephalic (optic) group with involvement of the optic nerve, retina, parieto-temporal-occipital lobes, thalamus and maxilla, i.e. AVM are noted at multiple sites along this pathway. A somatic mutation developing in the region of the neural crest or adjacent cephalic mesoderm before migration causes AVM with a segmental distribution.[9] The various angiographic acquisitions in this case demonstrate the capability of the present-day technology.

Case 3

A 25-year-old male presented with left-sided proptosis, conjunctival congestion (Fig. 7A), and watering of eyes 3 weeks following a road traffic accident. His cerebral angiogram revealed a direct CCF (Figs. 7B and C).

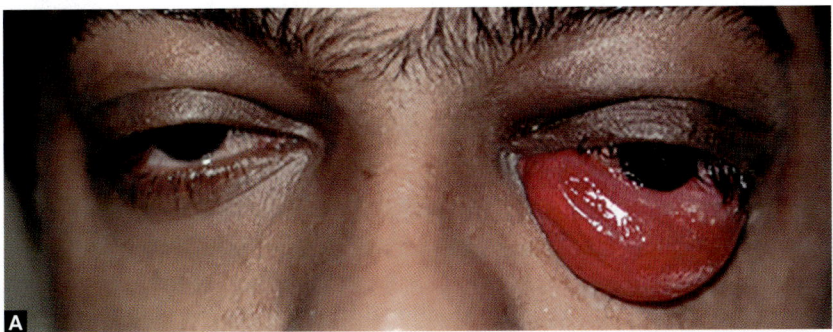

Fig. 7A

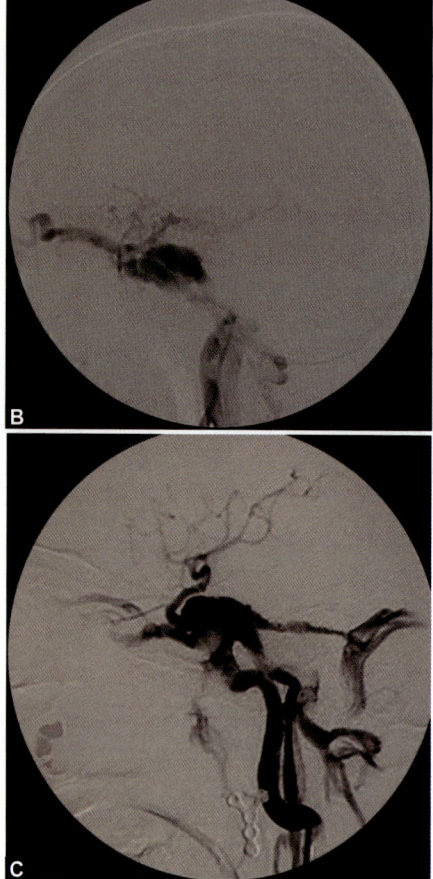

Figs. 7B and C

Figs. 7A to C: (A) A patient with left direct carotid-cavernous fistula (CCF) has proptosis and lower lid conjunctival congestion; (B) Left internal carotid artery (LICA) lateral view: a direct CCF with venous drainage to the superior ophthalmic vein as also to the inferior petrosal sinus. Note the paucity of forward flow intracranially suggesting this to be a high-flow fistula; (C) Right internal carotid artery (RICA) lateral view in a patient with a direct CCF after placing a balloon across the rent demonstrates the venous drainage to the superior ophthalmic vein, inferior petrosal sinus (IPS), and superior petrosal sinus (SPS). If additional balloons do not occlude the fistula, any of the venous routes demonstrated here may be used to place coils in the cavernous sinus and close the fistula.

Diagnostic CA is mandatory in patients with CCF to evaluate the anatomy and plan the access route for endovascular embolization.

Case 4

A 40-year-old female patient with a pineal mass was referred for a cerebral angiogram. Immediate postprocedure she had aphasia. MRI revealed an acute infarct in left MCA territory (Figs. 8A to D). At times thrombus may get dislodged into the intracranial circulation during angiogram causing vascular occlusion.

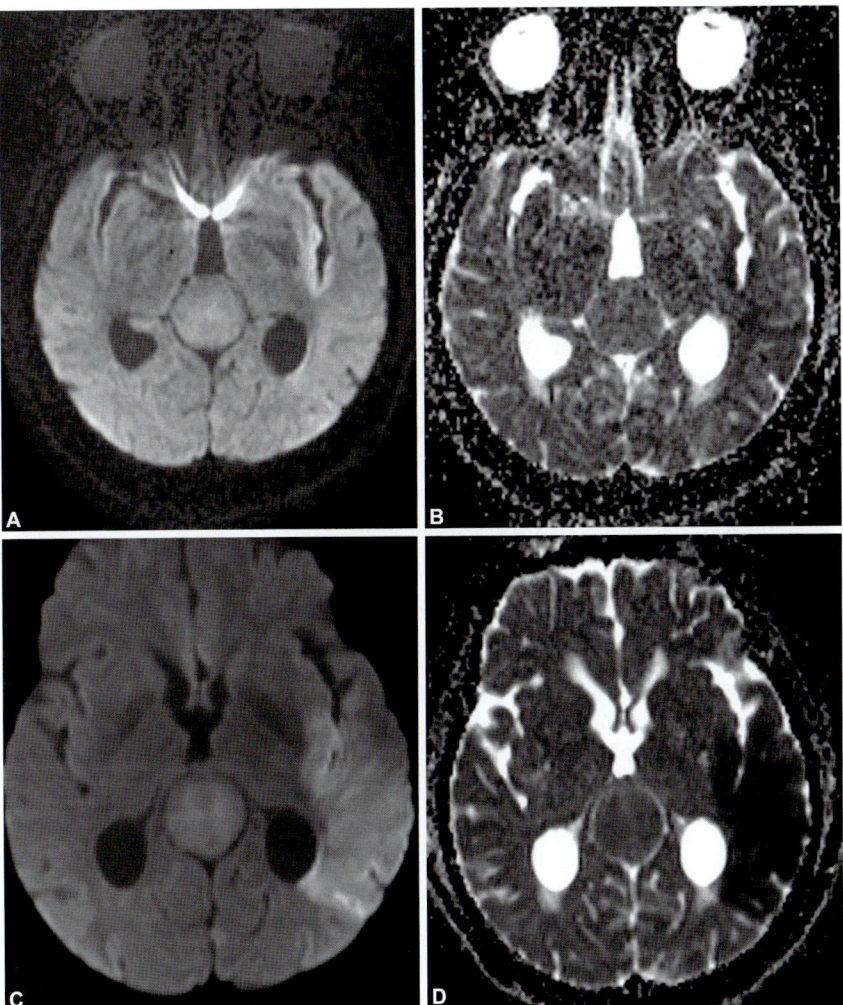

Figs. 8A to D: Preprocedure diffusion weighted imaging (DWI) trace images; (B) Preprocedure apparent diffusion coefficient (ADC) map revealed no diffusion restriction in the pineal mass and no parenchymal abnormality; (C) Postcerebral angiogram: diffusion weighted imaging (DWI) trace image; (D) Postcerebral angiogram apparent diffusion coefficient (ADC) image after aphasia was noticed reveals hyperintensity on trace image with corresponding hypointensity on ADC maps suggesting diffusion restriction implying an acute infarct in left middle cerebral artery (MCA) territory.

CONCLUSION

Cerebral angiogram is indispensable for evaluation of vascular lesions as discussed. It is important to understand the need for dedicated neuro-radiologists for best results. An integrated approach toward the diagnosis and management in these patients is absolutely essential. Equally important is the after care of these patients. Optimal use of the ever-advancing technology and refined human skills can be used for the advantage of the mankind.

REFERENCES

1. Seibert JA. Flat-panel detectors: how much better are they? Pediatr Radiol. 2006;36(Suppl 2):173-81.
2. Willinsky RA, Taylor SM, TerBrugge K, et al. Neurologic Complications of Cerebral Angiography: Prospective Analysis of 2,899 Procedures and Review of the Literature. Radiology. 2003;227:522-8.
3. North KN, Whiteman DAH, Pepin MG, et al. Cerebrovascular complications in Ehlers-Danlos syndrome type IV. Ann Neurol. 1995;38:960-4.
4. Gailloud P, Oishi S, Murphy K. Three-dimensional Fusion Digital Subtraction Angiography: New Reconstruction Algorithm for Simultaneous Three-Dimensional Rendering of Osseous and Vascular Information Obtained during Rotational Angiography. AJNR Am J Neuroradiol. 2004;25:571-3.
5. van Rooij WJ, Peluso JPP, Sluzewski M, et al. Additional Value of 3D Rotational Angiography in Angiographically Negative Aneurysmal Subarachnoid Hemorrhage: How Negative is Negative? AJNR Am J Neuroradiol. 2008;29:962-6.
6. Hochmuth A, Spetzger U, Schumacher M. Comparison of three-dimensional rotational angiography with digital subtraction angiography in the assessment of ruptured cerebral aneurysms. AJNR Am J Neuroradiol. 2002;23:1199-205.
7. Hirai T, Korogi Y, Suginohara K, et al. Clinical usefulness of unsubtracted 3D digital angiography compared with rotational digital angiography in the pretreatment evaluation of intracranial aneurysms. AJNR Am J Neuroradiol. 2003;24:1067-74.
8. Abe T, Hirohata M, Tanaka N, et al. Clinical benefits of rotational 3D angiography in endovascular treatment of ruptured cerebral aneurysm. AJNR Am J Neuroradiol. 2002;23:686-8.
9. Krings TS, Geibprasert CB, Luo JJ, et al. Segmental Neurovascular Syndromes in Children. Neuroimag Clin N Am. 2007;17:245-58.

Index

Page numbers followed by 'f' and 't' indicate figures and tables, respectively.

A

Abbott Medical Optics 117
Aberrometry-guided devices 125, 132
Ab-externo
    continuous loop fixation 190
    four-point fixation with haptic looping 191
    insertion of suture 189
    scleral fixation 190
    technique, subsequent variations 189
    two-point fixation 190
Ablation
    depth 8
    ratio 8
Acetylcysteine 303
AcrySof IQ PanOptix IOL 117
Acute retinal necrosis syndrome 276
Adeno-associated viral vectors 297
Aflibercept 217, 227, 228
    after ranibizumab intravitreal injections 2 226
    treated cases 269
Age-related eye disease study 227
Age-related fibrillopathy 135
Age-related macular degeneration 53, 116, 211, 222, 226, 227
    trials of treatment 224t, 226t, 227t
Ahmed
    capsule tension segment 173, 174, 174f, 175
    CT segment 176f
    glaucoma valve 80, 80f, 84f
        various models of 80t
    segment, steps of scleral fixation of 182f
Air pump assisted technique 29f
Akreos lens 195
Aladdin HW3.0 95, 96f
Albinism 46
Alpostadil 228
American Academy of Ophthalmology 1
American Society of Cataract and Refractive Surgery 1, 108

Amniotic membrane application 304f
Anacetrapib evaluation effects of 215
Angioanalytics 242, 243f
    use of 248f
Angioarchitecture of fistulous lesions 310
Angiography
    in retinal diseases 236
    machine 310
AngioVue OCT angiography software 240, 240f
Aniridia 76f
    with glaucoma 77
Anterior assisted levitation 165
Anterior chamber 135
    depth 90, 112, 136
    intraocular lens 167f
    sudden deepening of 160f
Anterior lamellar keratoplasty, recent advances in 32
Anterior segment optical coherence tomography 5f, 150, 151f
Anterior vitrectomy 185
Antiangiogenic factor 264
Anti-infective agents 283
Anti-vascular endothelial growth factor drugs 214
Aphakia 91
Aphakic
    eye blocked 87f
    glaucoma 76
    refraction 108
Arcuate
    incision 119f, 120
    keratotomies 123
Argon laser trabeculoplasty, treated eyes 67
Argos 97, 97f
Arrestin gene 291
Arterial
    access 311
    and vein occlusions 53
    dissections, causing 312
    thrombosis 312

Arteriovenous
   fistula 312
   malformation 310, 317*f*, 319*f*
   passage time 55
Artifact 241
   corrected by software 242*f*
   correction of motion 241
   movements 242*f*
   projection 242
   white line 242*f*
Artificial
   intelligence-based formulae 103
   pupil 50
Aspirin 280
Assisted levitation
   anterior 169*f*
   posterior 169*f*
Assort toric calculator 105
Astigmatic effect of surgical incision 126
Astigmatism
   correct preexisting 117
   location of incision to reduce 118*t*
   management in cataract surgery 123
   minimize postoperative 117
Astigmatismfix.com 107
Atherosclerotic disease, severe 310
Aurolab aqueous drainage implant 78, 79*f*, 83*f*
Autoimmune diseases 12
Autologous 303
   limbal transplantation 306
Autosomal recessive 288

B

Baerveldt implant 78, 85
   various models of 78*t*
Balanced salt solution 28
Barrett
   formula 130
   toric calculator 106
   True-K formula for IOL power calculation 109
   universal 2 102
Baylor nomogram 130
Beiko and Steinert technique 202
Belin/Ambrósio enhanced ectasia 9, 10*f*
Bevacizumab 217, 222, 224, 227
   eliminates the angiogenic threat 224
   treated cases 269
Bimanual irrigation and aspiration 164
Binkhorst regression 97
Bioimaging biomarkers 268-269
Biomechanical elasticity theory 11
Biometry 90, 112
Bioptics 123, 131
Blood-retinal barrier, outer 264

Blunt trauma 171
Branch retinal vein occlusion 211, 222, 246, 248
   evaluation of efficacy and safety 222
Branched retinal artery occlusion 247
   vascular network 255*f*
Brimonidine 228
Brown's syndrome 85
Bruch's membrane 239
Bubble, types of 25*f*
Burst mode power modulation 114*f*

C

Calcium channel blockers 64
Callisto 93*f*
Camellin-Calossi for postrefractive eyes 97
Candesartan 213
Cannula-based intrascleral tuck 203
Capillary dropout 239
   nonperfusion 277
   phase 315*f*
Capsular bag 172*f*
   devices 174*f*
   fibrosis 199*f*
   IOL complex, late spontaneous dislocation of 199*f*
   support, choice of 77*f*
Capsular hooks 172
   with long blunt loop 173*f*
Capsular support device 179
   for subluxated lenses 171
Capsular tension ring 141, 177
   insertion steps 181*f*
Capsule
   assessment of 166*f*
   careful assessment of 164
   retractors 143
   tension ring 173
      different sizes of 175
      insertion, technique of 180
   tension segment 142
Capsulorhexis 140, 178
   construction 127*f*
   strategies for 179
Carcinoma-associated retinopathy 287
Cardiovascular risk in type 2 diabetes 213
Carotid artery
   external 311, 313
   internal 311
   left internal 320*f*
   right external 313
   right internal 314, 315, 316, 317, 317*f*
Carotid-cavernous fistula 310, 320*f*
Cataract
   density 136
   postvitrectomy 159*f*
   surgery 90, 112, 121, 123, 156, 320

Index

Cell division theory 68
Central
  anterior vitrectomy 164
  corneal thickness 96
  macular subfield thickness 216
  permanent tarsorrhaphy 304
  retinal vein occlusion 211, 221, 222, 246-247, 249
  serous chorioretinopathy 254
    case of 256f
  subfield thickness 217, 218, 268
  subfoveal 262
  vein occlusion study 222
Cerebral angiography 312f, 321
  3D-digital subtraction angiography 315
  advances in 315
  case studies 317-321
  complications 312
  contraindications 310
  in neuro-ophthalmology 309
  indications for 310
  preprocedural workup 310
  procedure 311
  role of 309
  used for 312
Cerebral arterial metameric syndrome 319f
Cerebral artery, left middle 321f
Champagne bubbles 70f
Chemical burns 76
Chikungunya retinitis 282
  mimic herpetic 282
Choriocapillaries 241, 254
Chorioretinal lesions 283
Choroid 250f
Choroidal dystrophies choroideremia 288
Choroidal effusion 85
Choroidal neovascular membrane 226-228, 254
  complex, size of 254f
Choroidal neovascularization 226-227, 239, 253, 283
  type I, type II, type III 253
Choroideremia 293, 296
  with stellate macula 294f
Cicatricial pemphigoid 76
Ciliary neurotrophic factor 228, 297
Ciliary processes 135
Ciliary sulcus 189
  fixation 186
  position of 197
  sclerotomy 200
Cilioretinal artery 249f
Cionni ring 173, 174f, 175
Coaxial irrigation aspiration 164f

Collagen cross-linking 12
  for management of 14f
Collateral formation 246
Color Doppler imaging 55
  advantages 56
  limitations 56
  imaging machine 55f
Cone-rod dystrophy 292
Congenital
  chorioretinal scarring 283
  glaucoma 45
  stationary night blindness 287, 288, 290
Conjunctiva 88f, 302
  mobility 80
  limbal autografting 306
Conjunctival peritomy 200
Contact lenses 13
Continuous curvilinear capsulorhexis 140
Continuous mode power modulation 113f
Contrast-induced renal failure 312
Copaxone 228
Cornea for severe ocular burns 304f
Corneal
  asphericity 6
  astigmatism 123
    preoperative assessment 123
    surgical methods for treating 126
  calcification 45
  edema 205
    severe 24
  endothelial cell 199
  evaluation 135
  hydrops, acute 32
  incisions 127f
  infection 12
  irregularities 49
  neovascularization 45
  pachymetry 47
  patch graft 82f
  power 112
  stroma in isotonic 12
  thickness spatial profile 9
  tomography measures global corneal astigmatism 124
  topography 4f, 6, 7f, 16, 18f, 47
  touch and decompensation 89
  vascularization 305
Cortical
  aspiration 180
  cleaving hydrodissection 179
  material, removal of 140
Cosmetic keratopigmentation 45
  case 45, 48f
Cultivated limbal epithelial transplantation 306

Cycloplegic agents 303
Cyclotorsion 124
Cylindrical correction of toric IOL 121
Cystitome depresses 178f
Cystoid macular edema 89, 156, 157f, 195, 205
   development of 196
Cytomegalovirus 274, 275, 276, 279
   intravitreal therapy 282
   retinitis 274, 280, 281f
   treatment 282

D

Debris, tube blocked 88f
Deep anterior lamellar keratoplasty 23
Deep capillary plexus 241
Deep inner retina OCT angiogram segmentation 241
Deep layer 249
Deeper *en face* angiograms 242
Dengue
   ophthalmic complications 283
   related foveolitis 283
   virus retinopathy 283
Deoxyribonucleic acid viruses 274
Descemet's membrane 35
   endothelial keratoplasty 23
Descemet's stripping automated endothelial keratoplasty 23
Diabetes control and complications trial 213
Diabetes mellitus
   control of 212
   prevalence of 260
Diabetic macular edema 211, 213, 214, 215, 216, 220, 269, 269f, 270f
   antivascular endothelial growth factor 214t
   bilateral 218
   bioimaging biomarkers in 268
   lasers in 214t
   patient compliance 219
   SD-OCT-based morphological classification of 266
   trials with corticosteroids in 216t
Diabetic maculopathy 214
Diabetic patient with moderate NPDR 245f
Diabetic retinopathy 211, 212, 213, 243, 260
   candesartan trials 213
   clinical research 214, 215, 216, 220, 221
   occurrence/progression of 213t
   study 220
   study, early treatment for 214
   systemic factors 213t
   vitrectomy study 221

Diamond calibrated knife 41f
Diffuse corneal opacity 46
Diffuse slit lamp examination 137f
Diffuse subarachnoid hemorrhage 316f
Diffusion weighted imaging 321f
Digital
   image-guided systems 126
   subtraction angiography 310
Disability affected life years 17
Dislocated capsular bag-IOL complex 199f
Donor
   corneoscleral graft 24
   scleral patch graft 84f
   tissue for allogeneic limbal transplantation 306
Doppler optical coherence tomography 59
   advantages 59
   limitations 59
Doppler velocimetry 53
Drainage devices, current 77
Drug toxicity 295
Dry age-related macular degeneration 223, 252
Duke-Elder's classification 147
Dural arteriovenous fistula 310

E

Ectasia cases 7
Ectropion 305
Edema, resolution of 36
Efficacy *versus* effectiveness 211
Ellipsoid zone 263
Ellipsoid zone, classification of 263
Emphysema 34
En face OCT 247f
Enalapril 213
End-diastolic volume 55
Endocapsular placement 184
Endoilluminator-assisted descemet's membrane endothelial keratoplasty 24, 26f
Endophthalmitis 89, 156, 157f, 195, 197, 205
Endoscopy-assisted scleral-fixated IOL 191
Endothelial keratoplasty 23
   recent advances in 23
Endovascular procedures 317
Enface optical coherence tomography 267, 268f
   advantages of 267
Enface thickness maps 267
Entropion 305
Epinuclear plate 154
Episcleritis 277
Epithelial downgrowth 77

Index

Epstein-Barr virus 274
Ethylenediaminetetraacetic acid 45
Excessive conjunctival scarring 76
External limiting membrane 263, 265f, 270
Extraocular
    blood 196
    needle-guided haptic insertion technique 203
Exuberant vascular proliferation 246
Eyelid malpositions 305
EyePro application 109
Eyes
    chronic rubbing of 9
    undergoing penetrating keratoplasty 197
Eyestar 900 98, 99f

F

Famciclovir 279
Femto laser-assisted arcuate keratotomy 119f
Femtodelineation technique 152, 153f
Femtosecond laser 112, 128
Femtosecond laser-assisted
    arcuate keratotomy 117, 118, 129f
    cataract surgery 147, 149, 150
    intrastromal keratopigmentation technique 43f, 44f
    LASIK 132
Fenofibrate 213
    intervention 213
Fetal posterior cerebral artery 313f
Fibrinous membrane 87f
Fibronectin 131
Fibrovascular pannus formation 305
Finesse flex loop 203
Fish-tail technique 173
Flaccid bag taut 175f
Flap replacement surgery 16
Fluocinolone acetonide intravitreal implant 216t
Fluorescein angiography 244-246, 248
Fluorescein staining of ocular surface 304f
Focal disruption 264f
Foci of retinal necrosis 275
Food and Drug Administration 60
Fornix based conjunctival flap sutured 84
Foscarnet 279
Foveal
    avascular zone 246
    retinal inner layers 269
Fuchs' dystrophy 45, 116
Fundus
    albipunctatus 291
    evaluation 46
    fluorescein angiography 249, 277
    typical retinitis pigmentosa 289f
    xerophthalmicus 292

G

Galilei G6 97f, 98
Ganciclovir 282
Ganglion cell
    complex 61f
    layer 241, 262
Gaussian optics assumes 104
Gene therapy 297
Glaucoma
    in pregnancy 68
    primary 138
    secondary 156
Glaucoma drainage devices 74, 75, 86f, 87f
    choosing 81
    indications of 76f
    types of 74
Glaucomatous eyes 55
Global disruption 264f
Glued
    intraocular lens 168f
    intrascleral haptic fixation 200
    IOL, sutureless 201f
Goldmann three-mirror goniolens 69
Gore-Tex suture 192f
Graft injected into anterior chamber 30f
Gyrate atrophy 293, 294f, 296

H

Haigis 101
Haigis-L formula 107
Handshake technique 200, 202f
Haptic
    double suture fixation to 190
    eyelet 192f
    looping method 190
    tucked, tunnel 201f
Headache, sudden severe 317
Hemoglobin A1C 213
Henderson capsule tension ring 174f
Hepatitis B surface antigen 310
Herpes simplex viruses 274
Herpetic phase, acute 277
Herpetic retinitis 274
Herpetic retinopathies 275
    features of 279t
Hill-RBF calculator 103
Hoffer-Savini LASIK IOL power tool 108
Hoffman elbow 85
Hoffman's pouch 194f
    dissection of 194f
Holladay
    IOL consultant toric preoperative planner 106
    Schema-9, types of eyes 103t

Homocystinuria 171
Host Descemetic scaffolding 31, 31*f*, 32*f*, 33*f*
Human immunodeficiency virus 274, 310
Hybrid lens 13*f*
Hydrodelineation 149*f*
Hydrodissection 140, 179
Hypertension in diabetes study 213
Hyphema 85
Hypotony 85
   early postoperative 79
   maculopathy 89
   postoperative 204

I

Iluvien acetonide 228
Implants, functioning of 74
Indocyanine green 53
   angiography 236
   investigations with 223
Inferonasal quadrant 86*f*
Inferotemporal BRVO, case of
Inflammation, types of 274
   necrotizing 274
   non-necrotizing 274
Informed consent 310
Injectable suture device 190
Internal limiting membrane 239
Interventional radiology 309
Intracameral
   gas 32
   tube 81
Intracapsular cataract extraction 186
Intracorneal ring
   segments 14
   segments management of 15*f*
Intractable glaucoma shunts 74
   complications 85
   management of 74
   placement of tube 85
   preoperative evaluation 80
   site of implantation 85
   surgical procedure 81
   use of antifibrotics 85
Intralamellar keratoplasty 16
Intraocular ab-externo suture fixation 190
Intraocular inflammation 282
Intraocular lens 184, 288
   first implanted in 1949 90
   fixation 143
   implantation 95, 164
      sutured scleral-fixated 168*f*
   insertion 181
   Master 500 93, 93*f*
   Master 700 94, 95*f*
   positioning 127*f*
   power 186
      calculation 130
      classification 101
      formulae 100
      in eyes 107
      recent advances in 90
   secondary 23
   selection 115, 143, 199
      for scleral fixation 185
   single piece 167*f*
   three piece 167*f*
   types of 185
Intraocular pressure 53, 67, 74, 199
   lowering drugs 64
Intraoperative aberrometry 99, 108
   floppy iris syndrome 115
Intrascleral
   sutureless haptic fixation, surgical technique of 199
   tunnel 200
Intrastromal
   corneal dissectors 41*f*
   keratopigmentation 42
      instruments of 41*f*
   tunnel 50
Intravitreal
   antiviral therapy 280
   triamcinolone acetonide 214, 216, 222
   vascular endothelial growth factor 253
Iridocorneal endothelial syndrome 46, 76
Iridodialysis 46
Iris
   claw lens 143, 168*f*
   coloboma 39, 46, 49
   cysts, progressive 46
   hooks 171, 172*f*
   retractors 180*f*
Ischemic maculopathy 283
Ischemic retinopathies, cases of 242

J

Jacob technique 32
   for primary pre-descemetic deep anterior lamellar keratoplasty 36*f*
Joseph valve 74

K

Keratitis 277
Keratoconus 5
Keratocyte density, loss of 11
Keratometry 93, 124
Keratopigmentation 45-46
   complications 49
   contraindications to 47
   device for superficial automated 40*f*

functional therapeutic 47f
indications 45
innovative surgical option for 39
instruments 40
pigment selection 40
practice of 39
surgical techniques 42
technologies 40
therapeutic functional 46
Keratoplasty 16
Keratoprosthesis, type-1 307f
Knot erosion 193
    intraocular lens tilt 193
    use of scleral flaps 193
    use of scleral grooves 193
Koch nomogram 118
Krupin
    implants 79
    valve 74
Kyriele's plaques 281

L

Ladas super formula 102
Lagophthalmos 305
Lamellar keratoplasty, recent advances in 23
Lamellar scleral flaps 189, 202f
    dissection of 201f
Lamellar scleral graft 196f
Lampalizumab 228
Laser Doppler flowmetry 53, 58
    advantages 58
    limitations 58
Laser Doppler velocimetry 57
    advantages 57
    limitations 58
Laser *in situ*-keratomileusis 131
Laser photocoagulation 223
Laser speckle flowgraphy 54
Laser-assisted *in situ* keratomileusis 1, 112
Lasers in glaucoma, role of 67
Lens fragmentation 152
Lens touch 87f
Lenstar LS 900 94, 94f
Leukomatous corneas, management of 39
Lid margins 302
Limbal groove 199f
    incision 190
Limbal relaxing incision 123, 117-118, 125, 128
Limbal stem cell deficiency 302, 305f
Limbal transplants visible on ocular surface 306f
Lipid-modification 215
Lisinopril 213
Loading dosage 217
Lock-and-lead technique 203
Losartan 64, 213
Low-density lipoprotein 213
Lutein antioxidant supplementation trial 227
Lymphoma 276

M

MacTel stage 5 252f
Macular edema
    assessment of implantable dexamethasone 216
    due to retinal vein occlusion 222
Macular telangiectasia type 2 248
Macular thickness map 270f
Magnetic resonance imaging 49
Malyugin ring 140
Manual intrastromal keratopigmentation 42
Manual small incision cataract surgery 140
Marfan syndrome 171
Masket method 107
    modified 108
Matrix metalloproteinase 11
Maximum intensity projection 316
McCarthy post refractive IOL calculator 109
Mean dye velocity 55
Melanoma-associated retinopathy 287
Melles technique of optical recognition 35f
Mesenchymal stem cells 297
Michelson interferometer 92
Microaneurysms and vascular beading 244f
Microaneurysms development of 243
Microbial contamination 195
Microcatheters, use of 203
Microincisional cataract surgery
    advantages in difficult situations 115
    in customization, role of 115
Microkeratome-assisted LASIK 132
Microkeratome intraocular pressure 132
Micronized mineral pigments 41
    advantages of 41
Microrhexis forceps 158
Microsurgical technology 172
Microvascular abnormalities 246
Microvitreoretinal forceps, using 23-gauge 194f
Middle cerebral artery 313
Migraine 63
Minimal pre-descemetic stroma 35
Missed ectatic pathologies 16
Mitomycin-C 85
Mixed keratopigmentation 43
Miyake-Apple view 175f
Mizuo phenomenon 291, 292f

Molteno implant 77
  various models of 77t
Morcher capsule tension ring 174f
Motility disturbances 85
Moxaverine 228
Multifocal intraocular lens 116, 116f
Multifocal IOLs 117
Myopia, high 8

N

Necrotizing retinopathies 274
  clinical features 276
  etiology 276
Neodymium:yttrium aluminum garnet laser 67
Neovascular
  age-related macular degeneration 211, 223
  complex 243f
  glaucoma 68, 76
    case of 85
  tuft 245f
Nerve fiber layer 239
Neural progenitor cells 297
Neuroprotective agent 297
Neuroprotector 228
Neuroretinal changes, signs of 262
Nidek claims 96
Nifedipine 64
Night blindness 297
Nitinol flex loop 203
Noncontrast computed tomography 316f
Nonfoldable polymethylmethacrylate 129
Nonproliferative diabetic retinopathy 243-244
Nonsteroidal anti-inflammatory drug 71, 143
Normal tension glaucoma 55
Nuclear layer, inner 239, 241
Nuclear sclerosis, grade of 114
Nucleus drop 165, 169f
Nucleus management 170
Nuijts-Solomon bubble marker 125f
Nyctalopia 287
  approach to patient of 296
  classification and causes of 287
  clinical features of specific disorders causing 288
  etiology 287
  pathophysiology 295
  treatment 296

O

OA 2000 99, 99f
Occlusive vasculopathy 275
OCTA machines 237t
Ocular blood flow
  assessment of 53
  factors affect 62
    pharmacological 64
    physiologic 62
    systemic disease 63
  in glaucoma 53
  techniques for measuring 54t
Ocular burns
  acute 304f
  classification of 303t
  emergency 302
  management of 302
  practical approach 302
  vision restoration after severe 305
Ocular
  examination 296
  hypertension 64, 68
  infections 45
  surface
    check-up for dry eye 46
    diseases 76
    reconstruction 305
  vascular dysregulation 63
Oguchi's disease 291, 292f
Ohta Y-fixation technique 202
Okulix
  ray-tracing methods 94
  uses ray tracing optics 104
Olsen formula 104
Open angle glaucoma 68, 77
  primary 68
  secondary 68
Ophthalmic
  artery, right 317
  viscosurgical device 178
Ophthalmological assessment 46
Optic
  atrophy 283
  disk 61f, 281f
  nerve head 53
    blood flow of 64
Optical biometers 91, 92
  advantages of 91
  disadvantages of 91
Optical coherence tomography 199, 226, 236, 250, 289f
  angiography 59, 236, 240f, 244, 246, 248-250f, 254-256
  advantages 62
  amplitude-based 238
  complex signal-based 238
  correlation 61
  development timeline 60f
  image processing 239
  limitations 62
  normal eyes 240

phase-based 237
principle of 236
quantification of 239
retinal disorders 243
in diabetic retinopathy 260
signal 241
Optical low coherence reflectometry 91-92, 123
Optical microangiography 60
Optiwave
refractive analysis 100
quantification tool 242
Orbital region, right 317
Oregon Health and Science University 60
Ozurdex study 217

P

Pachymetry, preoperative 7
Panretinal photocoagulation 220, 222
Paraneoplastic retinopathy with carcinoma 294
Parenchymal abnormality 321f
Pars plana
clip 85
infusion cannula 200
phacoprosthesis 191
20-gauge vitrectomy 202f
vitrectomy 166f, 270
Partial coherence interferometry 91-92, 112
Patent iridotomy 68
Peak systolic velocity 55
Pegaptanib sodium 227
Pellucid marginal degeneration 5
Penetrating keratoplasty 23
Pentacam AXL 97, 98f
Peribulbar block 81
Periocular skin 302
Peripapillary retina 281f
Peripheral
cornea 199f
corneal 128
relaxing incisions 117
iridectomy 29
retina 275, 281
zone 137
Periphlebitis 277
Perivascular retina 278
Persistent epithelial defects 305
Petrosal sinus, superior 320
Phaco probe 163
removal of 163f
Phacodonesis 137, 176
Phacoemulsification 138, 176, 177, 179, 184
in subluxated lenses 171
stage of 114

surgery, development of 112
technique 140
Phacooptics 105
Phakic intraocular lenses 45
Phosphodiesterase inhibitor 228
Photic phenomena 49
Photodynamic therapy 223, 226
Photorefractive keratectomy 8
Phthisis bulbi 46
Pial arteriovenous fistula 310
Pigment clumps 251f
Pigment epithelial detachment 253, 256
Pigment epithelium derived factor 264
Placido-disc measure 124
Plate erosion 85
Plexiform layer
inner 239, 241, 262
outer boundary of 239, 241
Pluripotent
cells 68
stem cells 297
Pneumodescemetopexy 34
Polymerase chain reaction 276
Polymethyl methacrylate intraocular lens 192f
Polymethylmethacrylate rings 173
Polypoidal choroidal vasculopathy 223, 254
Post corneal refractive surgery 107
Postcerebral angiogram 321f
Posterior assisted levitation 165
Posterior capsular
defect 151f
rupture 156
anticipation of 158
early signs of 156
important clinical pearls 158
improperly managed 156
management 156
prevention of 158
recognition of 156, 158
stages 156
tear 162f
Posterior capsule rent 115
Posterior capsulorhexis 160f
Posterior chamber intraocular lens 199, 200
Posterior corneal astigmatism 124
Posterior fossa parenchyma 313f
Posterior polar cataract 147, 150, 159f
case of 152
classification of 147
phacoemulsification in 148
timing of surgery 148
Post-laser-assisted *in situ* keratomileusis ectasia 2f, 4f, 5f, 13
Post-LASIK ectasia
common clinical findings 2
epidemiology 1

grading system for 6*t*
histopathology 11
investigations 2
management 12
management of 1
pathogenesis 9
presenting features 2
prevention 16
risk factors for 5
Power modulation 113
    burst mode 113
    continuous mode 113
    pulse mode 113
Precise capsulotomy, creation of 150
Pre-Descemet's endothelial keratoplasty 23, 24
    air pump assisted 27, 29*f*
    graft 31*f*, 33*f*
Pre-Descemetic
    DALK for acute hydrops, modified tecnique 32
    dissection for acute hydrops 35*f*
Pregnancy period 12
Premacular hyaloid growth factor reservoir 261
Premium intraocular lenses 123
Proliferative diabetic retinopathy 213, 219, 245*f*
    clinical trials on 220*t*
Prophylactic laser 280
Pseudoaneurysm 312
Pseudodispersive viscoelastics 139
Pseudoexfoliation 68, 171
    and cataract surgery 138
    cataract: management 135
    deposits on
        intraocular lens 144*f*
        pupil 137
    endothelial deposits of 135
    eyes 138
    glaucoma 76
    postoperative complications 143
    preoperative evaluation 135
    syndrome 135
Pseudonight blindness 287
Pseudophakia 91
Pseudophakic
    eye 85
    glaucoma 76
Pseudoplasticity phenomenon 178
Pulsatile ocular blood flow 54
Puncture site hematoma 312
Pupil optic zone markers 41*f*
Pupil size 136
Pupillary
    constriction 150
    margin 135
    ruff 136
    stretch with Kuglen hooks 139*f*

R

Radial keratotomy 112
Radial superior incision 44*f*
Radiation therapy for age-related macular degeneration 226
Randleman's ectasia
    risk factor score system 6*t*
    score 8, 17
Randomized controlled trial 221
Ranibizumab 220, 221, 222, 226, 227, 228
    for choroidal neovascularization 222
    for diabetic macular edema 215
    for the treatment of macular edema 222
    treated cases 269
Rapamycin 228
Rapid progression 275
Real-life situation 212
Refraction-based formulae 101
Refractive targeting 112
Refractory infantile glaucoma 77
Reftinal detachment 157*f*
Regression formulae 101
Renin-angiotensin
    inhibitor 64
    system study 213
Residual stromal bed 5-6
Retina, outer 252
Retinal
    angiomatous proliferation 253
    arteriovenous malformation 318
    artery occlusion 247
    detachment 89, 156, 195, 205
        mechanism of 278
    secondary 276
    hemorrhage, large areas of 275
    implants 297
    layer: inner 262*f*
        disorganization of 261
    outer, disruption of 263
    macular degeneration, late-onset 294, 287
    necrosis: acute 274, 275, 276, 279
        active herpetic phase of 275*f*
        surgical management of 280
    necrosis: outer, progressive 274-277, 279
        diagnosis 278
        treatment 279

nerve fiber layer 60, 262
    defect 61f
    loss, inferior 64f
    layer thinning of 268
oximetry 53, 58
    advantages 59
    limitations 59
pigment epithelium 53, 239, 251f, 264f, 288
thickness 262
transvitreal oxygenation, improvement of 261
vascular disorders
    message from clinical trials 211
    real life situations management of 211
vasculitis 282
vein occlusion 211, 220, 246
vessel analyzer 53, 54, 58
    advantages 58
    limitations 58
Retinitis pigmentosa 287, 288
    atypical form of 290, 291f
    typical 289, 289f, 290f
Retinopathy of prematurity 211, 223, 224, 224t
Retrobulbar hemodynamics 64
Retrogeniculate damage 283
Rheological factors 63
Rhexis in weak zonules 178f
Rhodopsin gene 288
Rhodopsin kinase 291
Riboflavin solution 12
Riggs type 290
Rigid gas permeable 12
Rod photoreceptors 287, 288

S

Scanning laser ophthalmoscopic angiography 53, 54
    advantages 55
    limitations 55
Scarred limbal area 81
Scharioth
    forceps 200
    technique 200
Scheimpflug imaging 96
    dual 98
Schlemm's canal 68
Schocket procedure 77
Schroeder classification 148
Schubert-Bornschein type 290
Sclera-corneal incision 128
Scleral fixation
    devices 173
    Gore-Tex suture for ab-externo four-point 194f
    in small eyes 197
    intraocular lens 184
        implantation in children 196
        modification in materials for 192
    sutures, techniques of 188t
    two-point ab-externo 192f
    with Cionni ring, technique of 180
Scleral
    flaps 190
    lens 13f
    sutured IOLs, surgical techniques 187
Scleritis 277
Sclerocornea 46
Sclerotomies 200
Segmental retinal periarteritis 281
Selective laser trabeculoplasty 67, 69, 71, 72
    advantages 68
    complications 71
    contraindications 68
    disadvantages 68
    indications 68
    laser 70f
    mechanism of action of 68
    principle of 67
    technique 69
Setons, glaucoma drainage devices 74
Shaded surface display 316
Shunts nonrestrictive 74
Shunts nonvalved 74
Siderosis 295
Silicone oil-filled eyes 91
Silicone tube 77
Simple limbal epithelial transplantation 306
Singh's classification 148
Single-piece rigid polymethyl methacrylate lens 186
Sinskey hook 28
    using 194f
Slit lamp
    examination 137f
    marking 125f
Slit scanning corneal topography 123
Small incision cataract surgery 140-141
    steps of 141
Small incision technique 189
Small posterior capsular tear 158
Small pupil 139
Spectral domain-optical coherence tomography 260, 261f, 262f, 264f, 265f, 266f
    analysis in diabetic retinopathy 260
Spinal vascular malformations 310
Split-spectrum amplitude-decorrelation 249
    angiography 60

Staar Toric IOL 119
Standard care *vs* corticosteroid for retinal vein occlusion 222
Static zonulopathy 141
Steroid induced 68
Steven-Johnson syndrome 76
Stromal lamellae 11
Sturge-Weber syndrome 77
Subconjunctival hemorrhage 282
Subluxated lens 142*f*
   surgical procedure 176, 177
Suboptimal visual 130
Subretinal hemorrhages 253
Subtenon's anesthesia 81
Subtle retinal edema 281
Superficial and deep layers 251*f*
Superficial anterior lamellar keratoplasty 23, 42
   technique 43*f*
Superficial capillary plexus 243, 244
Superficial keratopigmentation 42
Superficial manual keratopigmentation 42
Superficial vascular plexus 241
Superotemporal quadrant 85
Suprachoroidal hemorrhage 85, 195-196
Surface ablation, advanced 8
Suture erosion 195
Suture knot erosion 196*f*
Suture-assisted sutureless technique 202
Sutured scleral fixation 184
   intraocular lenses 165, 195, 197
Sutured *vs* sutureless scleral fixation 205
Sutureless intrascleral haptic fixated 197
   developed technique of 197
Sutureless scleral fixation
   intraoperative complications 204
   postoperative complications of 204
Suture-related modification 192
Swept-source OCT 60, 92
Sylvian fissure, right 316
Systemic corticosteroids 280

T

Tandospirone 228
Tecnis
   multifocal IOL 117
   toric IOL 119
Telangiectasia 246
Telecentric keratometer 95
Tenon's
   cyst 89
   tissue growth 77
Tissue necrosis factor, administration of 303
Topcon's Aladdin HW3.0 95

Toric
   calculators 106
   intraocular lens 119, 129
      calculators 105
      implantation 120
      stability of 130
Torn zonules 171
Torsional (OZil) 114
Trabecular meshwork 67, 135
Trabeculectomy 77
Trabeculoplasty lens 69*f*
Tracey technologies 126
Tractional retinal detachment 283
Transient
   loss of consciousness 317
   vitreous hemorrhage 205
Translucent
   iris 46
   rendering 316
Transmission electron microscope 11
Transscleral fixation 186
   in children 198*t*
Traumatic
   cataract 158, 159*f*
   glaucoma 68, 76
Triamcinolone, uses stain vitreous 165*f*
Trimetazidine 228
Tube exposure 88
Tube retraction 85
Tucked-in lamellar keratoplasty 16, 23
Tunica vasculosa lentis 147
Two-handed technique 201
Two-instrument iris stretch 139

U

Ultrasound
   amplitude scan, first performed in 1956 90
   biomicroscopy examination 187
   customization 114
United Kingdom Prospective Diabetes Study 213
Universal Serial Bus 93
Universiol calculator 105
Urrets-Zavalia syndrome 46, 49
Utrata forceps 158
Uveitic glaucoma 68, 76
Uveitis 85
Uyemura's syndrome 292

V

Valganciclovir 282
Valved implants 79
Varicella zoster virus 274

Vascular
    access 311
    congestion 246
    density 59
    en face angiograms, percentage of 242
    endothelial growth factor 220, 254, 264
    lesion 310
    sheathing 283
    system visualization of 309
Vasospasm 63
Venous looping 246f
Vergence formulae 101
Verion planner 106
Vertebral artery 319f
    right 318
Verteporfin in photodynamic therapy 226
Viral keratitis 16
Viscoelastic, injecting 163f
Visual
    acuity 213
    field 289f
Vitamin A deficiency 292, 293f
Vitrectomy 23
    bimanual 161f
    cutter 166f
    for diabetic retinopathy-related
            vitreous haemorrhage 221t
    technique 161

Vitreomacular
    adhesion 261
    interface analysis 260
    traction 261, 261f
Vitreous hemorrhage 89, 195, 283

W

Wang-Koch modification for IOL formulae
            105t
Warfarin 280
WaveTec Vision Systems 100
Waxy disk pallor 289f
Weak zonules 171
West Nile virus 282
    retinopathy 282
Wet age-related macular degeneration 253

Y

Yamane's technique 203

Z

Zernike coefficient for spherical
            aberration 6
Zonular
    instability, signs of 138
    weakness, adjunctive devices for 141
Zonulodialysis 171
Zonulopathy 171